AF712494

RECENT DEVELOPMENTS IN AUTISM RESEARCH

RECENT DEVELOPMENTS IN AUTISM RESEARCH

MANUEL F. CASANOVA
(EDITOR)

Nova Biomedical Books
New York

Copyright © 2005 by Nova Science Publishers, Inc.

All rights reserved. No part of this book may be reproduced, stored in a retrieval system or transmitted in any form or by any means: electronic, electrostatic, magnetic, tape, mechanical photocopying, recording or otherwise without the written permission of the Publisher.

For permission to use material from this book please contact us:
Telephone 631-231-7269; Fax 631-231-8175
Web Site: http://www.novapublishers.com

NOTICE TO THE READER

The Publisher has taken reasonable care in the preparation of this book, but makes no expressed or implied warranty of any kind and assumes no responsibility for any errors or omissions. No liability is assumed for incidental or consequential damages in connection with or arising out of information contained in this book. The Publisher shall not be liable for any special, consequential, or exemplary damages resulting, in whole or in part, from the readers' use of, or reliance upon, this material.

This publication is designed to provide accurate and authoritative information with regard to the subject matter covered herein. It is sold with the clear understanding that the Publisher is not engaged in rendering legal or any other professional services. If legal or any other expert assistance is required, the services of a competent person should be sought. FROM A DECLARATION OF PARTICIPANTS JOINTLY ADOPTED BY A COMMITTEE OF THE AMERICAN BAR ASSOCIATION AND A COMMITTEE OF PUBLISHERS.

Library of Congress Cataloging-in-Publication Data
Available upon request

ISBN: 1-59454-497-2

Published by Nova Science Publishers, Inc. ✦ New York

Contents

Preface	*Benedetto Vitiello*	**vii**
Introduction	*Manuel F. Casanova*	**ix**
Chapter I	The Epidemiology of Pervasive Developmental Disorders *Eric Fombonne*	**1**
Chapter II	The Savant Syndrome in Autistic Disorder *Darold A. Treffert*	**27**
Chapter III	The Brain During Life in Autism: Advances in Neuroimaging Research *Janet E. Lainhart, Mariana Lazar, Erin D. Bigler and Andrew Alexander*	**57**
Chapter IV	EEG in Autism: Is There Just Too Much Going on in There? *Caroline Brown*	**109**
Chapter V	Gabaergic Dysfunction in Autism *S. Hossein Fatemi*	**127**
Chapter VI	Minicolumnar Pathology in Autism *Manuel F. Casanova*	**133**
Chapter VII	The Use of Animal Models to Understand Autism Spectrum Disorder *Elizabeth M. Powell*	**145**
Chapter VIII	Neural Network Modeling of Autism *Lennat Gustafsson and Andrew P. Paplinski*	**171**
Chapter IX	Autism Research: Future Directions *Eric London*	**195**
Index		**211**

Preface

Benedetto Vitiello
Child and Adolescent Treatment and Preventive Intervention
Research Branch National Institute of Mental Health

Autism Research: A High Public Health Priority

Autism is one of the most severe and impairing developmental disorders. In spite of advances in studying the structural and functional abnormalities associated with this disorder, its pathogenesis remains unknown. Although both psychosocial and pharmacological interventions are available that can improve behavior and overall functioning, no effective cure of autism is on hand. The burden of this illness on the affected children and their families is simply enormous. With recent estimates of prevalence between 2 and 6 per 1000 children, autism is more common than previously thought. Thus, it is not surprising that autism research is currently a high public health priority.

At the National Institutes of Health (NIH), funding for autism research was $93 millions in fiscal year 2003, which is a 4-fold increase over the 1997 level. As a reference, the entire NIH doubled during this period of time. In addition, other governmental agencies, such as the Centers for Disease Control and Prevention, as well as private foundations fund research in autism. An NIH-funded network of centers for Studies to Advance Autism Research and Treatment (STAART) has been recently established. This initiative adds to the Collaborative Programs of Excellence in Autism (CPEA) network, which is funded by the National Institute of Child Heath and Human Development and focused on the pathogenesis of autism, and the Research Units on Pediatric Psychopharmacology and Psychosocial Interventions (RUPP-PI) autism network, which is funded by the National Institute of Mental Health and is focused on treatment.

Major efforts are underway to try to identify vulnerability genes and environmental factors contributing to autism. A rational approach to developing a cure for the disorder must be built on the understanding of its pathogenesis. Hence the prominence that genetic and basic neuroscience research have at this stage. As in other areas of medicine, to be clinically relevant, basic research findings will have to be translated into novel diagnostic and therapeutic applications. The challenges of the bench-to-bedside translation cannot be underestimated. For certain disorders, such as Fragile X syndrome and cystic fibrosis, the genes have been identified a number of years ago, but no specific treatment has been thus far derived from this knowledge. Indeed, research to turn basic science findings into clinically useful discoveries has become a top priority across the biomedical field, with implications also for autism research.

While research efforts to understand the pathogenesis of autism are in progress, patients and their families are confronted with making treatment decisions now, and often have to choose among options that have not been adequately tested for efficacy and safety. Hence the importance of autism clinical trials and services research to test the therapeutic value of both psychosocial and pharmacological interventions in improving overall functioning and reducing the burden of the illness.

Given the high public health relevance of autism research, the publication of a volume devoted to this topic is clearly a timely and welcome contribution.

In: Recent Developments in Autism Research
Editor: Manuel F. Casanova, pp. ix-xiii
ISBN 1-59454-358-5
© 2005 Nova Science Publishers, Inc.

Introduction

*Manuel F. Casanova**

Gottfried and Gisela Kolb Endowed Chair in Psychiatry University of Louisville Department of Psychiatry, Louisville, KY

One writer has defined autism as "a developmental disorder…whose core features…are impairment in socialization, communication and imagination." [1] However, no phrases or sentences by themselves define autism. One may argue that longer descriptions are more defensible, are better able to detail the complexity of the syndrome, and provide a better basis for diagnosis. Still, after all is said and done, definitions usually fail to describe the part autism plays in the behavior of the afflicted individual: how it affects their beliefs, the way they perceive the world, and the way the world perceives them. In similar fashion, textbooks will cite a number of reasons to study autism: the number of affected patients, degree of social impairment, and chronicity. They fail; nevertheless, to stress its inextricable links to other areas of human thought and conduct. We can't talk about autism without discussing cognitive psychology, memory, or intelligence.

Autism is a condition that hits the patient in places that can't be hidden; in his/her behavior. It is a condition worn for public scrutiny, blending personal aspects of the patient's life with his/her social environment. It provides for guilt in patients and for Job-like ponderings in their parents. How do you measure the extent of damage to a patient's life or that of the parent's?

Present day thinking portrays the problem of autism in the context of a triangle. In this triangle each interconnected vertex alternatively represents the autistic person, pathophysiological theories on causation, and symptoms. This faulty "syllogism" inadequately represents the autistic person. In this context, medical theories extend piety to the patients. They tend to be denominationally driven and self-referential. Ultimately, theories may serve as decorative art if they are not clinically relevant. How can these ideas be reconciled with the tremendous gifts observed in some patients? In danger of mixing metaphors: how can we square the triangle? How can we reconcile those positive aspects of the condition, the charisma of autism, with its shortcomings?

* Email: M0CASA02@louisville.edu; Tel: (502)852-4077; Fax: (502)852-4978

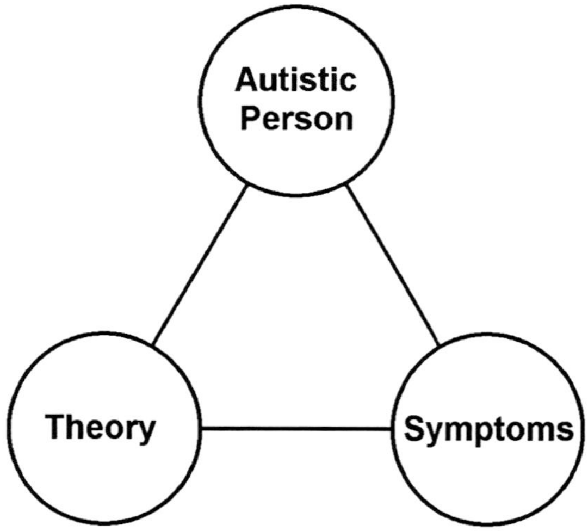

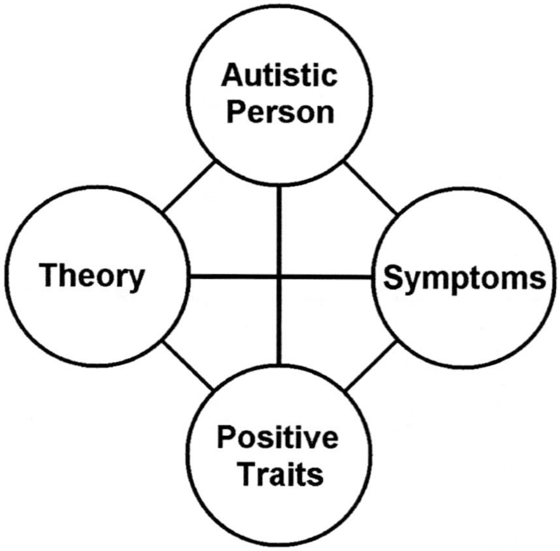

Like previous attempts, this book does not fairly represent autism. A handful of chapters could not possibly do so. Rather this book will focus on certain themes: those physical aspects which make an individual autistic. Although we are willing to entertain both psychological and biological explanations, this book will deal primarily with the biological. Even when these explanations overlap, ultimately, they perform different functions; one biased towards the need to know and the other towards the need to cure.

Clinicians have proposed different psychological theories to explain mental illnesses from the perspective of the mind. Some of them are imaginative explanations of facts that have not or can not be explained neurobiologically. Ultimately such explanations blur the line between cause and effect. Unsurprisingly, the number of psychological theories about a condition is a direct reflection on how little is known about its etiology. When little is know about a condition, theories proliferate, become grouped, and are publicized as new developments. Theories, stemming from this perspective, are difficult to falsify. Are they dogma or scientific explanations? In psychology, the more compelling the description, the more persistent is the underlying presumption. Moreover, psychological explanations have become fair game for the opinion of anybody who is willing to espouse a trendy name, e.g., refrigerator mothers, catch 22. These theories are not the end of psychoanalytic ruminations but rather represent a return to the same.

One could not argue, however, that only the biological perspective is correct or that it has escaped neuroscientific inquiry unscathed. The lack of reproducible findings has allowed for a proliferation of biological theories. In this regard, neuropathology echoes Dostoyevsky's unsettling remark that if there is no God, then everything is allowed. [2] If we do not have pathology, we should favorably consider every inquiry and every result. Unfortunately, this approach preserves falsehoods by building tale upon tale. Maybe finding pathology for autism is akin to existential horror. Finding pathology would locate the workings of minds in the brain. This approach leads to the astonishing hypothesis that "You, your joys and your sorrows, your memories and ambitions, your sense of personal identity and free will are in fact no more than the behavior of a vast assembly of nerve cells and their associated molecules." [3] This thesis undermines humans' tendency to flatter themselves, to assert their uniqueness. Desmond Morris once said that we tend to think of ourselves as fallen angels, not risen apes. [4]

Physicians are unwilling to accept a diminished role in fixing neurological and psychiatric problems akin to that of car mechanics. Yet no such qualms deter us from accepting organic explanations to deafness or hemiplegia. We take for granted that a steam shovel and a crane will dig faster and lift more weight than a human. However, the eyebrow of the world goes up when a computer beats the world chess champion. Broaching the subject of the mind makes the difference.

In the last decade a series of discoveries has destabilized the dominant image of autism within the medical and lay community. One of the better developments has been the introduction of two complementary diagnostic instruments, the ADI-R [5] and the ADOS. [6] In both instruments domain scores indicate severity of impairment based on symptom frequency and degree of interferences with daily living. ADI-R is better at fulfilling DMS-IV diagnostic criteria while ADOS is a briefer scale that takes into account developmental level.

Core deficits are now defined in terms of information processing impairment. At present there is enough scientific evidence to accord the status of "theory" to three different psychological conjectures on autism: deficits in theory of mind, executive function, and central coherence. First, deficits in theory of mind can be seen as exaggerations of gender based differences that are seemingly hard-wired into our brains. Asperger [7] was the first brave soul to suggest that his syndrome was the extreme of the male personality. Simon Baron-Cohen [8] has publicized this theory based on his own pioneering research spanning the spectrum from gossip to aggression, from evolution to everyday life, and from brain sciences to theory of mind. These differences reflect the way we systematize and develop empathy. Second, executive functions have a locus within the prefrontal cortex. Experimental work by Goldman-Rakic [9] indicates that, according to the anatomical area involved, the frontal lobe exhibits different working-memory domains. Visuospatial processing is performed by the dorsolateral prefrontal cortex. Working memory for the features of objects and faces occurs in the more lateral and inferior cortices, while semantic encoding and retrieval involves still more inferior and insular regions. It is easy to envision how a defect in working memory/executive functions can provide for abnormalities in language, thinking, and behavior. Lastly, central coherence is analogous to the binding phenomena studied in neurosciences. Weak central coherence, a pattern typical of autism, is a cognitive style that emphasizes low-level features in lieu of high-level integrative processing. Higher level integrative processing appears to be mediated by the synchronization of neuronal discharges on high- (gamma-) frequency EEG. Unsurprisingly investigators have recently reported a disorder of binding related gamma EEG oscillatory activity in autism.

It is noteworthy that Shakow, [10] working in the 1930's and 40's, generated a segmental set theory that seemingly joined both executive functions and central coherence. His theory stated that in order to successfully perform daily activities one needs to break down activities into segments while retaining the big picture or set. In some conditions, the big picture is easily lost. The underlying deficit appears related to hemispheric, rather than global, function. The right hemisphere interprets global patterns while the left hemisphere infers details of stimuli.

It is my biased opinion that the putative presence of minicolumnar abnormalities in the cortex of autistic patients offers an explanation to all of the previously mentioned core psychological theories. Thus no longer are there psychological theories nor neuropathological research; rather, there is an amalgam of ideas. Psychological research has now gained neuropathological underpinning while neuropathological research has significant psychological correlations.

Psychological theories now focus away from the inner life of emotions into action. They place an individual within the constraints of the environment, interacting with other people. Whenever evidence requires it, theories become malleable, confluent, and no longer painted into a corner. Theories have become commonsensical providing for easy and clear to enunciate observations. Arguments now rest on a bedrock; a starting point of further investigation.

We can now view autism as the result of a variation in the blueprint of the brain. Solving this enigma may partially map the mind's interior. The beauty of these recent findings lies, as E. O. Wilson [11] would say, in the way they trace causation through many levels of organization. They invite researchers of many disciplines to bring their own tools and expertise to the fray thus providing a multidimensional view of the condition. This book will describe the evolution of some of these discoveries. It will reconstruct their path and, in so doing, share in an amazing journey. The champagne is on ice; let's hope to uncork the bottle sometime in the near future.

References

[1] Frith U. *Autism and Asperger syndrome*. Cambridge, UK: Cambridge University Press; 1991.

[2] Dostoyevsky F. *The Brothers Karamazov*, book 2, chapter 6.

[3] Crick F. *The Astonishing Hypothesis: The Scientific Search for the Soul*. New York, NY: Scribner; 1994.

[4] Morris D. *The Naked Ape: A Zoologist's Study of the Human Animal*. London, UK: Jonathan Cape; 1967.

[5] Lord C, Rutter M, le Couteur A. Autism diagnostic interview—revised: A revised version of a diagnostic interview for caregivers of individuals with possible pervasive

developmental disorders. *Journal of Autism and Developmental Disorders.* 1994;24:659-685.

[6] Lord C, Risi S, Lambrecht L, et al. The autism diagnostic observation schedule—generic: a standard measure of social and communication deficits associated with the spectrum of autism. *Journal of Autism and Developmental Disorders.* 2000;30:205-223.

[7] Asperger H. Die "autistischen Psychopathen" im Kindesalter. *Archiv für Psychiatrie und Nervenkrankheiten.* 1944;117:76-136.

[8] Baron-Cohen S. *The Essential Difference.* New York, NY: Basic Books; 2003.

[9] Goldman-Rakic PS, Selemon LD. Functional and anatomical aspects of prefrontal pathology in schizophrenia. *Schizophrenia Bulletin.* 1997;23:437-458.

[10] Shakow D. *The Nature of Deterioration in Schizophrenic Conditions.* New York, NY: Coolidge Foundation; 1946. *Nervous and Mental Disorders Monographs* 70.

[11] Wilson EO. *Consilience: The Unity of Knowledge.* New York, NY: Alfred A. Knopf, Inc, 1998.

In: Recent Developments in Autism Research
Editor: Manuel F. Casanova, pp. 1-25
ISBN 1-59454-358-5
© 2005 Nova Science Publishers, Inc.

Chapter I

The Epidemiology of Pervasive Developmental Disorders

Eric Fombonne*
Canada Research Chair in Child Psychiatry
Director, Department of Psychiatry, Montreal Children's Hospital
Professor of Psychiatry, McGill University;
McGill University, Department of Psychiatry
The Montreal Children's Hospital, 4018 St. Catherine St. W. Montreal, Canada

Introduction

The aims of this chapter are to provide an up-to-date review of the methodological features and substantive results of published epidemiological surveys. This chapter updates our previous review[1] with the inclusion of 8 new studies made available since then. The specific questions addressed in this chapter are: a) what is the range of prevalence estimates for autism, and related disorders? b) what proportion of autism cases is attributable to specific associated medical disorders? c) is the incidence of autism increasing? d) what are the other correlates of autistic-spectrum disorders? e) what is the role, if any, of cluster reports in causal investigations of autism?

Selection of Studies

The studies were identified through systematic searches from the major scientific literature databases (MEDLINE, PSYCINFO) and from prior reviews.[1]–[35] Only studies published in the English language were included. Surveys which relied only on a questionnaire-based approach to define caseness were also excluded as the validity of the diagnosis is unsatisfactory in these studies. Overall, 42 studies published between 1966 and

* E-mail: eric.fombonne@mcgill.ca; Tel: (514) 412-4449; Fax: (514) 412-4337

2003 were selected which surveyed PDDs in clearly demarcated, non-overlapping samples. Of these, 36 studies provided information on rates of autistic disorder, 3 studies only provided estimates on all PDDs combined, and 2 studies provided data only on high-functioning PDDs. For several studies, the publication listed in the tables is the most detailed account or the earliest one; however, other published articles were used to extract relevant information from the same study, when appropriate.

Survey Descriptions

Surveys were conducted in 14 countries and half of the results have been published since 1997. Details on the precise socio-demographic composition and economical activities of the area surveyed in each study were generally lacking; most studies were, however, conducted in predominantly urban or mixed areas, with only 2 (studies 6 and 11) surveys carried out in predominantly rural areas. The proportion of children from immigrant families was generally not available and very low in 5 surveyed populations (studies 11, 12, 19, 23 and 26). Only in studies 4, 34, and 38 was there a substantial minority of children with either an immigrant or different ethnic background living in the area. The age range of the population included in the surveys is spread from birth to early adult life, with an overall median age of 8.0. Similarly, in 39 studies, there is huge variation in the size of the population surveyed, with a median population size of 63 860 subjects (mean = 255 000) and about half of the studies relying on targeted populations ranging in size from 15 870 to 166 860.

Study Designs

A few studies have relied on existing administrative databases [4], [5] or on national registers[6] for case identification. Most investigations have relied on a two-stage or multi-stage approach to identify cases in underlying populations. The first screening stage of these studies often consisted of sending letters or brief screening scales requesting school and health professionals to identify possible cases of autism. Each investigation varied in several key aspects of this screening stage. First, the coverage of the population varied enormously from one study to another. In some (i.e. studies 3, 17, 20, 24, 33), only cases already known from educational or medical authorities could be identified, whereas in other surveys an extensive coverage of the entire population, including children attending normal schools (studies 1, 25, 40) or children undergoing systematic developmental checks (studies 13, 19, 22, 32, 36) was achieved. In addition, the surveyed areas varied in terms of service development as a function of the specific educational or health care systems of each country and of the year of investigation. Secondly, the type of information sent out to professionals invited to identify children varied from simple letters including a few clinical descriptors of autism-related symptoms or diagnostic checklists re-phrased in non-technical terms, to more systematic screening based on questionnaires or rating scales of known reliability and validity. Thirdly, participation rates in the first screening stages provide another source of variation in the screening efficiency of surveys. Refusal rates were available for 13 studies and ranged from 0 % (study 25) to 35 % (study 40), with a median value of 14 %. Fewer studies could examine the extent to which refusal to participate or unco-operativeness in surveys is associated with the likelihood that the corresponding children have autism.

Although there is no consistent evidence that parental refusal to co-operate is associated with autism in their offspring, it appears that a small proportion of cases may be missed in some surveys as a consequence of non-co-operation at the screening stage. One survey included a weighting procedure to compensate for non-response (study 40).

Only two studies (studies 1 and 30) provided an estimate of the reliability of the screening procedure. The sensitivity of the screening methodology is also difficult to gauge in autism surveys. The usual approach which consists of sampling at random screened negative subjects in order to estimate the proportion of false negatives has not been used in these surveys for the obvious reason that, due to the very low frequency of the disorder, it would be both imprecise and very costly to undertake such estimations. As a consequence, prevalence estimates must be seen as underestimates of "true" prevalence rates. The magnitude of this underestimation is unknown in each survey.

Similar considerations about the methodological variability across studies apply to the intensive assessment phases. Participation rates in these second stage assessments were generally high, ranging from 76.1 % (study 12) to 98.6 % (study 25). The source of information used to determine caseness usually involved a combination of informants and data sources, with a direct assessment of the person with autism in 21 studies.

The assessments were conducted with various diagnostic instruments, ranging from a classical clinical examination to the use of batteries of standardized measures. The Autism Diagnostic Interview[7] and/or the Autism Diagnostic Observational Schedule[29] were used in the most recent surveys. The precise diagnostic criteria retained to define caseness vary according to the study and, to a large extent, reflect historical changes in classification systems. Thus, Kanner's criteria, Lotter's and Rutter's definitions were used in the first 8 surveys (all conducted before 1982), whereas DSM-based definitions took over thereafter as well as ICD-10 since 1990. However, most surveys have relied on the clinical judgement of experts to arrive at the final case groupings. It is worth underlining that field trials for recent classifications such as DSM-III-R[9] or DSM-IV/ICD-10[10] have also relied upon the judgement of clinical experts, taken as a gold standard to diagnose autism and calibrate diagnostic algorithms. Therefore, the heterogeneity of diagnostic criteria used across surveys is somewhat mitigated by reliance on expert clinical judgement to determine final caseness. It is furthermore difficult to assess the impact of a specific diagnostic scheme or of a particular diagnostic criterion on the estimate of prevalence since other powerful method factors confound between-studies comparisons of rates.

Characteristics of Autistic Samples

Data on children with autistic disorders were available in 36 surveys (studies 1–36; see Table 1). The number of subjects considered to suffer from autism ranged from 6 (studies 18 and 25) to 5038 (study 34) across studies (median: 48; mean: 209). An assessment of intellectual function was obtained in 21 studies. These assessments were conducted with various tests and instruments; furthermore, results were pooled together in broad bands of intellectual level which did not share the same boundaries across studies. As a consequence, differences in rates of cognitive impairment between studies should be interpreted with caution. The median proportion of subjects without intellectual impairment is 29.6 % (range:

0 %–60 %).[1] The corresponding figures are 29.3 % (range: 6.6 %–100 %) for mild to moderate intellectual impairments, and 38.5 % (range: 0 %–81.3 %) for severe to profound level of mental retardation. Gender repartition among subjects with autism was reported in 32 studies totaling 6963 subjects with autism, and the male/female sex ratio varied from 1.33 (study 7) to 16.0 (study 4), with a mean male:female ratio of 4.3:1. Thus, no epidemiological study ever identified more girls than boys with autism, a finding which parallels the gender differences found in clinically referred samples.[47] Gender differences were more pronounced when autism was not associated with mental retardation. In 13 studies (865 subjects) where the sex ratio was available within the normal band of intellectual functioning, the median sex ratio was 5.5:1. Conversely, in 12 studies (813 subjects), the median sex ratio was 1.95:1 in the group with autism and moderate to severe mental retardation.

Prevalence Estimations for Autistic Disorder

Prevalence estimates ranged from 0.7/10 000 to 72.6/10 000 (Table 1). Prevalence rates were negatively correlated with sample size (Spearman $r = -0.73$; $p < 0.01$); small-scale studies tended to report higher prevalence rates.

When surveys were combined in two groups according to the median year of publication (1994), the median prevalence rate for 18 surveys published in the period 1966–1993 was 4.7/10 000, and the median rate for the 18 surveys published in the period 1994–2004 was 12.7/10 000. Indeed, the correlation between prevalence rate and year of publication reached statistical significance (Spearman $r = 0.65$; $p < 0.01$); and the results of the 22 surveys with prevalence rates over 7/10 000 were all published since 1987. These findings point towards an increase in prevalence estimates in the last 15–20 years. In order to derive a best estimate of the current prevalence of autism, it was therefore deemed appropriate to restrict the analysis to 28 surveys published since 1987. The average rate was 16.2/10 000 and the median rate was 11.3/10,000. Similar values were obtained when slightly different rules and time cutpoints were used, with median and mean rates fluctuating between 10–13 and 13–18/10,000 respectively. From these results, a conservative estimate for the current prevalence of autistic disorder is most consistent with values lying somewhere between 10/10 000 and 16/10 000. For further calculations, we arbitrarily adopted the mid-point of this interval as the working rate for autism prevalence, i.e. the value of 13/10 000.

[1] Study 23, which relied upon different IQ groupings, has been excluded.

Table 1 Prevalence surveys of autistic disorder

No	Year of publication	Authors	Country	Area	Size of target population	Age	Number of subjects with autism	Diagnostic criteria	% with normal IQ	Gender ratio (M/F)	Prevalence Rate/ 10 000	95 % CI
1	1966	Lotter [11]	UK	Middlesex	78 000	8–10	32	Lotter	15.6	2.6 (23/9)	4.1	2.7; 5.5
2	1970	Brask [12]	Denmark	Århus County	46 500	2–14	20	Clinical	—	1.4 (12/7)	4.3	2.4; 6.2
3	1970	Treffert [13]	USA	Wisconsin	899 750	3–12	69	Kanner	—	3.06 (52/17)	0.7	0.6; 0.9
4	1976	Wing et al. [14]	UK	Camberwell	25 000	5–14	[1]17	Lotter	30	16 (16/1)	[2]4.8	2.1; 7.5
5	1982	Hoshino et al. [16]	Japan	Fukushima-Ken	609 848	0–18	142	Kanner	—	9.9 (129/13)	2.33	1.9; 2.7
6	1983	Bohman et al. [17]	Sweden	Västerbotten County	69 000	0–20	39	Rutter	20.5	1.6 (24/15)	5.6	3.9; 7.4
7	1984	McCarthy et al. [18]	Ireland	East	65 000	8–10	28	Kanner	—	1.33 (16/12)	4.3	2.7; 5.9
8	1986	Steinhausen et al. [19]	Germany	West Berlin	279 616	0–14	52	Rutter	55.8	2.25 (36/16)	1.9	1.4; 2.4
9	1987	Burd et al. [20]	USA	North Dakota	180 986	2–18	59	DSM-III	—	2.7 (43/16)	3.26	2.4; 4.1
10	1987	Matsuishi et al [21]	Japan	Kurume City	32 834	4–12	51	DSM-III	—	4.7 (42/9)	15.5	11.3; 19.8
11	1988	Tanoue et al. [22]	Japan	Southern Ibaraki	95 394	7	132	DSM-III	—	4.07 (106/26)	13.8	11.5;16.2
12	1988	Bryson et al. [23]	Canada	Part of Nova-Scotia	20 800	6–14	21	New RDC	23.8	2.5 (15/6)	10.1	5.8;14.4
13	1989	Sugiyama & Abe [24]	Japan	Nagoya	12 263	3	16	DSM-III	—	—	13.0	6.7;19.4
14	1989	Cialdella & Mamelle [25]	France	1 département (Rhône)	135 180	3–9	61	DSM-III like	—	2.3	4.5	3.4;5.6

[1] This number corresponds to the sample described in Wing & Gould.[15]
[2] This rate corresponds to the first published paper on this survey and is based on 12 subjects amongst children aged 5 to 14 years.

Table 1 Prevalence surveys of autistic disorder (Continued)

No	Year of publication	Authors	Country	Area	Size of target population	Age	Number of subjects with autism	Diagnostic criteria	% with normal IQ	Gender ratio (M/F)	Preva -lence Rate/ 10 000	95 % CI
15	1989	Ritvo et al. [26]	USA	Utah	769 620	3–27	241	DSM-III	34	3.73 (190/51)	2.47	2.1;2.8
16	1991	Gillberg et al.3	Sweden	South-West Gothenburg & Bohuslän County	78 106	4–13	74	DSM-III-R	18	2.7 (54/20)	9.5	7.3;11.6
17	1992	Fombonne & du Mazaubrun [30]	France	4 régions, 14 départements	274 816	9–13	154	Clinical ICD-10 like	13.3	2.1 (105/49)	4.9	4.1;5.7
18	1992	Wignyosumarto et al. [31]	Indonesia	Yogyakarita (SE of Jakarta)	5120	4–7	6	CARS	0	2.0 (4/2)	11.7	2.3;21.1
19	1996	Honda et al. [32]	Japan	Yokohama	8537	5	18	ICD-10	50.0	2.6 (13.5)	21.08	11.4;30.8
20	1997	Fombonne et al. [33]	France	3 départements	325 347	8–16	174	Clinical ICD-10-like	12.1	1.81 (112/62)	5.35	4.6;6.1
21	1997	Webb et al. [34]	UK	South Glamorgan, Wales	73 301	3–15	53	DSM-III-R	—	6.57 (46/7)	7.2	5.3;9.3
22	1997	Arvidsson et al. [35]	Sweden	Mölnlycke	1941	3–6	9	ICD-10	22.2	3.5 (7/2)	46.4	16.1;76.6
23	1998	Sponheim & Skjeldal [36]	Norway	Akershus County	65 688	3–14	34	ICD-10	[4]47.1	2.09 (23/11)	5.2	3.4;6.9
24	1999	Taylor et al. [37]	UK	North Thames	~490 000	0–16	427	ICD-10	—	—	8.7	7.9;9.5

[3] For the Göteborg surveys,[27]–[29] a detailed examination showed that there was overlap between the samples included in the 3 surveys; consequently only the last survey[29] has been included in this table.

[4] In this study, mild mental retardation was combined with normal IQ, whereas moderate and severe mental retardation were grouped together.

Table 1 Prevalence surveys of autistic disorder (Continued)

No	Year of publication	Authors	Country	Area	Size of target population	Age	Number of subjects with autism	Diagnostic criteria	% with normal IQ	Gender ratio (M/F)	Prevalence Rate/ 10 000	95 % CI
25	1999	Kadesjö et al. [38]	Sweden	Karlstad	826	6.7–7.7	6	DSM-III-R ICD-10 Gillberg[5]	[6]47.1	2.09 (23/11)	5.2	3.4;6.9
26	2000	Baird et al. [39]	UK	South-East Thames	16 235	—	50	ICD-10	60	15.7 (47/3)	30.8	22.9;40.6
27	2000	Powell et al. [40]	UK	West Midlands	25 377	—	62	Clinical ICD10 DSM-IV	—	—	7.8	5.8;10.5
28	2000	Kielinen et al. [41]	Finland	Oulu & Lapland	152 732	—	187	ICD-8 ICD-9 ICD-10	49.8	4.12 (156/50)	12.2	10.5;14.0
29	2001	Bertrand et al. [42]	USA	Brick Township, New Jersey	8896	—	36	DSM-IV	36.7	2.2 (25/11)	40.5	28.0;56.0
30	2001	Fombonne et al. [43]	UK	England & Wales	10 438	5–15	27	DSM-IV ICD-10	55.5	8.0 (24/3)	26.1	16.2;36.0
31	2001	Magnusson & Saemundsen [44]	Iceland	Whole Island	43 153	5–14	57	Mostly ICD-10	15.8	4.2 (46/11)	13.2	9.8;16.6
32	2001	Chakrabarti & Fombonne [45]	UK	Staffordshire	15 500	2.5–6.5	26	ICD10 DSM-IV	29.2	3.3 (20/6)	16.8	10.3;23.2
33	2001	Davidovitch et al. [46]	Israel	Haiffa	26 160	7–11	26	DSM-III-R DSM-IV	—	4.2 (21/5)	10.0	6.6;14.4
34	2002	Croen et al. [4]	USA	California	4 950 333	5–12	5,038	CDER[7]	[8]62.8	4.47 (4116/921)	11.0	10.7;11.3
35	2002	Madsen et al. [6]	Denmark	National register	63 859	8	46	ICD-10	—	—	7.2	5.0;10.0
36	2004	Chakrabarti & Fombonne	UK	Staffordshire	10 903	4–7	24	ICD-10 DSM-IV	33.3	3.8 (19/5)	22.0	14.4;32.2

[5] Gillberg's criteria for Asperger syndrome
[6] In this study, mild mental retardation was combined with normal IQ, whereas moderate and severe mental retardation were grouped together.
[7] Level 1—full syndrome
[8] This proportion is likely to be overestimated and to reflect an underreporting of mental retardation in the CDER evaluations.

Associated Medical Conditions

Overall the proportion of cases of autism which could be causally attributed to known medical disorders was low. Tuberous sclerosis and Fragile X disorder are the medical disorders with the strongest association with autism. The fraction of cases of autism with any known medical condition potentially etiologically significant ranged from 0 % to 16.7 %, with a mean value of 5.9 %. [1]

Rates of Other Pervasive Developmental Disorders

Unspecified PDDs—PDDNOS

Several studies have provided useful information on rates of syndromes similar to autism but falling short of strict diagnostic criteria for autistic disorder. [1] Because the screening procedures and subsequent diagnostic assessments differed from one study to another, these groups of disorders are not strictly comparable across studies. In addition, as they were not the group on which the attention was focused, details are often lacking on their phenomenological features in the available reports. Different labels have been used to characterize them such as the triad of impairments involving impairments in reciprocal social interaction, communication and imagination.[15] These groups would be overlapping with current diagnostic labels such as atypical autism and PDDNOS. Fourteen of the 36 surveys yielded separate estimates of the prevalence of these developmental disorders, with 10 studies showing higher rates for the non-autism disorders than the rates for autism. The ratio of the rate of non autistic PDD to the rate of autism varied between from 0.44 to 3.33 with a mean value of 1.6, which, assuming a 13/10 000 rate for autistic disorder, translates into an average prevalence estimate of 20.8/10 000 for PDDNOS. This group has been much less studied in previous epidemiological studies but progressive recognition of its importance and relevance to autism has led to changes in the design of more recent epidemiological surveys (see below) that are now designed to include these less typical children in the case definition adopted in surveys. It should be clear from these figures that they represent a very substantial group of children whose treatment needs are likely to be as important as those of children with autism.

Asperger Syndrome and Childhood Disintegrative Disorder

The reader is referred to recent epidemiological reviews for these two conditions.[48],[49]

In brief, epidemiological studies of Asperger syndrome (AS) are sparse, probably due to the fact that it was acknowledged as a separate diagnostic category only recently in both ICD-10 and DSM-IV. Only two epidemiological surveys (studies 25 and 41) have been conducted which *specifically* investigated its prevalence.[38],[50] However, only a handful ($N < 5$) of cases were identified in these surveys, with the resulting estimates of 28 and 48/10,000 being extremely imprecise. By contrast, other recent autism surveys have consistently identified smaller numbers of children with AS than those with autism *within* the same survey. In 7 such surveys (studies 23–27 and 32, reviewed elsewhere,[49] and study 36), the ratio of autism to AS rates in each survey was above unity, suggesting that the rate of AS was consistently *lower* than that for autism (Table 2). How much lower is difficult to establish from existing data, but a ratio of 5 to 1 would appear an acceptable, albeit conservative, conclusion based on this limited available evidence. This translates into a rate for AS which would be 1/5 that of autism. We therefore used for subsequent calculations an estimate of 2.6/10 000 for AS. A recent survey of high-functioning PDDs in Welsh mainstream primary schools (study 40) has yielded a relatively high (uncorrected) prevalence estimate of 14.5/10 000.[51] Of the 17 children contributing to this figure, 10 had either Asperger disorder or high-functioning autism as a primary diagnosis. Assuming than half of these would have Asperger disorder, we could extrapolate a 4.3/10 000 prevalence, a figure that is in line with other studies. However, much caution should be applied to this calculation as it is based on several assumptions that are impossible to verify.

Few surveys have provided data on childhood disintegrative disorder (CDD), also known as Heller syndrome, disintegrative psychosis (ICD-9) or late-onset autism.[52] In addition to the 4 studies (studies 9, 23, 31, 32) of our previous review,[48] another survey has provided new data on CDD (study 36). Taking the 5 studies into account (Table 3), prevalence estimates ranged from 1.1 to 9.2/100 000. The pooled estimate based on 7 identified cases and a surveyed population of 358 633 children, was 1.9/100 000. The upper-bound limit of the associated confidence interval (4.15/100 000) indicates that CDD is a very rare condition, with 1 case to occur for every 65 cases of autistic disorder. As cases of CDD were both rare and already included in the numerator alongside autism cases in most surveys, we do not provide separate estimates of the numbers of subjects suffering from CDD in subsequent calculations.

Prevalence for Combined PDDs

Taking the aforementioned *conservative* estimates, the prevalence for all PDDs is at least 36.4/10 000 (i.e. the sum of estimates for autism (13/10 000), PDDNOS (20.8/10 000), and AS (2.6/10 000)). This global estimate is derived from a conservative analysis of existing data. However, 8 recent epidemiological surveys yielded even higher rates in six instances (Table 4). The two surveys that did not might have probably underestimated the rates. In the Danish investigation (study 35), case finding depended upon notification to a National Registry, a method which is usually associated with lower sensitivity for case finding. The Atlanta survey by the CDC (study 38) was based on a very large population (which typically yields lower prevalence: see above) and age specific rates were in fact in the 40–45/10 000 range in some birth cohorts.[55] The common design features of the 4 epidemiological enquiries (studies 26, 29, 32, 36) that yielded higher rates are worthy of mention. First, the case definition chosen for these investigations was that of a pervasive developmental disorder (PDD) as opposed to the narrower approach focusing on autistic disorder typical of previous surveys. Investigators were concerned with any combination of severe developmental abnormalities occurring in one or more of the 3 symptomatic domains defining PDD and autism. Second, case finding techniques employed in these surveys were proactive, relying on multiple and repeated screening phases, involving both different informants at each phase and surveying the same cohorts at different ages, which certainly maximized the sensitivity of case identification. Third, assessment were performed with standardized diagnostic measures (i.e. ADI-R and ADOS) which match well the more dimensional approach retained for case definition. Finally, these samples comprised young children around their fifth birthday, thereby optimizing sensitivity of case finding procedures. Furthermore, the size of targeted populations was reasonably small (between 9000 and 16 000), probably allowing for the most efficient use of research resources. Conducted in different regions and countries by different teams, the convergence of estimates is striking. Two further results are worth noting. First, in sharp contrast with the prevalence for combined PDDs, the separate estimates for autistic disorder and PDDNOS vary widely in studies where separate figures were available, as if the reliability of the differentiation between autistic disorder and PDDNOS was mediocre at that young age, despite the use of up-to-date standardized measures. Secondly, the rate of mental retardation was, overall, much lower than in previous surveys of autism. While this should not be a surprise for children in the PDDNOS/AS groups, this trend was also noticeable within samples diagnosed with autistic disorder. To what extent this trend reflects the previously mentioned differential classification issues between autism and PDDNOS or a genuine trend over time towards decreased rate of mental retardation within children with autistic disorder (possibly as a result as earlier diagnosis and intervention) remains to be established.

In conclusion, the convergence of surveys around an estimate of 60/10 000 for all PDD combined is striking, especially when coming from studies with improved methodology. This estimate appears now to be the best estimate for the prevalence of PDDs currently available.

Time Trends

The debate on the hypothesis of a secular increase in rates of autism has been obscured by a lack of clarity in the measures of disease occurrence used by investigators, or rather in their interpretation. In particular, it is crucial to differentiate prevalence (the proportion of individuals in a population who suffer from a defined disorder) from incidence (the number of new cases occurring in a population over a period of time). Prevalence is useful to estimate needs and plan services; only incidence rates can be used for causal research. Both prevalence and incidence estimates will be inflated when case definition is broadened and case ascertainment is improved. Time trends in rates can therefore only be gauged in investigations which hold these parameters under strict control over time. These methodological requirements must be borne in mind whilst reviewing the evidence for a secular increase in rates of PDDs.

Five approaches to assess this question have been used in the literature.

Table 2 Asperger Syndrome (AS) in Recent Autism Surveys

Author	*Size of population*	*Age group*	Assessment	Autism	Asperger Syndrome	Autism		Asperger Syndrome		Autism/ AS Ratio
			Informants	*Instruments*	*Diagnostic Criteria*	*N*	*Rate/ 10 000*	*N*	*Rate/ 10 000*	
Sponheim & Skjeldal [36]	65 688	3–14	Parent Child	Parental Interview + direct observation, CARS, ABC	ICD-10	32	4.9	2	0.3	16.0
Taylor et al. [37]	490 000	0–16	Record	Rating of all data available in child record	ICD-10	427	8.7	71	1.4	6.0
Kadesjö et al. [38]	826	6.7–7.7	Child Parent Professional	ADI-R, Griffiths Scale or WISC, Asperger Syndrome Screening Questionnaire	DSM-III-R/ ICD-10 Gillberg's criteria (Asperger syndrome)	6	72.6	4	48.4	1.5
Baird et al. [39]	16 235	7	Parents Child Other data	ADI-R Psychometry	ICD-10 DSM-IV	45	27.7	5	3.1	9.0
Powell et al. [40]	25 377	1–4.9	Records	ADI-R Available data	DSM-III-R DSM-IV ICD-10	54	—	16	—	3.4
Chakrabarti & Fombonne [45]	15 500	2.5–6.5	Child Parent Professional	ADI-R, 2 wks multidisciplinary assessment, Merrill-Palmer, WPPSI	ICD-10 DSM-IV	26	16.8	13	8.4	2.0
Chakrabarti & Fombonne (2004)	10 903	2.5–6.5	Child Parent Professional	ADI-R, 2 wks multidisciplinary assessment, Merrill-Palmer, WPPSI	ICD-10 DSM-IV	24	22.0	12	11.0	2.0
Overall						**614**		**123**		**5.0**

Table 3 Surveys of Childhood Disintegrative Disorder (CDD)

	Country (Region/State)	Size of target population	Age group	Assessment	N	M/F	Prevalence estimate (/100 000)	95 % CI (/100 000)
Burd et al. [20]	USA (North Dakota)	180 986	2–18	Structured parental interview and review of all data available—DSM-III criteria	2	2/-	1.11	0.13;3.4
Sponheim & Skjeldal [36]	Norway (Akershus County)	65 688	3–14	Parental interview and direct observation (CARS, ABC)	1	?	1.52	0.04;8.5
Magnusson & Saemundsen [44]	Iceland (whole island)	85 556	5–14	ADI-R, CARS and psychological tests—mostly ICD-10	2	2/-	2.34	0.3;8.4
Chakrabarti & Fombonne [45]	UK (Staffordshire, Midlands)	15 500	2.5–6.5	ADI-R, two weeks multidisciplinary assessment, Merrill-Palmer, WPPSI—ICD-10/DSM-IV	1	1/-	6.40	0.16;35.9
Chakrabarti & Fombonne (2004)	UK (Staffordshire, Midlands)	10 903	2.5–6.5	ADI-R, two weeks multidisciplinary assessment, Merrill-Palmer, WPPSI—ICD-10/DSM-IV	1	1/-	9.20	0;58.6
Pooled estimates		*358 633*			*7*	*6/-*	*1.90*	*0.87;4.15*

Table 4 Newer epidemiological surveys of PDDs

Study #	Author	Age	AUTISM			PDDNOS + AS			All PDDs
			Rate/ 10 000	*Male/ Female Ratio*	*% IQ normal*	*Rate/ 10 000*	*Male/ Female Ratio*	*% IQ normal*	*Rate/ 10 000*
26	Baird et al. [39]]	7	30.8	15.7	60.0	27.1	4.5	—	57.9
29	Bertrand et al. [42]	3–10	40.5	2.2	37.0	27.0	3.7	51.0	67.5
32	Chakrabarti & Fombonne [45]	4–7	16.8	3.3	29.0	44.5	4.3	94.0	61.3
35	Madsen et al. [6]	8	7.7	—	—	22.2	—	—	30.0
36	Chakrabarti & Fombonne (2004)	4–7	22.0	4.0	33.3	35.8	8.7	91.6	58.7
37	Scott et al. [53]	5–11	—	—	—	—	—	—	[1]58.3
38	Yeargin-Allsopp et al. [54]	3–10	—	—	—	—	—	—	34.0
39	Gurney et al. [5]	6–11	—	—	—	—	—	—	52.0

[1] Computed by the author

Referral Statistics

Increasing numbers of children referred to specialist services or known to special education registers have been taken as evidence for an increased incidence of autism-spectrum disorders. However, trends over time in *referred* samples are confounded by many factors such as referral patterns, availability of services, heightened public awareness, decreasing age at diagnosis and changes over time in diagnostic concepts and practices, to name only a few. Failure to control for these confounding factors was obvious in some recent reports,[56] such as the widely quoted reports from California educational services.[57],[58] Firstly, these reports applied to numbers rather than rates, and failure to relate these numbers to meaningful denominators left the interpretation of an upward trend vulnerable to changes in the composition of the underlying population. For example, the population of California was 19 971 000 in 1970 and rose to 35 116 000 as per July 1st 2002, a change of 75.8 %. Thus, part of the increase in numbers of subjects identified with autism merely reflects the change in population size, but this has not or incompletely been taken into account in the DDS reports. Second, the focus on the year-to-year changes in absolute numbers of subjects known to California state-funded services detracts from more meaningful comparisons. For example, as per December 2002, the total of subjects with a PDD diagnosis was 17 748 in the 0–19 age group (including 16 108 autism codes 1 & 2 and 1640 other PDDs).[58] The population of 0–19 year olds of California was 10 462 273 in July 2002. If one applies a rather conservative PDD rate of 30/10 000, one would expect to have 31 386 subjects within this age group with a PDD living in California. These calculations do not support the "epidemic" interpretation of the DDS data. Rather, they suggest that children identified in the DDS database were only a subset of the population prevalence pool and that the increasing numbers reflect merely an increasing proportion of children accessing services. Third, no attempt was ever made to adjust the trends for changes in diagnostic concepts and definitions. However, major nosographical modifications were introduced during the corresponding years with a general tendency in most classifications to broaden the concept of autism (as embodied in the terms "autism spectrum" or "pervasive developmental disorder"). Fourth, age characteristics of the subjects recorded in official statistics were portrayed in a confusing manner where the preponderance of young subjects was presented as evidence of increasing rates in successive birth cohorts.[56] The problems associated with disentangling age from period and cohort effects in such observational data are well known in the epidemiological literature and deserve better statistical handling. Fifth, the decreasing age at diagnosis leads in itself to increasing numbers of young children being identified in official statistics or being referred to already busy specialist services. Earlier identification of children from the prevalence pool may result in increased service activity; however, it does not mean increased *incidence*.

Another study of this dataset was subsequently launched to demonstrate the validity of the "epidemic" hypothesis.[59] The investigation was, however, flawed in its design. The authors relied on DDS data and aimed at ruling out changes in diagnostic practices, immigration into California as factors explaining the increased numbers. While immigration was reasonably ruled out, the study comparing diagnoses of autism and mental retardation over time was impossible to interpret in light of the extremely low (< 20 %) response rates. Furthermore, a study only based on cases registered for services cannot rule out that the proportion of cases within the general population who registered with services has changed over time. For example, assuming a constant incidence and prevalence at 2 different time points (i.e. there is no epidemic), the number of cases known to a public agency delivering services could well increase by 200 % if the proportion of cases from the community referred to services rises from 25 % to 75 % in the interval. In order to rule out this (likely, see above) explanation, data over time are needed *both* on referred subjects *and* on non-referred (or referred to other services) subjects. Failure to address this possibility precludes any inference to be drawn from a study of the DDS database to the California population.[55] The conclusions of this report were therefore simply unwarranted.

A recent re-analysis of the California data has in fact strongly suggested that switches in diagnostic practices from mental retardation to autism could also account for increased numbers of subjects with an autism diagnosis in the California DDS datasets.[4] Similar data were obtained in the UK by Jick and Kaye,[60] who showed that the incidence of specific developmental disorders (including language disorders) decreased by about the same amount that the incidence of diagnoses of autism increased in boys born from 1990–1997.

On the whole, evidence from these referral statistics is therefore very weak and certainly does not deserve the media attention that has been orchestrated around them. Accordingly, proper epidemiological studies are needed in order to assess secular changes in the incidence of a disorder.

Comparison of Cross-Sectional Epidemiological Surveys

Due to their cross-sectional methodology, most epidemiological investigations of autism have all been concerned with prevalence. As shown earlier, epidemiological surveys of autism each possess unique design features which could account almost entirely for between-studies variations in rates, and time trends in rates of autism are therefore difficult to gauge from published prevalence rates. The significant correlation previously mentioned between prevalence rate and year of publication could merely reflect increased efficiency over time in case identification methods used in surveys as well as changes in diagnostic concepts and practices. Thus, changes in diagnostic practices were reported in Magnusson and Saemundsen's study,[44] where ICD-9 rates for the oldest cohorts born in the years 1964–1983 were lower than the ICD-10 rates of the most recent 1984–1992 birth cohorts. Similarly, lower rates in the oldest birth cohorts were thought to reflect changes in diagnostic practices and boundaries in the study of Webb et al.[34] One large survey recently conducted in the UK (study 24) also documented a steep rise in the number of cases diagnosed with autism or atypical autism, and a similar trend for AS. The interpretation of these trends is, however, unclear since there was control of neither drift, over time, in diagnostic practices nor of changes in service development.

The most convincing evidence that method factors could account for most of the variability in published prevalence estimates comes from a direct comparison of 8 recent surveys conducted in the UK and the USA (Table 5). In each country, 4 surveys were conducted around the same year and with similar age groups. As there is no reason to expect huge between-area differences in rates, prevalence estimates should therefore be comparable within each country. However, an inspection of estimates obtained in each set of studies (Table 5: right-hand column) shows a six-fold variation in rates for UK surveys, and a fourteen-fold variation in US rates. In each set of studies, high rates derive from surveys where intensive population-based screening techniques were employed whereas lower rates were obtained from studies relying on administrative methods for case finding. Since no passage of time was involved, the magnitude of these gradients in rates can only be attributed to differences in case identification methods across surveys, and the replication of the pattern in two countries provides even more confidence in this interpretation. Thus, following this analysis of recent and contemporaneous studies, it should become obvious that no inference on trends in the incidence of PDDs can be derived from a simple comparison of prevalence rates over time, since studies conducted at different periods are likely to differ even more with respect to their methodology.

The next two approaches are in essence comparable to this one although specific attempts are made to maintain some design features of surveys constant.

Table 5 Study design impact on prevalence

	Location	Size	Age Group	Method	PDD Rate /10 000
UK Studies					
Chakrabarti & Fombonne [45]	Staffordshire	15 500	2 ½–6 ½	Intense screening + assessment	62.6
Baird et al. [39]	South East Thames	16 235	7	Early screening + follow-up identification	57.9
Fombonne et al. [43]	England & Wales	10 438	5–15	National household survey of psychiatric disorders	26.1
Taylor et al. [37]	North Thames	490 000	0–16	Administrative records	10.1
US Studies					
Bertrand et al. [42]	Brick Township, NJ	8896	3–10	Multiple sources of ascertainment	67.0
Sturmey & James [61]	Texas	3 564 577	6–18	Educational services	16.0
DDS [57]	California	3 215 000	4–9	Educational services	15.0
Hillman et al. [62]	Missouri	—	5–9	Educational services	4.8

Repeat Surveys in Defined Geographical Areas

Repeated surveys, using the same methodology and conducted in the same geographical area at different points in time, can potentially yield useful information on time trends provided that methods are kept relatively constant. The Göteborg studies[27],[29] provided 3 prevalence estimates which increased over a short period of time from 4.0 (1980) to 6.6 (1984) and 9.5/10 000 (1988), the gradient being even steeper if rates for the urban area alone are considered (4.0, 7.5 and 11.6/10 000).[29] However, comparisons of these rates is not straightforward as different age groups were included in each survey. For example, the rate in the first survey for the youngest age group (which resembles more closely the children included in the 2 other surveys) was 5.1/10 000. Secondly, the increased prevalence in the second survey was explained by improved detection among the mentally retarded, and that of the third survey by cases born to immigrant parents. That the majority of the latter group was born abroad suggests that migration into the area could be a key explanation. Taken in conjunction with a change in local services and a progressive broadening of the definition of autism over time acknowledged by the authors,[29] these findings do not provide evidence for an increased incidence in the rate of autism.

Two separate surveys conducted on children born 1992-1995 and 1996-1998 in Staffordshire in the UK (Table 1: studies 32 and 36) were performed with rigorously identical methods for case definition and case identification. The prevalence for combined PDD was comparable and not statistically different in the 2 surveys (Chakrabarti and Fombonne, unpublished data, 2004), suggesting no upward trend in overall rates of PDD during the studies time interval.

Successive Birth Cohorts

In large surveys encompassing a wide age range, increasing prevalence rates among the most recent birth cohorts could be interpreted as indicating a secular increase in the incidence of the disorder, provided that alternative explanations can confidently be ruled out. This analysis was used in two French surveys (Table 1: studies 17 and 20) which derived from large sample sizes. The surveys included consecutive birth cohorts from 1972 to 1985, and, pooling the data of both surveys, age-specific rates showed no upward trend.[33] Some weight should be given to these results as they derive from a total target population of 735 000 children, 389 of whom had autism. However, the most retarded children with autism were reflected in these studies and, as a consequence, any upward trend which would apply specifically to high-functioning subjects might have gone undetected.

A recent analysis of special educational disability from Minnesota (study 39) showed a sixteen-fold increase in the number of children identified with a PDD from 1991–1992 to 2001–2002.[5] The increase was not specific to autism since during the same period an increase of 50 % was observed for all disability categories (except severe mental handicap), especially for the category including ADHD. The large sample size allowed the authors to assess age, period and cohort effects. Prevalence increased regularly in successive birth cohorts; for example, amongst 7 year olds, the prevalence rose from 18/10 000 in those born in 1989, to 29/10 000 in those born in 1991 and to 55/10 000 in those born in 1993, suggestive of birth cohort effects. Within the *same* birth cohorts, age effects were also apparent since for children born in 1989 the prevalence rose with age from 13/10 000 at age 6, to 21/10 000 at age 9 and 33/10 000 at age 11. As argued by the authors, this pattern is not consistent with what one would expect from a chronic non fatal condition diagnosed in the first years of life. Their analysis also showed a marked period effect that identified the early 1990s as the period where rates started to go up in all ages and birth cohorts. Gurney et al.[5] further argued that this phenomenon coincided closely with the inclusion of PDDs in the federal Individual with Disabilities Educational Act (IDEA) funding and reporting mechanism in the USA. A similar interpretation of upward trends had been put forward by Croen et al.[4] in their analysis of the California DDS data.

Incidence Studies

Only three studies provided recently incidence estimates[40],[63] (also Smeeth et al, unpublished data, 2004). All studies showed an upward trend in incidence over short periods of time. For example, in the largest study of 1410 subjects, there was a 10-fold increase in the rate of first recorded diagnoses of PDDs in United Kingdom general practice medical records from 1988–1992 to 2000–2001 (Smeeth et al, unpublished data, 2004). The increase was more marked for PDDs other than autism but the increase in autism was also obvious.

However, none of these studies investigations could determine the impact of changes over time in diagnostic criteria, improved awareness and service availability on the upward trend.

Conclusion on Time Trends

The available epidemiological evidence does not strongly support the hypothesis that the incidence of autism has increased. As it stands now, the recent upward trend in rates of *prevalence* cannot be directly attributed to an increase in the *incidence* of the disorder. There is some evidence that diagnostic substitution and changes in the policies for special education and the increasing availability of services are responsible for the higher prevalence figures. Most of the existing epidemiological data are inadequate to properly test hypotheses on changes in the incidence of autism in human populations. Moreover, due to the low frequency of autism and PDDs, power is seriously limited in most investigations and variations of small magnitude in the incidence of the disorder are very likely to go on undetected.

Other Correlates

Autism, Race and Immigrant Status

Some investigators have mentioned the possibility that rates of autism might be higher among immigrants.[29],[64][66] Five of the 17 children with autism identified in the Camberwell study (study 4) were of Caribbean origin,[66] and the estimated rate of autism was 6.3/10 000 for this group as compared to 4.4/10 000 for the rest of the population.[2] However, the wide confidence intervals associated with rates from this study (Table 1) indicate no statistically significant difference. In addition, this area of London had received a large proportion of immigrants from the Caribbean region in the 1960's and, under circumstances where migration flux in and out of an area are happening, estimation of population rates should be viewed with much caution. Only one child was born from British-born Afro-Caribbean parents in a recent UK survey,[34] providing little support to this particular hypothesis. Similarly, the findings from the Göteborg studies paralleled an increased migration flux in the early 1980s in this area[64]; they, too, were based on relatively small numbers (19 children from immigrant parents). In the same geographical area, Arvidsson et al.[35] (study 22) had 5 children out of 9 in their sample with either both parents ($N = 2$) or 1 parent ($N = 3$) having immigrated to Sweden; however, there were no systematic comparisons with rates of immigrants in the population. It is worth noting that a positive family history for developmental disorders was reported in 3 such cases and a chromosomal abnormality in 1 further case. In the Icelandic survey (study 31), 2.5 % of the autism parents were from non-European origin compared to a 0.5 % corresponding rate in the whole population, but it was unclear if this represented a significant difference. In study 23, the proportion of children with autism and a non-European origin was marginally but not significantly raised as compared to the population rate of immigrants (8 % versus 2.3 %) but this was based on a very small sample (2 children on non-European origin). A UK survey found comparables rates in areas contrasting for their ethnic composition.[40] In the Utah survey (study 15, Table 2), where a clear breakdown by race was achieved,[26] the autism parents showed no deviation from the racial distribution of this state; the proportion of non-whites in this study and state was, however, noticeably low, providing little power to detect departures from the null hypothesis. Unfortunately, other studies have not systematically reported the proportion of immigrant or ethnic groups in the areas surveyed. However, in four studies where the proportions of immigrant groups were low (studies 11, 12, 19, 21), rates of autism were in the upper range of rates. Conversely, in other populations where immigrants contributed substantially to the denominators (studies 14, 17 and 20), rates were in the rather low band. The analysis of a large sample ($N = 4356$) of Californian PDD children showed a lower risk of autism in children of Mexico born mothers and a similar risk for children of mothers born outside the USA as compared to California born mothers.[67] In this study, the risk of PDD was raised in African-American mothers with an adjusted rate ratio of 1.6 (95 % CI: [1.5,1.8]); by contrast, the prevalence was similar in white, black and other races in the population based survey of Atlanta,[54] where case ascertainment is likely to be more complete than in the previous study.

Taken altogether, the combined results of these reports should be interpreted in the specific methodological context of these investigations. Most studies had low numbers of identified cases, and especially small numbers of autistic children born from immigrant parents, and many authors in these studies relied upon broadened definitions of autism. Statistical testing was not rigorously conducted and doubts could be raised in several studies about the appropriateness of the comparison data which were used. Thus, the overall proportion of immigrants in the population may be an inappropriate figure to which to compare observed rates of children from immigrant parents amongst autistic series; fertility rates of immigrant families are likely to be different from those in the host populations and call for strictly age-adjusted comparisons of individuals at risk for the disorder. The proportion of immigrants in the entire population might seriously underestimate that for younger age groups, and, in turn, this could have given rise to false positive results. In addition, studies sampling children through services or clinical sources may be biased as ethnicity and race are likely to differentially affect access to these settings. In addition, studies were generally poor in their definition of immigrant status, with some unclear amalgamation of information on country of origin, citizenship, immigrant status, race and ethnicity. Finally, it is unclear what common mechanism could explain the putative association between immigrant status and autism, since the origins of the immigrant parents (especially in study 16; see also Gillberg and Gillberg[68]) were very diverse and represented in fact all continents. With this heterogeneity in mind, what common biological features might be shared by these immigrant families and what would be a plausible mechanism explaining the putative association between autism and immigrant status? The possibility of an increased vulnerability to intrauterine infections in non-immunized immigrant mothers was raised but not supported in a detailed analysis of 15 autistic children from immigrant parents.[68] These authors instead posited that parents, and in particular fathers, affected with autistic traits would be inclined to travel abroad in order to find female partners more naïve to their social difficulties. This speculation was based, however, on 3 observations only, and assessment of the autistic traits in two parents was clearly not independently obtained.

The hypothesis of an association between immigrant status or race and autism, therefore, remains largely unsupported by the empirical results. Most of the claims about these possible correlates of autism derived from *post-hoc* observations of very small samples and were not subjected to rigorous statistical testing. Large studies have generally failed to detect such associations.

Autism and Social Class

Twelve studies provided information on the social class of the families of autistic children. Of these, 4 studies (1, 2, 3 and 5) suggested an association between autism and social class or parental education. The year of data collection for these four investigations was before 1980 (Table 2), and all studies conducted thereafter provided no evidence for the association. Thus, the epidemiological results suggest that the earlier findings were probably due to artefacts in the availability of services and in the case finding methods, as already shown in other samples.[66],[69]

Cluster Reports

Occasional reports of space or time clustering of cases of autism have raised concerns in the general public. In fact, only one such report has been published in the professional literature,[70] which described 7 children with either autism or PDDNOS living within a few streets from each other in a small town of the Midlands (UK). The cluster was first identified by a parent and the subsequent analysis was uninformed with proper statistical procedures and inconclusive as to whether or not this cluster could have occurred by chance only. The comparison of the incidence or prevalence rate within the cluster to that of the general population (as performed by Baron-Cohen et al.[70]) is an inappropriate technique to assess cluster alarms since, by definition, a pre-selection bias occurs in the delineation of the cluster boundaries.[1] Thus, finding an increased incidence or prevalence rate ratio in a cluster does *not* prove anything; this erroneous approach has been referred to in the literature as the Texan sharpshooter effect, referring to the gunman who shot first and then painted a target around the bullet hole. On the other hand, a negative finding would certainly suggest a random phenomenon.

Cluster alarms are likely to represent random occurrence in most instances, as illustrated by several recent investigations of cluster alarms for other rare disorders of childhood. Cluster alarms in autism have not been investigated with scientific rigor whereas research strategies and ad hoc statistical procedures exist for that purpose. The approach to such cluster alarms should be to confirm the alarm in the first place, using the available techniques to assess the significance of clusters and to exclude random noise in spatial and time distribution of the disorder. It is only when an alarm has been confirmed that more complex epidemiological investigations should be set up to investigate risk factors and causal mechanisms.

Conclusion

Epidemiological surveys of autism and PDDs have now been carried out in several countries. Methodological differences in case definition and case finding procedures make between survey comparisons difficult to perform. Nevertheless, in spite of these differences, some common characteristics of autism and PDDs in population surveys have emerged with some consistency. Autism is associated with mental retardation in about 70 % of the cases and is overrepresented amongst males (with a male/female ratio of 4.3:1). Autism is found in association with some rare and genetically determined medical conditions, such as tuberous sclerosis. A majority of surveys has ruled out social class as a risk factor for autism, a result once supported by studies of clinical, i.e. less representative, samples. The putative association of autism with immigrant status or race is, so far, not borne out by epidemiological studies. The conclusion of a lack of variation in the incidence of autism according to race or ethnicity is reached, however, from a weak empirical base and future studies might address this issue more efficiently. In fact, epidemiological studies of autism and PDDs have generally been lacking sophistication in their investigation of most other risk factors.

The same considerations apply to the issue of secular changes in the incidence of autism. The little evidence which exists does not support this hypothesis but power to detect time trends is seriously limited in existing datasets. The debate has been largely confounded by confusion between prevalence and incidence. Whilst it appears that prevalence estimates have gone up over time, this increase most likely represents changes in the concepts, definitions, service availability and awareness of autistic-spectrum disorders in both the lay and professional public. To assess whether or not the incidence has increased, method factors which account for an important proportion of the variability in rates must be tightly controlled.

Taking 35/10 000 and 60/10 000 as two working rates for the combination of all PDDs, and using population estimates for the USA of July 1st 2002, it can be estimated that about 284 000 and up to 486 000 subjects under the age of 20 suffer from a PDD in the USA. These figures carry straightforward implications for current and future needs in services and early educational intervention programs.

References

[1] Fombonne E. Epidemiological surveys of autism and other pervasive developmental disorders: an update. *Journal of Autism and Developmental Disorders.* 2003; 33:365-82.

[2] Wing L. The definition and prevalence of autism: A review. *European Child and Adolescent Psychiatry.* 1993; 2:61-74.

[3] Fombonne, E. The epidemiology of autism: A review. *Psychological Medicine.* 1999; 29:769-786.

[4] Croen LA, Grether JK, Hoogstrate J, Selvin S. The changing prevalence of autism in California. *Journal of Autism and Developmental Disorders.* 2002; 32:207-215.

[5] Gurney JG, Fritz MS, Ness KK, et al. Analysis of prevalence trends of autism spectrum disorder in Minnesota. *Archives of Pediatrics & Adolescent Medicine.* 2003; 157: 622-627.

[6] Madsen KM, Hviid A, Vestergaard M, et al. A population-based study of measles, mumps, and rubella vaccination and autism. *New England Journal of Medicine.* 2002; 347: 1477-1482.

[7] Le Couteur A, Rutter M, Lord C, et al. Autism Diagnostic Interview: A standardized investigator-based instrument. *Journal of Autism and Developmental Disorders.* 1989; 19: 363-387.

[8] Lord C, Risi S, Lembrecht L, et al. The Autism Diagnostic Observation Schedule—Generic: A standard measure of social and communication deficits associated with the spectrum of autism. *Journal of Autism and Developmental Disorders*. 2000; 30: 205-223.

[9] Spitzer RL, Siegel B. The DSM-III-R field trial of pervasive developmental disorders. *Journal of the American Academy of Child and Adolescent Psychiatry*. 1990; 6: 855-862.

[10]Volkmar FR, Klin A, Siegel B, et al. Field trial for autistic disorder in DSM-IV. *American Journal of Psychiatry*. 1994; 151: 1361-1367.

[11]Lotter V. Epidemiology of autistic conditions in young children, I: prevalence. *Social Psychiatry*. 1966; 1: 124-137.

[12]Brask BH. A prevalence investigation of childhood psychoses. In: Barnepsykiatrisk forening i Norge. *Nordic Symposium on the Care of Psychotic Children*. Oslo, Norway: Universitetsforlagets Trykningssentral; 1972: 145-153.

[13]Treffert DA. Epidemiology of infantile autism. *Archives of General Psychiatry*. 1970; 22: 431-438.

[14]Wing L, Yeates SR, Brierly LM, Gould J. The prevalence of early childhood autism: Comparison of administrative and epidemiological studies. *Psychological Medicine*. 1976; 6: 89-100.

[15]Wing L, Gould J. Severe impairments of social interactions and associated abnormalities in children: Epidemiology and classification. *Journal of Autism and Developmental Disorders*. 1979; 9: 11-29.

[16]Hoshino Y, Yashima Y, Ishige K, et al. The epidemiological study of autism in Fukushima Ken. *Folia Psychiatrica et Neurologica Japonica*. 1982; 36: 115-124.

[17]Bohman M, Bohman IL, Björck PO, Sjöholm E. Childhood psychosis in a northern Swedish county: Some preliminary findings from an epidemiological survey. In: Schmidt MH, Remschmidt H, eds. *Epidemiological Approaches in Child Psychiatry*. Stuttgart, Germany: Georg Thieme Verlag; 1983: 164-173.

[18]McCarthy P, Fitzgerald M, Smith MA. Prevalence of childhood autism in Ireland. *Irish Medical Journal*. 1984; 77: 129-130.

[19]Steinhausen H-C, Göbel D, Breinlinger M, Wohlloben B. A community survey of infantile autism. *Journal of the American Academy of Child Psychiatry*. 1986; 25: 186-189.

[20]Burd L, Fisher W, Kerbeshan J. A prevalence study of pervasive developmental disorders in North Dakota. *Journal of the American Academy of Child and Adolescent Psychiatry*. 1987; 26: 700-703.

[21]Matsuishi T, Shiotsuki M, Yoshimura K, Shoji H, Imuta F, Yamashita F. High prevalence of infantile autism in Kurume City, Japan. *Journal of Child Neurology*. 1987; 2: 268-271.

[22]Tanoue Y, Oda S, Asano F, Kawashima K. Epidemiology of infantile autism in Southern Ibaraki, Japan: Differences in prevalence in birth cohorts. *Journal of Autism and Developmental Disorders*. 1988; 18: 155-166.

[23]Bryson SE, Clark BS, Smith IM. First report of a Canadian epidemiological study of autistic syndromes. *Journal of Child Psychology and Psychiatry*. 1988; 4: 433-445.

[24]Sugiyama T, Abe T. The prevalence of autism in Nagoya, Japan: A total population study. *Journal of Autism and Developmental Disorders*. 1989; 19: 87-96.

[25]Cialdella P, Mamelle N. An epidemiological study of infantile autism in a French départment. *Journal of Child Psychology and Psychiatry*. 1989; 30: 165-175.

[26]Ritvo ER, Freeman BJ, Pingree C, et al. The UCLA-University of Utah epidemiologic survey of autism: Prevalence. *American Journal of Psychiatry.* 1989; 146: 194-199.

[27]Gillberg C. Infantile autism and other childhood psychoses in a Swedish region: Epidemiological aspects. *Journal of Child Psychology and Psychiatry.* 1984; 25: 35-43.

[28]Steffenburg S, Gillberg C. Autism and autistic-like conditions in Swedish rural and urban areas: A population study. *British Journal of Psychiatry.* 1986; 149: 81-87.

[29]Gillberg C, Steffenburg S, Schaumann H. Is autism more common now than ten years ago? *British Journal of Psychiatry.* 1991; 158: 403-409.

[30]Fombonne E, du Mazaubrun C. Prevalence of infantile autism in 4 French régions. *Social Psychiatry and Psychiatric Epidemiology.* 1992; 27: 203-210.

[31]Wignyosumarto S, Mukhlas M, Shirataki S. Epidemiological and clinical study of autistic children in Yogyakarta, Indonesia. *Kobe Journal of Medical Sciences.* 1992; 38: 1-19.

[32]Honda H, Shimizu Y, Misumi K, Niimi M, Ohashi Y. Cumulative incidence and prevalence of childhood autism in children in Japan. *British Journal of Psychiatry.* 1996; 169: 228-235.

[33]Fombonne E, du Mazaubrun C, Cans C, Grandjean H. Autism and associated medical disorders in a large French epidemiological sample. *Journal of the American Academy of Child and Adolescent Psychiatry.* 1997; 36: 1561-1569.

[34]Webb EVJ, Lobo S, Hervas A, Scourfield J, Fraser WI. The changing prevalence of autistic disorder in a Welsh health district. *Developmental Medicine and Child Neurology.* 1997; 39: 150-152.

[35]Arvidsson T, Danielsson B, Forsberg P, Gillberg C, Johansson M, Kjellgren G . Autism in 3-6 year-old children in a suburb of Goteborg, Sweden. *Autism.* 1997; 2: 163-173.

[36]Sponheim E, Skjeldal O. Autism and related disorders: epidemiological findings in a Norwegian study using ICD-10 diagnostic criteria. *Journal of Autism and Developmental Disorders.* 1998; 28: 217-227.

[37]Taylor B, Miller E, Farrington CP, et al. Autism and measles, mumps, and rubella vaccine: no epidemological evidence for a causal association. *The Lancet.* 1999; 353: 2026-2029.

[38]Kadesjö B, Gillberg C, Hagberg B. Autism and Asperger syndrome in seven-year old children: A total population study. *Journal of Autism and Developmental Disorders.* 1999; 29: 327-331.

[39]Baird G, Charman T, Baron-Cohen S, et al. A screening instrument for autism at 18 months of age: A 6 year follow-up study. *Journal of the American Academy of Child and Adolescent Psychiatry.* 2000; 39: 694-702.

[40]Powell J, Edwards A, Edwards M, Pandit BS, Sungum-Paliwal SR, Whitehouse W. Changes in the incidence of childhood autism and other autistic spectrum disorders in preschool children from two areas in the West Midlands, UK. *Developmental Medicine and Child Neurology.* 2000; 42: 624-628.

[41]Kielinen M, Linna SL, Moilanen I. Autism in Northern Finland. *European Child and Adolescent Psychiatry.* 2000; 9: 162-167.

[42]Bertrand J, Mars A, Boyle C, Bove F, Yeargin-Allsopp M, Decoufle P. Prevalence of autism in a United States population: the Brick Township, New Jersey, investigation. *Pediatrics.* 2001; 108: 1155-1161

[43]Fombonne E, Simmons H, Ford T, Meltzer H, Goodman R. Prevalence of pervasive developmental disorders in the British nationwide survey of child mental health. *Journal of the American Academy of Child and Adolescent Psychiatry.* 2001; 40: 820-827.

[44]Magnusson P, Saemundsen E. Prevalence of autism in Iceland. *Journal of Autism and Developmental Disorders.* 2001; 31: 153-163.

[45]Chakrabarti S, Fombonne E. Pervasive developmental disorders in preschool children. *Journal of the American Medical Association.* 2001; 285: 3093-3099.

[46]Davidovitch M, Holtzman G, Tirosh E. Autism in the Haifa area—an epidemiological perspective. *Israeli Medical Association Journal.* 2001; 3: 188-189.

[47]Lord C, Schopler E, Revecki D. Sex differences in autism. *Journal of Autism and Developmental Disorders.* 1982; 12: 317-330.

[48]Fombonne E. Prevalence of childhood disintegrative disorder (CDD). *Autism.* 2002; 6: 147-155.

[49]Fombonne E, Tidmarsh L. Epidemiological data on Asperger disorder. *Child and Adolescent Psychiatric Clinics of North America* 2003 ; 12: 15-21.

[50]Ehlers S, Gillberg C. The epidemiology of Asperger syndrome: A total population study. *Journal of Child Psychology and Psychiatry.* 1993; 34: 1327-1350.

[51]Webb E, Morey J, Thompsen W, Butler C, Barber M, Fraser WI. Prevalence of autistic spectrum disorder in children attending mainstream schools in a Welsh education authority. *Developmental Medicine and Child Neurology.* 2003; 45: 377-84.

[52]Volkmar FR. Childhood disintegrative disorder: Issues for DSM-IV. *Journal of Autism and Developmental Disorders.* 1992; 22: 625-642.

[53]Scott FJ, Baron-Cohen S, Bolton P, Brayne C. Brief report: Prevalence of autism spectrum conditions in children aged 5-11 years in Cambridgeshire, UK. *Autism.* 2002; 6: 231-237.

[54]Yeargin-Allsopp M, Rice C, Karapurkar T, Doernberg N, Boyle C, Murphy C. Prevalence of autism in a US metropolitan area. *JAMA* 2003; 289: 49-55.

[55]Fombonne E. The prevalence of autism. *JAMA* 2003; 289: 1-3.

[56]Fombonne E. Is there an epidemic of autism? *Pediatrics.* 2001; 107: 411-413.

[57]Department of Developmental Services. *Changes in the population of persons with autism and pervasive developmental disorders in California's Developmental Services System: 1987 through 1998.* Sacramento, CA: California Department of Developmental Services; 1999. Available at:
<http: //www.dds.ca.gov/autism/pdf/autism_report_1999.pdf>.

[58]Department of Developmental Services. *Autism Spectrum Disorders: Changes in the California Caseload—an Update 1999 through 2002.* Sacramento, CA: California Department of Developmental Services; 2003. Available at:
<http: //www.dds.ca.gov/Autism/pdf/AutismReport2003.pdf>.

[59]Byrd R, Sage AC, Keyzer J, et al. *Report to the Legislature on the Principal Findings from The Epidemiology of Autism in California. A comprehensive pilot study.* Sacramento, CA: UC Davis M.I.N.D. Institute; 2002. Available at:
<http: //www.ucdmc.ucdavis.edu/mindinstitute/html/news/pdfs/study_final.pdf>

[60]Jick H, Kaye JA. Epidemiology and possible causes of autism. *Pharmacotherapy.* 2003; 23: 1524-1530.

[61]Sturmey P, James V. Administrative prevalence of autism in the Texas school system. *Journal of the American Academy of Child and Adolescent Psychiatry.* 2001; 40: 621.

[62]Hillman R, Kanafani N, Takahashi T, Miles J. Prevalence of autism in Missouri: Changing trends and the effect of a comprehensive State autism project. *Missouri Medicine.* 2000; 97: 159-163.

[63]Kaye J, del Mar Melero-Montes M, Jick H. Mumps, measles, and rubella vaccine and the incidence of autism recorded by general practitioners: a time trend analysis. *British Medical Journal.* 2001; 322: 460-463.

[64]Gillberg C. Infantile autism in children of immigrant parents: A population-based study from Göteborg, Sweden. *British Journal of Psychiatry.* 1987; 150: 856-858.

[65]Gillberg C, Schaumann H, Gillberg IC. Autism in immigrants: children born in Sweden to mothers born in Uganda. *Journal of Intellectual Disability Research.* 1995; 39: 141-144.

[66]Wing L. Childhood autism and social class: A question of selection? *British Journal of Psychiatry.* 1980; 137: 410-417.

[67]Croen LA, Grether JK, Selvin S. Descriptive epidemiology of autism in a California population: who is at risk? *Journal of Autism and Developmental Disorders.* 2002; 32: 217-224.

[68]Gillberg IC, Gillberg C. Autism in immigrants: a population-based study from Swedish rural and urban areas. *Journal of Intellectual Disability Research.* 1996; 40: 24-31.

[69]Schopler E, Andrews CE, Strupp K. Do autistic children come from upper-middle-class parents? *Journal of Autism and Developmental Disorders.* 1979; 9: 139-151.

[70]Baron-Cohen S, Saunders K, Chakrabarti S. Does autism cluster geographically? A research note. *Autism.* 1999; 3: 39-43.

[71]Kulldorff M. Statistical evaluation of disease cluster alarms. In: Lawson AB, Biggeri A, Böhning D, Lesaffre E, Viel J-F, Bertollini R, eds. *Disease mapping and risk assessment for public health.* Chichester, UK: Wiley & Sons; 1999:143-149.

In: Recent Developments in Autism Research
Editor: Manuel F. Casanova, pp. 27-55
ISBN 1-59454-358-5
© 2005 Nova Science Publishers, Inc.

Chapter II

The Savant Syndrome in Autistic Disorder

Darold A. Treffert, M.D. *
W4065 Maplewood Lane Fond du Lac, Wisconsin 54935 Clinical Professor,
Department of Psychiatry University of Wisconsin Medical School, Madison, Wisconsin

Introduction

Savant Syndrome is a rare, but spectacular, condition in which persons with various developmental disabilities, including Autistic Disorder, have astonishing areas of brilliance, ability or talent—"islands of genius"—that stand in jarring, marked contrast to overall handicap. Savant syndrome is of special interest in autistic disorder however because as many as 10 % of autistic persons can have these extraordinary abilities, a much higher incidence than any other CNS disorders such as mental retardation, other developmental disabilities, brain injury or disease.[1] Why should that be so? What is it about autistic disorder that produces this fairly common linkage in an otherwise rare disorder?

While the first cases of savant abilities were described as long as 150 years ago, the cases of the so-called "calculating twins"—identical twin brothers with autism—brought the *autistic savant* to new attention. At the 1964 American Psychiatric Association Annual meeting Horwitz and his co-workers[2] presented a paper describing the phenomenal calendar calculating and memory abilities of these twin brothers. They are examples of savant syndrome occurring in autistic disorder. The brothers can identify on what day a particular date fell or will fall over a time-span of 80 000 years, or can tell, for example what date the second Tuesday of April will fall in the next 40 years, or what years, in the next 100, Easter will fall on March 18th. They also can remember the weather for each day of their adult life. Sacks[3] describes these two brothers swapping 20 digit prime number for amusement when they were hospitalized together, yet were unable to multiply the simplest of numbers. They

* dtreffert@pol.net

also were able to count matches as they fell to the floor instantly, almost before they hit the floor.

If those scenes sound familiar, they are, because those were some of the savant abilities incorporated into the composite autistic savant Raymond Babbitt, portrayed so accurately by Dustin Hoffman in the award winning movie *Rain Man* which made "autistic savant" a household term.

A discussant at that 1964 APA meeting noted: *"The importance then, of the Idiot Savant lies in our inability to explain him; he stands as a monument of our own ignorance and the phenomenon of the idiot savant exists as a challenge to our capabilities"*. Indeed he or she does still present a challenge for explanation and understanding, but no model of brain function will be complete until it can account for, and fully incorporate, this extraordinary phenomenon. The autistic savant may provide some special insights toward such understanding and this is what this chapter hopes to explore.

Some Early Descriptions

Dr. Benjamin Rush, the father of American Psychiatry, provided one of the earliest reports of savant syndrome in 1789 when he described in detail the lightning calculating ability of Thomas Fuller "who could comprehend scarcely anything, either theoretical or practical, more complex than counting."[4] When Fuller was asked how many seconds a man had lived who was 70 years, 17 days, and 12 hours old he gave the correct answer of 2 210 500 800 in 90 seconds, even correcting for the 17 leap years included.

The term *idiot savant*, however, was coined by Dr. J. Langdon Down in 1887 and remained the name for that condition in the medical literature for the next 100 years.[5] In a series of lectures that year before the Medical Society of London, Down, who is better remembered for having named Down's Syndrome, recounted his 30 year experience as Superintendent of the Earlswood Asylum during which time he had encountered some fascinating cases that demonstrated a striking juxtaposition of superiority and deficiency in the same patients. Among the 10 cases he described in colorful detail were the characteristic musical, artistic, mathematical and mechanical skills, coupled with phenomenal memory, which have so unfailingly typified the savant syndrome since that time. Dr. Down meant no harm by the term "idiot", and in fact apologized for having to apply it—"I have no liking for the term. It is so frequently a name of reproach," he cautioned. But at that time the term *idiot* was an accepted, official, scientific term in England for persons with an IQ below 25 and Down combined that with the word savant, or "knowledgeable person", derived from the French word *savoir* meaning "to know".

While descriptive, the term was actually a misnomer since almost all reported cases occur in persons with IQ above 40. In the interest of accuracy and dignity the term savant syndrome has been substituted and is widely used. The term savant syndrome is preferable to *autistic savant* because, as will be shown, only about 50 % of persons with savant syndrome have autistic disorder, and the other 50 % have other developmental disabilities or other forms of central nervous system injury or disease.

Of the 10 cases Dr. Down described in his lectures, it is not clear which might have had autistic disorder since that condition was not recognized at that time as such. The cases were all categorized simply as mental retardation or mental deficiency. While Down describes the particular skills his 10 patients possessed, he does not describe their overall status sufficient to reach any conclusions about diagnosis beyond mental retardation. But certainly, even from the brief descriptions of the various skills, one can presume that some of his cases may have had autistic disorder. One other observation by Down has stood the test of time—the rarity of female savants: "All these cases of idiot savants were males, I have never met with a female."

Twenty-seven years later it was Dr. A. F. Tredgold,[6] however, who wrote the first definitive work on this fascinating condition, devoting an entire chapter to the idiot savant in his 1914 textbook, *Mental Deficiency*, still available in revised editions today. Although more modern and sophisticated theories about the savant have emerged in the 90 years since that chapter was written, Tredgold's precise observations, and careful, colorful and detailed clinical descriptions have never been surpassed. It provides trailblazing, classic and insightful descriptions. Tredgold describes 20 patients "with special aptitudes which are quite phenomenal, not merely in comparison with aments, but often with the acquirements of ordinary persons," that had been brought to his attention by a number of his colleagues. Those cases are a catalog and index of the categories of skills—musical, artistic, mathematical, calendar calculating and mechanical/spatial—which simply are repeated over and over again, strikingly so, in cases reported by so many different investigators over these many years since that chapter was published. Several additional, special skills are reported as well however: the "gift of tongues"—a polyglot savant; a case of heightened "special senses"—olfactory and tactile abilities; and a case of "pronounced sense of locality"—spatial and directional skills. Each of those cases also document the prodigious memory so typical and uniform in present day cases, now nearly a century later. Tredgold was particularly intrigued with the case of The Genius of Earlswood Asylum and describes that remarkable savant in elaborate, and colorful detail.

Like Down, Tredgold noted that female savants were conspicuously few and only one of his cases was a female. Once again, however, there is not sufficient clinical detail about each case to reach a conclusion regarding how many of Tredgold's cases had autistic disorder, but certainly, without doubt, a number of his cases by present day standards would have a diagnosis of autistic disorder.

Recent Reviews of Savant Syndrome

After Tredgold's classic chapter, a number of anecdotal reports of individual savant cases continued to appear in the scientific literature. But it was more than six decades later that Hill[7] provided a comprehensive review article on the "special skills" of "savants," along with discussion on theories of causation. That review covered more than 60 reports from the late 1890's to the mid-1970's involving over 100 savants. That same year, Rimland[1] provided a summary of his data on "special abilities," as reported by parents, in 531 autistic children out of a total of a survey population which at that time numbered 5400 autistic children in the Institute for Child Behavior Research Data Bank (Rimland has over 34 000 such cases now in that data bank). A decade later the next review article, "The idiot savant: a review of the syndrome," appeared in the *American Journal of Psychiatry*,[8] and a year later the book, *Extraordinary People: Understanding Savant Syndrome*[9] was published. That book was re-issued later with an epilogue update.[10]

It is a comprehensive review of the history of the disorder, case reports since Down's original description, a summary of the theories of causation, and it documents recent advances and new research. In his 1989 book *Musical Savants*, Miller[11] provides an in-depth review of that topic, including a detailed description of a new case. An article which explores savant syndrome in autistic persons specifically was published by Kehrer[12] under the title *Savant capabilities of autistic persons*. The most recent in-depth, review article of savant syndrome, including an extensive bibliography, was published by Nettelbeck and Young,[13] in which they reviewed more than 100 publications between 1978 and 1999, as well as five books.[3]'[9]'[11]'[14]'[15] Dr. Beate Hermelin[16] recently summarized her personal story of research with autistic savants over a long time span in her book *Bright Splinters of the Mind.*

Savant Syndrome Today—What We Do Know

There are a number of things we do know about savant syndrome even though there is still much we need to explore further. But from the accounts and research over the past 150 years certain things can be said:

Incidence

Savant syndrome is rare. In Rimland's survey[1] of 5400 autistic children, 531 (9.8 %) were reported by parents to have special abilities. Hermelin[16] puts that figure much lower, however, stating, "It is now more realistically held that at most one or two in 200 of those within the autistic spectrum disorder can justifiably be regarded as having a genuine talent," although she goes on to point out, importantly, "though a reliable frequency estimate does not exist as yet." Hill[7] found that the incidence of savant skills was 1: 2000 (0.06 %) in an institutionalized population with a diagnosis of mental retardation. A recent study[17] in Finland, based on a survey of 583 facilities serving persons with developmental disabilities, found 45 cases of savant syndrome creating an incidence of 1.4 per thousand, or approximately double the Hill incidence estimate, but still very uncommon. It is not unusual to encounter a clinician who has not seen a person with savant syndrome throughout years of a busy practice in private or public settings even if seeing a substantial number of persons with developmental disabilities.

Whatever the exact figures, savant syndrome, although rare overall, is seen much more frequently, conspicuously so, in autistic disorder than in other developmental disabilities or in mental retardation. However since mental retardation particularly is much more common than autistic disorder, about 50 % of persons with savant syndrome have autistic disorder, and the other 50 % have other forms of developmental disability or mental retardation. Thus not all autistic persons are savants, and not all savants have autistic disorder.

Sex Ratio

Consistent in all the reports since Down's original description, males outnumber females in an approximate 6: 1 ratio. Of 103 persons classified as savants in 63 publications, Hill[7] reported 89 were male and 14 were female providing that 6: 1 male: female ratio. Part of the reason for the higher male incidence of savant syndrome is the relatively high incidence of savant syndrome in autistic disorder which itself has an already high 4: 1 male: female ratio. Contributing to the male: female discrepancy in both disorders are newer findings on the role of testosterone on cerebral lateralization, which will be discussed below.

Congenital vs. Acquired Etiology

The vast majority of savant syndrome cases occur in those conditions, including developmental disabilities, present from birth. But cases do occur where the special skill arises after injury or disease to the central nervous system in infancy, childhood or even adult life, including recent cases of striking savant abilities emerging as a fronto-temporal dementia proceeds. Other etiologies for acquired savant abilities have been head injury, encephalitis, epilepsy or stroke. These cases of 'acquired' savant abilities raise special questions about buried potential, perhaps, within us all and point out as well the plasticity, and compensatory potential, of the central nervous system in some persons.

Mental Handicap, Blindness and Musical Genius

Conspicuously prominent in all the cases of savant syndrome in the past, and present cases as well, is the recurrent, curious triad of developmental disability, blindness and musical genius. While this musical genius and blindness can sometimes be linked with mental retardation or other forms of developmental disability, the link with autism has been particularly striking, and seemingly disproportionate.

The link of music with mental handicap and blindness has a long history. Tredgold[6] (1914) described of a case of a blind, musical savant at the Salpetriere in 1861 and he made observed that "most aments are fond of music." Later that century Thomas Greene Wiggins, known more popularly as "Blind Tom" Buthune[18] became internationally well known, and may have been the highest paid black performer of that era. He was described by some as "the eighth wonder of the world." A number of recent cases, with autism as the basic disability, have become particularly prominent and well known.[10] In a closer look at these cases two additional factors almost always surface—premature birth and blindness is usually from retinopathy of prematurity (retrolental fibroplasias). Keeler[19] pointed out the frequent occurrence of infantile autism in patients blinded from retrolental fibroplasias, compared to blindness from other causes, and raised the question of whether some vascular capillary process similar to that which occurs in the retina (which is brain tissue) might occur elsewhere in the brain and lead to the characteristic autistic symptoms seen in these patients. Rimland[20] also raised that same possibility commenting on the high frequency of premature births in autistic children, some of whom developed retrolental fibroplasia suggesting the same process on the retina may be duplicated in the reticular activating system particularly.

The relationship of blindness, premature birth, autistic disorder and musical genius is discussed in more detail by Treffert.[9]

More recently a second cause visual impairment with links to mental handicap and musical genius has begun to surface. Optic Nerve Hypoplasia (ONH), or underdevelopment of the optic nerves, was once considered rare but is now a leading cause of pediatric congenital vision loss in the U.S. Septo-optic Dysplasia (SOD), sometimes known as DeMorsier's Syndrome, is a form of ONH with many associated structural abnormalities of the brain, including absence of the corpus callosum and/or septum pellucidum, abnormalities of the pituitary gland and other endocrine abnormalities. A number of parents of ONH and SOD children have noted autistic-like behaviors in their children along with musical expertise. A web site at www.focusfamiliesl.org serves as a valuable resource on the manifestations and management of SOD and ONH. On that site there is a very interesting, and helpful link to a chart entitled *Autism Spectrum Disorder in Learners with Blindness/Vision Impairments—A Comparison of Characteristics.* This chart compares and contrasts "typical development", "Blind/Vision Impaired Development", and "Autism Spectrum Disorder Development" on several scales including communication; responses to sensory information; and restricted, repetitive and stereotyped patterns of behavior. These comparisons are important because there are a number of skills and behaviors that children with visual impairment can have that are similar to, but not the same as, skills and behaviors seen in autism spectrum disorders.

The overlap of certain behaviors in children with vision impairment or loss with those of autism are well known and reported, and in comprehensive evaluations of children with vision impairment or loss it is vital to make those differentiations.

The link between vision loss or impairment and musical genius is sufficiently common that a special facility—Soundscape—opened in London in November, 2003 totally devoted to persons, a number of whom have autistic disorder, who have loss of sight coupled with musical ability, and in some cases, musical genius. One such autistic savant, Derek, has become quite well known in England, and internationally as well, as a very accomplished jazz piano musician. A publication by Ockelford[21] describes the use of music in the education of children and young people who are visually impaired and have learning disabilities.

The Nature of the Special Skills

Considering all the skills in the human repertoire, it is striking savant skills, through all the reports this past 150 years, occur within a consistent and intriguingly narrow range. Those are generally in five areas: music; art; calendar calculating; lightning calculating and mechanical or spatial skills. Calendar calculating is often the most frequently reported skill. Why this obscure ability appears with such regularity among almost all savants is a particularly intriguing question. The musical skill is most often performance, and usually piano playing although complex composing has been reported as well as facility with as many as 20 instruments. Art skills are usually drawing or painting although sculpting is reported as well. Lightning calculating includes rapid calculation of complex equations or fascination and facility with prime numbers, for example. Mechanical or spatial skills include the ability to measure distances precisely without benefit of instruments, for example, or the ability to construct complex models or structures with painstakingly fine accuracy.

Other skills have been reported less often. They include prodigious language facility—polyglot savants[15]; unusual sensory discrimination in smell, touch or vision; perfect appreciation of passing time without knowledge of clock face; superior coordination and balance skills and athletic ability; and outstanding knowledge in specific fields such as neurophysiology, statistics or navigation, for example. In Rimland's[1] sample of 543 autistic children in whom special skills were reported musical ability was the most frequently reported skill followed by memory (which he listed as a special skill), then art, pseudo verbal abilities, mathematics, maps and directions, coordination, calendar calculating and extrasensory perception in that order.

Generally a single, special skill exists but in some savants several skills exist simultaneously. Rimland and Fine[22] noted that the incidence of multiple skills appeared to be higher in autistic savants than in savants with other developmental disabilities. Sometimes the multiple skill surfaces with the same enormity, and surprise, as the original skill.

While right brain/left brain terminology is an oversimplification, because of cross connections and cross representations, the two brain hemispheres do tend to specialize in certain functions. Savant skills tend to be those associated with the right hemisphere—non-symbolic, artistic, concrete, directly perceived—in contrast to those associated with the left hemisphere which are more sequential, logical, symbolic and including language specialization. Whatever the skills they are always associated with prodigious memory within the skill area itself. It is a memory of special type—vastly deep but exceedingly narrow—as will be described later. Some observers list prodigious memory as a special skill, adding it as a skill in addition to the five general areas listed above. However prodigious memory ability is, in my view, a skill all savants possess cutting across all of the skill areas a shared, integral part of the syndrome itself. That is, the special skill + prodigious memory *is* the savant syndrome.

Finally, these skills exist over a *spectrum of abilities*. The most common savant abilities are called *splinter skills*. These include behaviors such as obsessive preoccupation with, and memorization of, music and sports trivia, license plates numbers, maps, historical facts, or obscure items such as vacuum cleaner motor sounds, for example. *Talented savants* are those persons in whom musical, artistic, mathematical or other special skills are more prominent and highly honed, usually within an area of single expertise, and are very conspicuous when viewed against their overall handicap. The term *prodigious savant* is reserved for those very rare persons in an already uncommon condition where the special skill or ability is so outstanding that it would be spectacular even if it were to occur in a non-handicapped person. There are probably fewer than 50 prodigious savants living worldwide at the present time who would meet this very high threshold of special skill. The placement on this spectrum is admittedly subjective but there does seem to be a natural division between these three levels of ability and expertise.

The Extraordinary Memory of the Savant

Whatever the special skills the savant demonstrates, a remarkable memory of a unique and uniform type welds the condition together.[23] Terms such as automatic, mechanical, concrete and habit-like have been applied to this extraordinary memory of the savant by clinicians and researchers alike this past century. Down[5] used the term "verbal adhesion" to describe a memory adept at remembering facts without comprehension of their meaning. Critchley[24] described savant memory as "exultation of memory" or "memory without reckoning." Tredgold[6] used the term "automatic" and Barr[25] characterized his patient with prodigious memory as "an exaggerated form of habit."

Such unconscious memory—memory without reckoning—suggests what Mishkin and Petri[26] referred to a non-cognitive "habit" formation system rather than a "cognitive" memory system. They proposed two different neural circuits for these two different types of memory, a higher level cortico-limbic circuit for so called semantic or cognitive memory, and a lower level, cortico-striatal circuit for the more primitive habit memory which is sometimes referred to as procedural memory. It may be that the same factors that produced left hemisphere damage, including prenatal hormonal influences in some cases, are instrumental in producing damage to the higher level cognitive memory circuits leaving the savant to rely on the more primitive, but spared, habit memory circuits and thus producing the characteristic right brain skills coupled with habit memory capabilities.

Others have suggested defects and dysfunction in the hippocampus and amygdala may produce the uniform type of memory that savants display. Rimland and Fine[22] suggested that defects in amygdala function produced over-reliance on the hippocampus in memory function and retrieval, producing the extraordinary memory in the savant. In support of that hypothesis Bauman and Kemper[27] found histopathologic changes in the hippocampus, amygdala, cerebellum and other areas of the forebrain in a post-mortem examination of a 25 year old autistic patient. They concluded such pathology occurred early in the prenatal period and included neuron destruction in the affected areas. They further suggested "although defects in memory have been little studied in autism, they may well underlie the pronounced difficulties in social interaction, language function, and learning that characterize these patients."

Some Well Known Autistic Savants

Six of Kanner's[28] original 10 cases of Early Infantile Autism had musical abilities specifically mentioned. Most had a broad repertoire of songs by age 3. One child at age 1½ was able to name the composers of symphonies played to him and all the children were able to reproduce accurately songs they had heard only a few times. Kanner was struck in general by the overall heightened memory capacity of all of his 10 Early Infantile Autism cases.

The identical twin brother calendar calculators have been extensively described by Horwitz[2] and more recently by Sacks[3]. One of the twins was featured on the 1983 *60 Minutes* program on savant syndrome that featured three remarkable and memorable savants—a pianist, a sculptor and calendar calculator. Many persons remember that program vividly, entitled *Genius,* as their first exposure to savant syndrome on national television. Several of the twins' special abilities were incorporated into the savant skills of Raymond Babbitt in the movie *Rain Man*. Viscott[29] after four years of therapy with a female musical savant described her case in great detail with special attention to the psychodynamics of the case and how those factors impacted on the acquisition of her remarkable musical skills. Selfe[30] documented the case of Nadia who, at age 3 had phenomenal drawing ability but lost that astonishing ability at age 7 when she entered a school for language development. As her language skills increased, her special drawing ability disappeared. Questions have arisen as to whether that was merely a temporal coincidence, or whether there was, in her case, a costly trade-off of the special skills for language and social skills development.

Stephen Wiltshire's phenomenal art ability has been well publicized by two very successful art books by, and about him: *Drawings* and *Floating Cities*.[31],[32] Sacks[33] wrote a very informative introduction to the *Floating Cities* book and has written extensively elsewhere about Stephen as well. To the surprise of all those around him, Stephen rather suddenly showed a dramatic musical savant ability in addition to his already well demonstrated art ability. A BBC documentary underscores his extraordinary drawing and memory skills when, after a 12 minute helicopter ride over London, three hours later he has produced a drawing of his vision from the sky, extraordinarily accurate, containing 4 square miles, 12 major landmarks and 200 other buildings. The President of the Royal Academy in London said, of Stephen as a child artist, "Happily, every now and then, a rocket of young talent explodes and continues to shower us with his sparks. Stephen is one of those rockets…I've never seen in all my competition drawing such a natural and extraordinary talent this child seems to have…Stephen is possibly the best child artist in Britain."[31]

Richard is a well-known Scottish artist whose drawings are internationally renowned and collected by Margaret Thatcher and Pope John Paul II, among others.[10],[34] A London art professor was "thunderstruck" by the oil crayon drawings that Wawro did as a child, describing them as an "incredible phenomenon rendered with the precision of a mechanic and the vision of a poet." A 1983 videotape entitled *With Eyes Wide Open,* and a 1989 videotape entitled *A Real Rain Man: Portrait of an Autistic Savant* document his outstanding abilities and growth as an artist.

Joseph is a person with whom Dustin Hoffman spent a great deal of time preparing for his role depicting both autism, and savant skills. The movie opened in Joseph's hometown as a thank you to Joseph and his mother for all their help in that preparation. Joseph has lightning calculating abilities and extensive memorization capacity. There have been two excellent documentaries about Joseph, a 1967 film called *The Invisible Wall*, and a 1986 film entitled *Portrait of an Autistic Young Man,* both projects of the UCLA Behavioral Sciences Media Laboratory. Mr. Hoffman not only viewed those films in preparing for his role in *Rain Man*, but viewed some 16 hours of outtakes from the 1986 production as well.

Tony, blind and autistic, is an extremely gifted jazz pianist whose skills, at age 17, were so impressive to allow him to be admitted to the prestigious Berklee College of Music in Boston from which he graduated magna cum laude. Films of Tony at age 6 provided evidence of his already massive talent and on March 2, 1997, the CBS Sunday Night Movie, *Journey to the Heart*, told his remarkable story. Tony presently is proficient on 20 musical instruments and has released three CDs.[10]

Most recently Matt, age 11, has gained a great deal of notoriety nationally and internationally as a jazz piano performer, and composer. He heads his own group—The Matt Savage Trio—joining with two professional musicians in a group he leads. As a tribute to his talent, the Bosendorfer Piano Company has honored him as a Bosendorfer Piano Artist. He is the youngest such artist, and the only child, be so named in the 175 year history of the company. He and his group have played at the New Orleans Jazz Festival, The Blue Note Jazz Club in New York, among many other venues, and have had three appearances to date on the *Today* show. He has released four CDs, the more recent ones consisting generally of all his own compositions.

Jonathan Lerman: Drawings by an Artist with Autism[35] was published as a very insightful book about Jonathan and his extraordinary art. A critic describes Jonathan's art as "working with the assurance of a Matisse, the speed of a Picasso, and the humor of a born cartoonist." Of particular interest is the fact that Jonathan's art includes interpretation, rather than just replication, and includes fascination with faces, a trait very unique among autistic artists. Also, the emotional tone of Jonathan's pictures is very evident and striking, a characteristic also usually not the focus of other savant artists.

Female savants continue to be rare in this already rare condition. But the most well known case is that of Nadia described in detail by Selfe,[30] whose case has triggered considerable discussion about a "dreaded trade-off," perhaps, of special skills for language and social skills acquisition. I will address that question later. Viscott[29] documented in great detail, including considerable psychodynamic detail, a female musical savant whom he followed for a number of years. Ellen is a blind, autistic musician described in detail by Treffert.[9] Along with her musical ability Ellen demonstrates very precise spatial location abilities, and precise time keeping without access to a clock face or other time instruments.

Rain Man, the Movie: Rain Man, Real Life

For most persons the autistic savant they know best is Raymond Babbitt as depicted so realistically by Dustin Hoffman in the Academy Award winning movie *Rain Man*. That film, while not a documentary, did a great public service in educating a whole nation about autistic savants, making that term a household word. The inspiration for the original script of that movie was based on a real life person, Kim, with a massive encyclopedic memory. But the story is not based on Kim's life or abilities alone. Instead, the autistic characteristics, and the savant abilities grafted on to that autism, that Raymond Babbitt possesses represents a composite of abilities from a number of real life autistic savants, some of whom are described above. Dustin Hoffman spent time with several savants, and their families, to learn the characteristics of autism, and the types of special abilities savants demonstrate. He did a marvelous job then depicting both autism, and savant skills. As mentioned, while not a documentary, that movie turned out to be a tremendous public education tool regarding autism, and savant abilities, as embodied in the autistic savant. The producers were interested in maintaining accuracy, and sensitivity. In my view both goals were met. There was no "cure" of autism in a six-day cross-country trip. And Raymond Babbitt did not end up changing drastically in those six days. Rather, it was the brother who changed from at first dismissing Raymond's special abilities as a deterrent or nuisance, to seeing them as special gifts, and from seeing his brother as a weird person to appreciating his brother as a very special person. There is a message in that change for all of society—it is we who need to change our stereotyping and classifying rather than always expecting the autistic savant to somehow change and conform to our idea of what shape their soul should be.

The only reservation about the movie is that some in the audience may come away with the impression that all autistic persons are savants, or that all savants are autistic. As pointed out above, neither is true. Not all autistic persons are savants, and not all savants have autistic disorder.

More information about each of the savants above, and examples of some of their special skills and abilities can be found on the savant syndrome web site at www.savantsyndrome.com. There is much more information about the movie *Rain Man* on that site as well.

Theories to Explain the Savant

Over the past century numerous theories have been put forth in an attempt to explain the savant syndrome phenomenon by various investigators. Those theories have included eidetic imagery or the related but separate phenomenon generally called photographic memory; inherited skills; sensory deprivation and social isolation; highly developed rote memory; compensation and reinforcement to offset lack of more generalized skills; and concrete thinking and an inability to think abstractly.[8] There are problems with each of those theories. For example, formal testing for eidetic imagery shows that phenomenon to be present in some, but certainly not all savants, and when present it may exist more as a marker of brain damage then being central to savant syndrome. With respect to family history, two studies, one with 25 savants[36] and another with a sample of 51 savants,[37] showed relatives with special skills or abilities in *some* cases but certainly not all; another study of 23 relatives[38] of carefully studied savants found only one family member with special skills. A number of studies, particularly by Hermelin[16] and her co-workers, have shown that savant skills in calendar calculating and music extend well beyond memorization alone as accounting for the special abilities such that literal, rote memory alone does not provide an explanation for savant skills. Nettlebeck and Young[13] concur with that conclusion in their extensive review article.

There have been three recent neuropsychological theories regarding the origins of autism generally, with some applicability to savant syndrome in autism more specifically. These three theories are discussed in depth in Hermelin's *Bright Splinters of the Mind.*[16] The "theory of mind" construct derives from the difficulty autistic children have relating to others. This cognitive inability to acquire "theory of the mind" leaves autistic child unable to understand that persons around him or her have their own thoughts, beliefs and feelings (a "mind") that is different from the autistic child's own self. The autistic child is unable to "mind read" and cannot understand, therefore, the intentions, ideas and actions of others, which produces a profound social ineptness.

"Weak central coherence" theory proposes that autistic children see parts of a stimulus, rather than the whole Gestalt as their chief cognitive defect. Hermelin describes it this way: "this term refers to a bias of those with autism towards focusing attention on parts and details of information rather than on integrated perception, cognition and memory. Thus those with autism do tend not to see the woods for the trees." While this cognitive defect permeates the whole world of the autistic child, including language, such attention to detail and this style of information processing might provide, Hermelin proposes, a unique pathway toward achievement and success in the autistic savant within their area of giftedness that does have some specific applicability, at least, to savant syndrome.

"Executive dysfunction" theory proposes autistic children suffer from difficulties with executive functions such as planning, attention shifting, and flexible thinking, for example, all of which are functions necessary for normal social interaction. These defects, however, appear in a number of conditions other than autistic disorder and as such have no specific application to savant syndrome.

All of these theories—their promise and their shortcomings—are discussed in greater detail elsewhere.[10] Suffice it to say *to date no single theory can account for all instances of savant syndrome.*

Left Brain Injury with Right Brain Compensation

One theory that consistently provides an increasingly plausible explanation for savant abilities in many cases however, is *left brain injury with right brain compensation*, particularly as demonstrated with recent advances in functional brain imaging and other newer techniques. Brink[39] presented a case of a normal 9-year old boy who was left mute, deaf and paralyzed by a gunshot wound to the left hemisphere. Following that injury an unusual savant-like mechanical skill emerged, presumably from the undamaged right hemisphere. Tanguay[40] pointed out that the skills most often seen in autistic savants are those associated with right hemisphere functioning. Rimland[20] reached that same conclusion highlighting the simultaneous nature of right brain activities in contrast to the sequential nature of the left brain activities. Reports of two cases, one by Steel, Gorman and co-workers[41] and the other by Charness, Clifton and MacDonald,[42] documented findings of left hemisphere damage on neuropsychological tests and imaging studies. The imaging and NP test results on Leslie, a prodigious musical savant, likewise demonstrate left brain damage.[9]

Evidence of Left Hemisphere Dysfunction in Autistic Disorder

In 1999 DeLong[43] reported low serotonin synthesis in the left hemisphere of persons with autistic disorder and neuropsychological tests also confirmed left hemisphere deficits in these individuals. Even before CAT scans and MRI techniques were available, pneumoencephalographic abnormalities in the left temporal lobe and dilatation of the left temporal horn of the left ventricle were found in 15 out of 17 autistic patients,[44] and 4 of the 17 persons had savant skills in music or mechanical areas. These investigators concluded that motor and language functions were "taken over" by the right hemisphere because of deficits in the left hemisphere.

In more recent work, Sussman and Lewandowski[45] compared 15 autistic children with 15 mentally retarded youngsters matched for age, IQ and other measures sensitive to neuropsychological dysfunction. This sample of autistic children showed bilateral NP involvement affecting left hemisphere functioning predominantly, but not exclusively. Boddaert and co-workers[46] demonstrated in five autistic youngsters and eight controls, at rest and while listening to speech-like sounds, that the volume of activation was larger on the *right* side in the autistic youngsters with less activation on the *left* side; the reverse pattern was found in the control group. A study by Escalante and Minshew[47] demonstrated that autistic persons with a history of early language disturbance showed more atypical cerebral dominance than both healthy participants and autistic persons with normal early language skills.

A Significant New Discovery: "Acquired" Savant Skills in Dementia Patients

Perhaps the most powerful confirmation of the left brain damage/right brain compensation comes from the work of Dr. Bruce Miller of the University of California at San Francisco. Miller[48] reported the unexpected emergence of artistic savant skills in five elderly patients with fronto-temporal dementia (FTD). That report described five elderly patients with fronto-temporal dementia (FTD) who acquired *new* artistic skills with the onset and progression of this particular form of dementia. Consistent with characteristics and traits in savants, the creativity in these five patients was visual, not verbal; the images were meticulous copies that lacked abstract or symbolic qualities; episodic memory was preserved but semantic memory was devastated; and there was intense, obsessive preoccupation with the art skills. Imaging studies showed a predominance of dominant-hemisphere (left brain) injury consistent with the studies outlined above.

The authors of this study hypothesized that selective degeneration of the anterior temporal and orbitofrontal cortex (particularly in the left hemisphere) decreased inhibition of visual systems involved with perception, thereby enhancing artistic interest and abilities. Kapur[49] called this process "paradoxical functional facilitation," and he speculated it is this process which accounts for unexpected behavioral improvement in some persons following brain injury. This represents a particular form of brain function compensation in undamaged areas of the cortex and other areas and could be a part of the right brain compensatory process in savants as well as in these five dementia patients.

In an expansion of that work, Miller[50] then described seven additional such FTD patients who acquired or sustained new *visual* or *musical* talents despite the progression of their dementia. No Alzheimer's patient with that form of dementia observed during the same period of time exhibited similar talents. The total of 12 FTD patients with these newly emerged or sustained savant-like talents were compared on SPECT imaging and neuropsychological tests to FTD patients without such talent. Nine of the twelve showed asymmetric left-sided SPECT defects, one had bilateral abnormalities (left on MRI, right on SPECT), while two had asymmetric right-sided dysfunction (one of whom was left handed). The talented group performed better on tasks assessing right frontal lobe functions, but worse on verbal abilities. The authors conclude, "Loss of function in the left anterior temporal lobe may lead to the "paradoxical functional facilitation" of artistic and musical skills. Patients with the left-sided temporal lobe variant of FTD offer an unexpected window into the neurological mediation of visual and musical talents."

SPECT Imaging in a 9 Year Old Autistic, Artistic Savant

But what application do these findings have to autistic savants? A great deal because Miller's team[51] carried out these same imaging and neuropsychological studies on a newly diagnosed nine-year old autistic, artistic savant, DB. The researchers also describe in detail the "striking parallels" of DB with other autistic savants, particularly Nadia. DB showed an obsession for one art medium (felt-tipped pen) and one type of subject (cartoon figures). In addition of his extraordinary drawing skill DB also showed exceptional memory. MRI scan was normal but SPECT functional imaging showed bilateral increased frontal perfusion with bilateral *anterior temporal lobe* hypo fusion which was worse on the *left* than on the right. This of course is the same site of pathology implicated in the 12 elderly FTD patients with newly emerged savant-like skills described above. They conclude: "*The anatomic substrate for the savant syndrome may involve loss of function in the left temporal lobe with enhanced function of the posterior cortex.*"

The Right Hemisphere and Compensatory Process: New Capacity vs. Released Capacity

As there has been more reflection on the role of a compensatory process to left brain injury in savants, some have pointed out, usefully, that rather than thinking in terms of the right hemisphere being newly stimulated in some manner, it may be rather than the left brain injury simply releases the right brain capacity from what Silberman[52] called the "benevolent tyranny of the left hemisphere." In other words, the compensatory process is a freeing up of dormant right brain capacity by reducing intrinsic left hemisphere domination rather than the right brain somehow developing new capacity. This new way of viewing the compensatory process has much relevance when one considers the possibility of dormant potential, perhaps, within us all. Recently Dr. Allan Snyder[53] and others have been using rTMS applied to the left-brain to temporarily immobilize a portion of the hemisphere function to see if some savant abilities in normal persons might emerge. He recently published his initial findings and in that report points out that what is being done here is not 'stimulation' of the right hemisphere, but rather 'inhibition' of left hemisphere function on a temporary basis allowing dormant lower level circuitry to emerge.

A Plausible Hypothesis

While no single theory can as yet explain all savants, in my view, based on observations and studies to date summarized above, a plausible explanation for many cases of savant syndrome can be summarized thus: *In the savant, there is disruption of typical left hemisphere functions as a result of prenatal influences, sometime sex linked (testosterone), or prenatal or subsequent injury or disease, even later in life, which, in turn, leads to a compensatory migration of capability and dominance of right hemisphere function. A predilection for simultaneous, non symbolic, literal skills and functions results. Such left hemisphere cortical abnormality is coupled with damage to the higher level cortico-limbic (cognitive) memory circuits, probably arising from those same influences, causing the savant to rely upon and largely be limited to more primitive, lower level cortico-striatal (habit) memory circuits. These cortical and memory circuit injuries together produce the savant's characteristic cluster of symptoms, capabilities, and unique memory. In talented savants, concreteness and impaired ability to think abstractly are locked in a very narrow band but with constant repetition and practice, the savant is able to produce sufficient coding so that access to some unconscious algorithms can be automatically attained. In the prodigious savant some genetic factors may be operative as well, since practice alone cannot account for access to the vast rules and syntax of music, art and mathematics, which is innate (like software installed) in these individuals. Once established, intense concentration, practice, compensatory drives and reinforcement from family, therapists and caretakers, play important roles in further developing and polishing the extraordinary mix of skill and memory made possible by the unique and idiosyncratic brain functioning.*

Young[37] carried out the largest study on savants (51 persons) in which, in addition to obtaining family histories, each savant was interviewed and given standardized psychological and neuropsychological tests. She concluded, based on this single largest sample studied in a uniform manner, that the savant is a neurologically impaired individual who shows language and intellectual impairments consistent with autism. Skills are generally rule based, rigid, and highly structured lacking critical aspects of creativity and cognitive flexibility. Preserved neurological capacity to process information related to their skills, a well developed declarative memory, a familial disposition toward high achievement and support, plus the opportunities for encouragement and support provide a climate for savant skills to develop. In a more recent summary of that work Young and Nettelbeck[13] conclude that literal rote memory capacity alone does not provide a basis for savant skills, nor do they represent "separate intelligences" outside the concept of overall general intelligence.

Why Are there More Male than Female Savants?

Throughout all the past and more recent cases, male savants continue to outnumber female savants in an approximate 6: 1 ratio. Of 103 individuals classified as savants in 63 publications, 89 were male and 14 were female providing this 6: 1 ratio.[7] In part this discrepancy is contributed to by the fact that autistic disorder is frequently the underlying developmental disability on to which the savant skills are grafted, and autistic disorder itself has a 4: 1 male: female ratio. But work by Geschwind and Galaburda[54] on cerebral lateralization provides added insight into the cause of that discrepant ratio. Citing a wide variety of human and animal studies, these researchers have pointed out that the left hemisphere normally completes its development later than the right and thus is subjected to prenatal influences, some of which are detrimental, for a longer period of time. In the male fetus, circulating testosterone, which can reach very high levels, can slow growth and impair neuronal function in the more vulnerably exposed left hemisphere, with an actual enlargement and shift of dominance favoring talents associated with the right brain, the kind of skills seen in savants. This same high male: female ratio is seen in dyslexia, delayed speech, stuttering, hyperactivity and indeed autistic disorder itself. It also accounts for the higher incidence of left-handedness in males. A "pathology of superiority" was postulated, with compensatory growth in the right brain as a result of impaired development or actual injury to the left brain. Although a left-brain injury/right brain compensation theory is not new, earlier theories could not explain why such injury would be more frequent in males than females. This hormonal influence finding may account for that difference, and it adds more impetus to the left-brain injury/right brain compensation data outlined above.

The Concept of Ancestral Memory

Leslie Lemke is a musical virtuoso. At age 14 he played back flawlessly Tchaikovsky's Piano Concerto No. 1 having heard it for the first time while listening to a television movie several hours earlier. Leslie has never had a piano lesson in his life. He is blind so he cannot read music. He is also developmentally disabled and has cerebral palsy. Yet he has a seemingly endless repertoire of pieces and has given concerts internationally. Professional musicians who have met Leslie marvel at his innate access to the rules of music and vast syntax of musical "language" given his otherwise severe limitations. How it is possible for prodigious savants to have *innate* access to and knowledge of the vast rules and syntax of mathematics, art or music with no prior exposure or formal teaching or training is one of the most puzzling, and challenging questions surrounding the prodigious savant particularly.

In order to fully explain the prodigious savant, it seems to me, one has to invoke a third type of memory capacity that must exist along side the generally accepted cognitive-semantic and habit-procedural memory capacities described above. I call that third type of memory *ancestral memory*. One way of defining ancestral memory is the genetic transmission of knowledge.

Brill[55] quoting Dr. William Carpenter in comparing savant Zerah Colburn's calculating powers to Mozart's mastery of musical composition, defined these "congenital gifts" as "intuitions": "In each of the foregoing cases, then, we have a peculiar example of the possession of an extraordinary congenital aptitude for certain mental activity, which showed itself at so early a period as to exclude the notion that it could have been acquired by the experience of the individual. To such congenital gifts we give the name of intuitions; it can scarcely be questioned that like the instincts of the lower animals, they are the expression of constitutional tendencies embodied in the organism of the individuals who manifest them."

Carl Jung used the term "collective unconscious" to define his even broader concept of inherited traits, intuitions and collective wisdom of the past.

Wilder Penfield[56] in his pioneering book *Mystery of the Mind*, also refers to three types of memory-that associated with "conditioned reflexes"; a type he called "experiential" and "racial." "Animals," he states, "particularly show evidence of what might be called racial memory."

Whether called ancestral or racial memory, intuitions, or even collective unconscious, the concept of a genetic transmission of knowledge of a complex type is necessary to explain how the prodigious savant particularly *can* remember things they never learned. We tend to think of ourselves as being born with an intricate and magnificent piece of organic machinery, i.e. the brain and a huge blank disk. What we become, it is commonly believed, is the accumulation of learning, experiences and emotions embedded on that blank disc. But the prodigious savant apparently comes already programmed with a vast amount of skill and knowledge within his or her area of expertise—"software installed" one might say—which accounts for the innate, extraordinary abilities over which the savant shows such mastery. It is an area of memory function worthy of much more study, and a type of memory function, it seems to me, necessary to be able explain particularly the prodigious savant.

A Gene for Savant Syndrome?

In my view, and the view of many other observers, autistic disorder is not a single entity with a single cause any more than mental retardation is a single disorder with only one cause. The beginning of wisdom is to call things by their right names.

So the search for the sub-groups that make up what is called in the aggregate autistic disorder is underway in the hopes such more precise sub-grouping will provide clues to specific causes, and interventions, for the individual sub-groups. Dr. Ericka Nurmi et al.[57] at Vanderbilt University recently were searching for such sub-groups using *genetic* exploration and methods. Interestingly, one such sub-group that they could identify was a subset of persons who shared savant skills that did separate out, using their genetic methodology, from a larger group of autistic persons who did not have such skills. In their paper, they point out that as many as 20 genes may contribute to autism risk. Over-representation of certain genes on Chromosome 15q11-q13 has been thought previously to perhaps contribute to autism risk.

In this study 94 multiplex families (multiple affected members; mainly affected sibling pairs and their parents) were included. 21 families were identified as "savant-skills-positive" and 73 families were identified as "savant-skills negative." This corresponds generally with the relative scarcity of savant skills in autism. The study found "the subset of 21 savant-skills positive families yielded significantly increased evidence for linkage to 15q11-q13…families in which probands had few or no savant skills ($n = 73$) showed no evidence of linkage."

Since savant abilities are sometimes seen in autism, but also occur in other conditions, the investigators point out that their results indicate that savant abilities and autism may be genetically linked, but not exclusively so since savant skills (rote memory, arithmetic, calendar calculating, musical ability, visual-spatial and mechanical ability) can be seen in other disorders, and even in non-disabled persons. Prader-Willi syndrome is due to a deletion on this same 15q11-13 chromosome, and some of the features of Prader-Willi syndrome and autism (including exceptional puzzle skills for example) overlap. From these observations the researchers conclude: "These data could be explained by a gene (or genes) in the chromosome 15q11-13 region that, when perturbed, contributes to predisposition to a particular cognitive style or pattern on intellectual impairments and relative strengths. Precisely how those skills are manifested in a given individual may be influenced by a variety of environmental, and possibly, genetic factors." The authors of this study point out that the presence or absence of savant skills was by parent reporting only without specific testing for those skills qualitatively or quantitatively. But the finding that savant skills did separate out a particular sub-group from the larger aggregate group is particularly interesting. The fact that "these results may suggest the possibility that the 15q11-13 locus that contributes to autism may also be relevant to savants who are not autistic" is also interesting and challenging.

Head Size, Autism, and (?) Savant Syndrome

In his original description of autism, Kanner[58] commented on the conspicuously large heads in some of his first 11 cases. Fifty years later Bailey[59] and colleagues reintroduced the possibility of a relationship between abnormalities in head size and brain volume in autistic disorder. Stevenson,[60] after studying 100 patients under age 21 with autism stated that "macrocephaly appears to be the single most consistent physical characteristic of children with autism," and subsequent other researchers have reached that same conclusion. Courchesne, Carper and Akshoomoff[61] examined history, clinical indices and MRI results in 48 children ages 2–5 who were diagnosed as having Autistic Spectrum Disorder in comparison to typically developing, non-autistic controls. Brain development in the autism group, compared to normal controls, showed slight undergrowth of brain before birth; sudden and excessive increase in head size between 1–2 months and 6–14 months; a gradual slowing in rate of brain growth between ages 2–4 so that by ages 4–5 brain size in autism reaches its near maximum (8 years sooner than that of non-autistic children); and a gradual decline in overall brain size extending from middle or late childhood to adulthood so that by those ages brain size in autism is not significantly different from the healthy average.

This is an important study for a number of reasons. First, it correlates well with a number of earlier studies on head size and autism, but goes beyond those to include measures of head size and brain volume in the same individuals over time. Second, apparently this proliferation in brain size occurs early in post-natal life, either some time before or concurrent with the typical time that behavioral symptoms appear in autistic children and would argue against later environmental or vaccine-related causes, for example, as being primary etiologic factors in autism. Third, these findings, if confirmed, could be an "early warning risk factor for autism," or perhaps more accurately an early marker of the condition. Fourth, as the authors point out, such brain changes, if they are significant in the etiology of autistic disorder would argue for as early an intervention as possible as one way of ameliorating damage and fostering compensatory and remedial pathways taking advantage, perhaps, of the extreme plasticity of the brain in these early months and years.

There are several caveats, and reassurances, that need to be pointed out concerning this study. First, the sample is small, only 48 individuals, and the results need to be replicated in larger studies of both head circumference and brain volume. Second, by way of reassurance to all parents, not all children with extreme head circumference increase turn out to have autistic disorder. Such increases sometime occur in healthy developing infants (6 %) who do not go on to develop autistic spectrum disorder. Third, not all children with autistic spectrum disorder demonstrate these changes. According to the study 88 % showed early postnatal brain overgrowth with head circumference measurements exceeding the 87th percentile by 6–14 months, and 59 % showed extreme (> 2.0 SD) increases in the first year. But 88 % and 59 %, while impressive, are not 100 %.

Lainhart[62] commenting on this study points out that increased rate of head circumference perhaps should not be viewed as a "risk factor" as the authors suggest, because a risk factor must precede the onset of a disorder. Instead in these cases the increased head size early in these children would be more accurately characterized as a concomitant or marker of autism rather than a "risk factor."

What might be happening during this early brain enlargement? Courchesne[61] suggests several possibilities: excessive numbers or rates of growth of neurons and/or glial cells; excessive number of minicolumns; excessive and premature expansion of dendritic and axonal arbor; excessive numbers of axonal connections; and/or premature myelination. Delong[43] takes this one step further by pointing out that autistic children produce far less serotonin than normal children and in male autistic children lower serotonin synthesis is left-sided, compared to the normal right hemisphere synthesis, coupled with increased serotonin synthesis in the right dentate nucleus of the cerebellum. He concludes: "These PET images indicate that the concept of idiopathic autism as a left-hemisphere syndrome is not over-simplified." This article presents other data in support of the left-hemisphere serotonin deficit hypothesis, and its neuropsychological manifestation of complex left-hemisphere dysfunction with sparing of right hemisphere (complex visual-spatial) function. He postulates, "Serotonin deficiency, by permitting excessive neuronal growth, might account for the postnatal brain enlargement seen in some autistic children."

So what does this have to do with savant syndrome? Clearly some persons with savant syndrome who do not have autistic disorder (approximately 50 %) show definite evidence of left brain damage on NP testing and imaging studies, with apparent right hemisphere compensatory changes as pointed out earlier. But in persons with autistic spectrum disorder (the other approximately 50 %) usually left brain damage of the characteristic type seen in this other group, is not as apparent on imaging studies. Could it be that the 'brain damage' in the autistic spectrum disorder persons is occurring, from whatever causes, during this early life period of excessive, and apparently disorganized, brain growth? And could it be that the 'brain damage' is not just left hemisphere, but also includes the connecting system of the brain—the corpus callosum and other structures—which otherwise are the mediator, modulators, and connectors between the two hemispheres and their more harmonious interaction?

Why that possibility? Taking DeLong's[43] findings one step further, Gazzaniga[63] has written a paper in which he points out that split-brain patients confirm and re-emphasize the importance of hemispheric specialization regarding left brain/right brain function, and split memory function as well. The role of the corpus callosum and allied structures "as a great communicator" between the two hemispheres is particularly critical to integration of brain function overall. In some savants, corpus callosum abnormalities, including absence of that structure entirely, are evident on imaging studies. It may be that the "brain damage" of *non-autistic* savants from pre-, peri-, or postnatal causes which is evident on many of their imaging studies shows up instead, in the *autistic* savant, as "damage" of a different type involving not so much just the hemispheres themselves, but also as a lack of coordination or integration between them because of dysfunction in the corpus callosum and allied structures. And it may be also that it is this period of rapid and excessive brain growth in autistic disorder that occurs during, and accounts for, the reported head size changes in autistic children in those early years. In short, the search for the cause of savant syndrome which does involve some of the left brain/right brain damage and compensation outlined earlier is going to have to extend beyond the brain hemispheres themselves to other allied structures. Correspondingly, the period of rapid, excessive and disorganized brain growth described in this section will need to be studied closely as the possible cause of the unique brain circuitry and altered brain function seen in savant syndrome. Some newer techniques such as fiber tracking, described below, might be useful in that search.

Prodigy and Savant Syndrome: Are they Related?

Questions are often raised as to what are the differences in brain mechanisms, if any, between (a) prodigies with certain musical or mathematical skills, for example; (b) persons with savant syndrome with similar skills and abilities; and (c) the rest of us who function normally overall but lack some special area of expertise. The most obvious difference is, of course, that savants, by definition, have their special skill or skills *in spite of* some basic mental disability, generally with low IQ scores overall, while prodigies are persons also with special abilities but *without* such mental disabilities who generally function at a normal or very high level overall and whose IQ scores generally reflect that level of function.

Mauro Pesenti and co-workers,[64] using PET imaging, studied brain mechanisms between a German calculating prodigy (Rudiger Gamm) and normal control subjects as they perform mental calculations. Commenting on that work Butterworth[65] points out, "Gamm is remarkable in that he is able, for example, to calculate 9th powers and 5th roots with great accuracy, and he can find the quotients of 2 primes to 60 decimal places." He called Gamm the "expert" and the control group "non-experts." Several important findings emerged. When doing calculations in a typical manner, both the expert and non-expert showed calculation processes activated in the brain bi-laterally but with a clear *left-sided* predominance in a number of specific brain areas. When Gamm did the more complex calculations so accurately and quickly compared to controls however, he "recruited" a system of brain areas implicated in episodic memory including *right* medial frontal and parahippocampal areas, and utilized as well as unique method of exploiting the unlimited storage capacity of long-term memory to maintain the sequence of steps and intermediate results needed for the more complex calculations whereas controls relied on more typical very limited span of short-term working memory. The "expert" seemed to develop a long term episodic memory by borrowing from other areas of long term memory, just as a computer extends the capacity of RAM by using swap space on the hard drive to create a larger "virtual memory," and recruited much of that from *right* sided structures.

This study is of interest for several reasons. It compares PET images of the expert prodigy with those of non-expert calculators and points out the unique brain mechanisms in the expert when doing his special skill, providing some neural insights into at least this form of prodigy function. But of interest to savant syndrome is the fact that when doing these special skills, the prodigy is relying on some *right* brain capacities, and some special memory recruitment. It will be interesting to compare the prodigy neural function with the neural function of a savant performing the same task to see if these same areas are involved, or recruited, in the savant as in the prodigy. I suspect they are. These findings are consistent with the right-brain nature of savant "unconscious" skills, and are consistent as well with the special unconscious "memory without reckoning," which is an integral part of savant syndrome as well. Could it be that the same "recruiting" of unused long term memory space to provide long term working memory is operative in the savant as in the prodigy? Are prodigies and savants alike in that manner? From this study Butterworth raises the same question scattered throughout our inquiry about the savant: "This study, though focused on a remarkable individual, illuminates the unremarkable as well as the extraordinary skills we all possess." Another piece of the savant puzzle perhaps?

Savant Skills: a Conduit Toward Normalization

Etiologic considerations aside, what is the best approach to the savant and his or her special skills? Phillips[66] framed the controversy when he stated: "The problem of treatment comes next. The question that arises is one of method, whether it is better to *eliminate the defect*, or *train the talent*. Based on numerous case reports and my own experience, the answer to that important question is to train the talent and with it some of the "defect" subsides. The special talent or skill, in fact, can become a conduit toward normalization, using the unique savant skills to increase language acquisition, social skills and independence overall. And further, in my experience with a number of savants and from reports of many other clinicians and investigators, this increase in language and social skills can be done *without* any tradeoff or loss of special abilities for those valuable gains in other areas, the case of Nadia notwithstanding. The so-called "dreaded trade-off," in my experience and that of many other researchers and clinicians, overwhelmingly does *not* occur; instead the special skills act as a unique and valuable conduit toward normalization.

Nettlebeck and Young,[13] after studying and following the largest single sample of savants in a standardized manner conclude that the interests of the savant are best served by a balanced educational approach that includes social skills, training, counseling and opportunities for interactions with others, together with encouraging savant skills but not letting them dominate the individual's life. The goal of dealing with the special skills in the savant is not to eradicate them, monotonous, impractical and frivolous as they might sometimes seem. The goal rather is to put them to good use, creatively and patiently, without fear they will either take over the savant's life or disappear from it. The skills instead can remain as modes of expression through which others can reach and relate to the savant. Such communication and mentoring can lead to the development of other related skills.

There are now a number of well-known savants that demonstrate impressively, particularly over the last decades, how well that conduit toward normalization works and the amazing success that training the abilities can have on lessening the dis-abilities without having to sacrifice any of the unique special capacities.[10]

Dr. Trevor Clark[67] of the Autism Association of New South Wales in Sydney, Australia developed The Savant Skill Curriculum using a combination of successful strategies currently employed in the education of gifted children (enrichment acceleration and mentorship) and autism education (visual supports and social stories) in an attempt to apply, usefully, the often non-functional obsessive savant and splinter skills of a group of students with autism. The design and implementation of a differentiated curriculum for a group of autistic savants was the first formal, documented study to do so. This Savant Skills Curriculum proved highly successful in the functional application of savant skills and an overall reduction in the level of autism behaviors in many subjects.

Gains in behavior, social skills and academic self-esteem were observed. Improvements in the communication skills of some subjects were also reported.

In November, 2002, Soundscape Centre began operating as a unique facility for some musical savants. Soundscape Centre is the only specialized educational facility in the world uniquely dedicated to the needs, and potential, of persons with sight loss and special musical abilities—including some musical savants. Located at Redhill College in Surrey, England, it is a joint initiative between The Royal National Institute for the Blind and the Amber Trust that specializes in helping persons who have learning disabilities, sight loss and special musical abilities or needs.

Hope University in Anaheim, California was the first institution of its kind to offer "arts-infused" curricula for developmentally challenged adults with special skills in the fine arts. Its motto is "train the talent and diminish the disability." While the student body is not limited to musical savants, some do attend with the goal of using musical or other fine art skills to broaden other academic abilities, language and social skills.

New Findings, New Techniques, and Future Directions

No model of brain function, including memory, will be complete until it can account for, and fully incorporate, the rare but spectacular condition of savant syndrome.

In the past decade particularly, there has been a great deal of progress in helping to explain this jarring juxtaposition of severe mental disability and prodigious mental ability. Many questions remain unanswered, but interest in this fascinating condition is accelerating especially since the discovery of savant skills in previously non-disabled older persons with the onset and progression of frontotemporal dementia. This finding has far-reaching implications regarding buried potential in some, or perhaps, all of us.

New functional imaging techniques such as PET, SPECT, and functional MRI will help provide insights into brain function, not just brain architecture, not only in savant syndrome but in autistic disorder and other developmental disabilities as well. Those findings can then be correlated with detailed and standardized neuropsychological testing in larger samples of savants, comparing and contrasting those findings with data from both disabled and non-disabled control groups, including prodigies. The interface between genius, prodigies and savants is especially intriguing and these studies can shed light also on the important debate regarding general intelligence vs. separate intelligences. Some researchers suggest that savants provide a unique window into the creative process itself. Certainly from these studies, some of which are already underway, important information can emerge regarding brain function, brain plasticity, and CNS compensation, recruitment and repair.

Some New Techniques

Fiber tracking is one such new technique.[68] Using MRI scans which measure random movements of water inside and outside nerve cells, actual nerve fiber bundles can be individually identified and visualized, documenting the specific, direct connections between particular areas of the brain. While PET scans can measure activity in certain designated areas of the brain when certain tasks are performed, and from that activity certain assumptions can be made about connections of brain areas, fiber tracking provides detailed maps of the actual connections—the specific "wiring"—of the brain and its interconnections via these fibers. Such fiber tracking will have considerable usefulness in studying the "wiring"' of a number of brain disorders such as Alzheimer's, Schizophrenia, and a number of other neurological disorders providing a better understanding of the neuropathology involved as well as leads to better remedial methods in those disorders such as some post-stroke "re-wiring" often commented on. Such fiber tracking holds promise as a less invasive procedure than PET scans and seems like a natural modality for further research in savant syndrome with some of the left hemisphere/right hemisphere and corpus callosum findings outlined above.

Event-related brain potentials (ERPs) are early components (up to 100 ms) of brain activity which reflect initial, "preconscious" stages of mental processing which are fast, low level elementary mental operations. Later measurements of ERPs reflect higher level mental processing such as the so-called "executive" functions of the brain that dominate normal information processing.

Birbaumer[69] describes his work comparing ERPs of a "human calculator"—a non-autistic arithmetic whiz—to same age, same intelligence, healthy controls. While the human calculator has the same stages of information processing as the slower control subjects, amplitudes of ERPs of the calculating whiz are increased early on "indicating enhanced automatic low-level processing." Birbaumer is attempting now to see whether this particular type of early, lower level processing in non-savant geniuses is the same as occurs in autistic savants. He is undertaking this study to investigate the neurophysiological basis of outstanding skills in autistic savants using magnetoencephalography and electroencephalography from scalp readings. Participants will be required to accomplish a variety of simple and complex tasks that are adapted to their exceptional skill. Birbaumer and his team are recruiting persons now for that study who have Autistic Disorder, Asperger's Disorder or pervasive developmental disorder using standardized criteria; who have an IQ > 85; and who have motivation to concentrate on the tasks for at least 1 hour. That study is underway but results of that work are not available as yet.

The significance of Birbaumer's work is, first of all, that he has discovered ERPs as another way of measuring brain function in normal persons and savants. Further, he has found that healthy controls and neurological patients can, with use of a computer screen to observe his or her own changes in slowing brain potentials and can modify such brain potentials with training:

> "After many training sessions, brain-damaged patients and healthy controls can learn to control their own brain activity—which we normally cannot consciously perceive—and become sensitive to the changes that underlie elementary, low-level processing. By bringing their brain activity under voluntary control, these patients can use it to communicate from the mysterious early state of non-consciousness. The result may ultimately be that we find we all possess behavioural and physiological strategies to modify the early stages of cortical processing, with unprecedented consequences for behaviour and self-awareness."

Transmagnetic Repetative Stimulation (rTMS) is being used by several investigators to test the hypothesis that savant skills may be dormant in some, or all, of us, buried by the more advanced circuitry on which we have come to rely in day to day life, and by what some have called "the tyranny" of the left hemisphere described above.

Allan Snyder and John Mitchell[70] argue that savant brain processes occur in each of us but are overwhelmed by more sophisticated conceptual cognition. Autistic savants, they conclude, "have privileged access to lower levels of information not normally available through introspection." Since some of the research outlined above points to the left anterior temporal lobe particularly as being perhaps dominating right hemisphere skills seen in the savant, several researchers are testing that hypothesis by temporarily immobilizing portions of the left hemisphere with rTMS, to see if savant-like skills emerge in otherwise non-disabled persons.

Morrell, Young and Ridding[71] used rTMS in 17 normal individuals, eight male and nine female. Only two of the participants experienced a series of short-lived skills, such as calendar calculating, artistic ability and enhanced habit memory. These researchers suggest that savant skills may be limited to a small percentage of the normal population, much as they are limited to a small percentage of the disabled population. But their work continues and we await more recent results.

Allan Snyder and his team from the Centre for the Mind in Sydney, Australia published their results[53] of using rTMS in 11 volunteer participants. The abstract of that article reads thus:

> "The astonishing skills of savants have been suggested to be latent in everyone, but are not normally accessible without a rare form of brain impairment. We attempted to simulate such brain impairment in healthy people by directing low-frequency magnetic pulses into the left fronto-temporal lobe. Significant stylistic changes in drawing were facilitated by the magnetic pulses in 4 of our 11 participants. Some of these 'facilitated' participants also displayed enhanced proofreading ability. Our conclusions are derived from eleven right-handed male university students, eight of whom underwent placebo stimulation. We examined performance before, during and after exposure to the stimulation."

The article provides a number of "before" and "after" illustrations both of the drawing, and proofreading, abilities. Snyder's work also continues and we await further results and confirmation of these early results by others as well.

In summary, new imaging techniques such as PET, SPECT, and fMRI provide dynamic looks at brain function, not just brain structure, and newer techniques of entirely different types such as Fiber Tracking, Event Related Potentials and rTMS provide tools to examine brain function even more intimately not only in savants, but in a number of other populations as well. By applying a combination of these newer techniques, along with more established tools such as sophisticated neuropsychological testing, in compare and contrast methods with various populations—disabled persons with special abilities (savants); disabled persons lacking special abilities (non-savants); normal persons without special abilities (most of us); and normal persons who show special abilities (prodigies and geniuses)—in carefully designed control study fashion, we can move beyond the anecdotal reporting that has characterized so much reporting in savant syndrome these past 150 years to a time when information can be gathered more carefully and analyzed more comprehensively. In so doing it will be possible to not only to better understand the origins of savant syndrome, but to better understand the underpinnings of human potential overall. And I believe savant syndrome provides a unique window to brain function, including memory and even creativity, not just in savants, but in the rest of us as well.

Summary

Savant syndrome is a rare and extraordinary condition in which persons with autistic disorder or other mental disabilities have spectacular islands of genius that stand in jarring, stark contrast to overall handicap. Curiously, considering all the skills in the human repertoire, savant skills typically narrow to only five areas—art, music, calendar calculating, mathematics and mechanical/spatial skills. These skills cover a spectrum of abilities ranging from splinter skills, to talented, to prodigious. Whatever the special skill, it is always linked with a memory of a particular variety—exceedingly deep but very narrow—within the confines of the special ability. While savant syndrome does occur in other developmental disabilities, it is seen as often as one in ten autistic persons, and we need to better understand why that is so.

There is no single over-arching theory to explain this curious capacity. But increasingly a variety of studies point toward left-brain (and associated communicating structures) damage and imbalance with right-brain (and associated communicating structures) compensation as an important mechanism not only in savant syndrome, but also in autistic disorder itself. By using established along with newer research tools and techniques in larger sample studies, with control populations, savant syndrome can provide a unique window to brain and memory function overall, not only in autistic savants, but in prodigies and geniuses as well, along with a better and even more global glimpse at the hidden potential that lies, perhaps, within us all.

But there is more to savant syndrome than neurons, circuits and synapses.

Just as we can learn much about human potential from this jarring contradiction and curious coexistence of deficiency and superiority within the same person, we can also learn more about the power of love, belief, determination and optimism that is so prominent in the families and caretakers of these extraordinary people. These families and caretakers teach us the importance of not only caring *for* the savant, but the importance of caring *about* him or her as well. In our efforts to unravel some of this marvelous mystery, we need to better understand not only the condition the savant has, but better understand, and appreciate, the savant who has that condition as well. We can also learn that in using and celebrating the special gifts that the autistic savant has, those magnificent abilities do not disappear. Rather they become a useful conduit toward normalization that can ameliorate some of the dis-ability of the autistic savant, while allowing the a-bility to flourish and grow. Just as Luria[72] was curious not only about the *mind* of the mnemonist, but he wondered about the *world* of the mnemonist he studied so carefully as well, we too need to be mindful of the *world* of the savant while trying to better understand and appreciate his or her savant *skills*. By doing both—studying and observing carefully *and* caringly—we can, I am convinced, be propelled further along than we have ever been before in better understanding both the brain *and* human potential.

References

[1] Rimland B. Savant capabilities of autistic children and their cognitive implications. In: Serban G, ed. *Cognitive Defects in the Development of Mental Illness*. New York, NY: Brunner/Mazel; 1978: 43-65.

[2] Horwitz WA, Kestenbaum C, Person E, Jarvick L. Identical twins—"idiot savants"—calendar calculators. *American Journal of Psychiatry*. 1965; 121: 1075-1079.

[3] Sacks O. The twins. *New York Review of Books*. 1985; 32(3): 16-20.

[4] Scripture EW. Arithmetical prodigies. *American Journal of Psychology*. 1891; 4: 1-59

[5] Down JL. *On Some Affections of Childhood and Youth*. London, UK: Churchill; 1887.

[6] Tredgold AF. *Mental Deficiency (Amentia)*. 2nd ed. New York, NY: William Wood; 1914.

[7] Hill AL. Savants: Mentally retarded individuals with special skills. In: Ellis N, ed. *International Review of Research in Mental Retardation.* New York, NY: Academic Press; 1978.
[8] Treffert DA. The idiot savant: A review of the syndrome. *American Journal of Psychiatry.* 1988; 145: 563-572.
[9] Treffert DA. *Extraordinary People: Understanding "Idiot Savants".* New York, NY: Harper and Row; 1989.
[10]Treffert DA. *Extraordinary People: Understanding Savant Syndrome.* Lincoln, NE: iUniverse.com, Inc.; 2000.
[11]Miller LK. *Musical Savants: Exceptional Skill in the Mentally Retarded.* Hillsdale, NJ: Laurence Erlbaum Associates; 1989.
[12]Kehrer WR. Savant capabilities of autistic persons. *Acta Paedopsychiatrica.* 1992; 55: 151-155.
[13]Nettelbeck T, Young R. Savant syndrome. *International Review of Research in Mental Retardation.* 1999; 22: 137-173.
[14]Howe MJA. *Fragments of Genius.* London, UK: Routledge; 1989.
[15]Smith N, Tsimpli I. *The Mind of a Savant: Language, Learning and Modularity.* Oxford, UK: Blackwell; 1995.
[16]Hermelin B. *Bright Splinters of the Mind: A Personal Story of Research with Autistic Savants.* London, UK: Jessica Kingsley Publishers; 2001.
[17]Saloviita T, Ruusila L, Ruusila U. Incidence of savant syndrome in Finland. *Perceptual and Motor Skills.* 2000; 91: 120-122.
[18]Southall G. *Blind Tom: The Post-Civil War Enslavement of a Black Musical Genius.* Minneapolis, MN: Challenge Productions; 1979.
[19]Keeler WR. Autistic patterns and defective communication in blind children with retrolental fibroplasia. In: Hoch P, Zubin J, eds. *Psychopathology of Communication.* New York, NY: Grune and Stratton; 1958: 64-83.
[20]Rimland B. *Infantile Autism: The Syndrome and Implications for a Neural Theory of Behavior.* New York, NY: Appleton-Century-Crofts; 1964.
[21]Ockelford A. *Sound Moves: Music in the Education of Children and Young People Who are Visually Impaired and Have Learning Disabilities.* London, UK: Royal National Institute for the Blind; 1998.
[22]Rimland B, Fine D. Special talents of autistic savants. In: Obler L, Fine DA, eds. *The Exceptional Brain.* New York, NY: Guilford Press; 1988: 472-492.
[23]Treffert DA. The mind of the savant: An "exultation of memory". In: Mazur GO, ed. *One Hundred Year Commemoration to the Life of A.R. Luria (1902–2002).* New York, NY: Semenenko Foundation; 2002: 96-118.
[24]Critchley M. *The Divine Banquet of the Brain.* New York, NY: Raven Press; 1979.
[25]Barr MW. Some notes on echolalia, with the report of an extraordinary case. *Journal of Nervous and Mental Diseases.* 1898; 25: 20-30.
[26]Mishkin M, Petri HL. Memories and habits: Some implications for the analysis of learning and retention. In: Squire LR, Butters N, eds. *Neuropsychology of Memory.* New York, NY: Guilford Press; 1984: 287-296.
[27]Bauman M, Kemper TL. Histoanatomic observations of the brain in early infantile autism. *Neurology.* 1985; 35: 866-874.
[28]Kanner L. Early infantile autism. *Journal of Pediatrics.* 1944; 25: 200-217.

[29]Viscott DS. A musical idiot-savant. *Psychiatry*. 1970; 33: 494-515.
[30]Selfe L. *Nadia: A Case of Extraordinary Drawing Ability in an Autistic Child*. London, UK: Academic Press; 1977.
[31]Wiltshire S. *Drawings*. London, UK: J.M. Dent and Sons; 1987.
[32]Wiltshire S. *Floating Cities*. New York, NY: Summit Books; 1991.
[33]Sacks O. *An Anthropologist on Mars*. New York, NY: Alfred A. Knopf; 1995.
[34]Treffert DA, Wallace GL. Islands of genius. *Scientific American*. 2002; 286(6): 76-85.
[35]Rexer L. *Jonathan Lerman: Drawings by an Artist with Autism*. New York, NY: George Braziller; 2002.
[36]Duckett J. *Idiot-savants: Super-specialization in Mentally Retarded Persons* [dissertation]. Austin, TX: University of Texas at Austin, Department of Special Education; 1976.
[37]Young R. Savant Syndrome: *Processes Underlying Extraordinary Abilities* [dissertation]. Adelaide, Australia: University of Adelaide; 1995.
[38]LaFontaine L. *Divergent Abilities in the Idiot Savant* [dissertation]. Boston, MA: Boston University, School of Education; 1974.
[39]Brink TL. Idiot savant with unusual mechanical ability: An organic explanation. *American Journal of Psychiatry*. 1980; 137: 250-251.
[40]Tanguay PE. A tentative hypothesis regarding the role of hemispheric specialization in early infantile autism. Paper presented at: UCLA Conference on Cerebral Dominance; 1973; Los Angeles, CA.
[41]Steel JG, Gorman R, Flexman JE. Neuropsychiatric testing in an autistic mathematical idiot-savant: Evidence for nonverbal abstract capacity. *Journal of the American Academy of Child Psychiatry*. 1984; 3: 469-487.
[42]Charness N, Clifton J, MacDonald L. Case study of a musical "mono-savant": A cognitive-psychological focus. In: Obler L, Fine DA, eds. *The Exceptional Brain*. New York, NY: Guilford; 1988: 474-492.
[43]DeLong RG. Autism: New data suggest a new hypothesis *Neurology*. 1999; 52: 911-916.
[44]Hauser SL, DeLong GR, Rosman NP. Pneumographic findings in the infantile autism syndrome. *Brain*. 1975; 9: 667-688.
[45]Sussman K, Lewandowski L. Left-hemisphere dysfunction in autism: What are we measuring? *Archives of Clinical Neuropsychology*. 2003; 5: 137-146.
[46]Boddaert N, Belin P, Chabane N, et al. Perception of complex sounds: abnormal pattern of cortical activation in autism. *American Journal of Psychiatry*. 2003; 160: 2057-2060.
[47]Escalante-Mead PR, Minshew NJ, Sweeney JA. Abnormal brain lateralization in high-functioning autism. *Journal of Autism and Developmental Disorders*. 2003; 33: 539-543.
[48]Miller BL, Cummings J, Mishkin F, et al. Emergence of artistic talent in frontotemporal dementia. *Neurology*. 1998; 51: 978-982.
[49]Kapur N. Paradoxical functional facilitation in brain-behavior research: A critical review. *Brain*. 1996; 119: 1775-1790.
[50]Miller BL, Boone K, Cummings LR, Mishkin F. Functional correlates of musical and visual ability in frontotemporal dementia. *British Journal of Psychiatry*. 2000; 176: 458-63.
[51]Hou C, Miller BL, Cummings JL, et al. Artistic savants. *Neuropsychiatry, Neuropsychology, and Behavioral Neurology*. 2000; 13: 29-38.
[52]Silberman S. The key to genius. *Wired* December 2003: 226-258.

[53]Snyder AW, Mulcahy E, Taylor JL, Mitchell DJ, Sachdev P, Gandevia SC. Savant-like skills exposed in normal people by suppressing the left fronto-temporal lobe. *Journal of Integrative Neuroscience.* 2003; 2: 149-158.

[54]Geschwind N, Galaburda AM. *Cerebral Lateralization: Biological Mechanisms, Associations and Pathology.* Cambridge, MA: MIT Press; 1987.

[55]Brill AA. Some peculiar manifestations of memory with special reference to lightning calculators. *Journal of Nervous and Mental Diseases.* 1940; 92: 709-726.

[56]Penfield W. *Mystery of the Mind.* Princeton, NJ: Princeton University Press; 1978.

[57]Nurmi EL, Dowd M, Tadevosyan-Leyfer O, Haines J, Folstein S, Sutcliffe JS. Exploratory sub setting of autism families based on savant skills improves evidence of genetic linkage to 15q11-q13. *Journal of the Academy of Child Adolescent Psychiatry.* 2003; 42: 856-863.

[58]Kanner L. Autistic disturbances of affective contact. *Nervous Child.* 1943; 2: 217-250.

[59]Bailey A, Luther P, Dean A, et al. A clinicopathological study of autism *Brain.* 1998; 121: 889-905.

[60]Stevenson R, Schroer R, Skinner C, Fender D, Simensen RJ. Autism and macrocephaly. *Lancet.* 1997; 349: 1744-1745.

[61]Courchesne E, Carper R, Akshoomoff N. Evidence of brain overgrowth in the first year of life in autism. *Journal of the American Medical Association.* 2003; 290: 337-344.

[62]Lainhart JE. Increased rate of head growth during infancy in autism. *Journal of the American Medical Association.* 2003; 290: 393-394.

[63]Gazzaniga MS. Cerebral specialization and interhemispheric communication: Does the corpus callosum enable the human condition? *Brain.* 2000; 123: 1293-1326.

[64]Pesenti M, Zago L, Crivello F, et al. Mental calculation in a prodigy is sustained by right prefrontal and medial temporal areas. *Nature Neuroscience.* 2001; 4: 103-107.

[65]Butterworth B. What makes a prodigy? *Nature Neuroscience.* 2001; 4: 11-12.

[66]Phillips A. Talented imbeciles. *The Psychological Clinic.* 1930; 18: 246-255.

[67]Clark T. *The Application of Savant and Splinter Skills in the Autistic Population Through Curriculum Design: A Longitudinal Multiple-Replication Case Study* [dissertation]. Sydney, Australia: The University of New South Wales, School of Education Studies; 2001.

[68]Conturo TE, Lori NF, Cull TS, et al. Tracking neuronal fiber pathways in the living human brain. *Proceedings of the National Academy of Sciences of the United States of America.* 1999; 96: 10422-10427.

[69]Birbaumer N. Rain Man's revelations. *Nature.* 1999; 399: 211-212.

[70]Snyder AW, Mitchell DJ. Is integer arithmetic fundamental to mental processing? *Proceedings: Biological Sciences.* 1999; 266: 587-592.

[71]Morrell TL, Young RL, Ridding MC. *Investigation of Latent Savant Skills Using Transcranial Magnetic Stimulation* [dissertation]. Adelaide, Australia: University of South Autralia; 2000.

[72]Luria AR. *The Mind of a Mnemonist.* Cambridge, MA: Harvard University Press; 1968.

Additional information

www.savantsyndrome.com

This is a web site maintained by the Wisconsin Medical Society Foundation and is a continually updated comprehensive resource for current as well as historical information on savant syndrome.

In: Recent Developments in Autism Research
Editor: Manuel F. Casanova, pp. 57-108

ISBN 1-59454-358-5
© 2005 Nova Science Publishers, Inc.

Chapter III

The Brain During Life in Autism: Advances in Neuroimaging Research*

Janet E. Lainhart[#]
Associate Professor, Department of Psychiatry, University of Utah,
Salt Lake City, Utah Utah Autism Research Program 421
Wakara Way, Suite 143 Salt Lake City, Utah 84108

Mariana Lazar
Laboratory for Brain Imaging and Behavior, The Waisman Center,
University of Wisconsin, Madison, Wisconsin

Erin D. Bigler
Professor, Department of Psychology and Neuroscience,
Brigham Young University, Provo, Utah
Adjunct Professor, Departments of Psychiatry and Radiology,
University of Utah, Salt Lake City, Utah.

Andrew Alexander
Associate Professor, Departments of Psychiatry and Medical Physics,
University of Wisconsin, Madison, Wisconsin

Introduction

During the past decade, advances in neuroimaging have given us an unprecedented opportunity to study the brain during life in children and adults with autism. In this chapter, we discuss what has been learned from the neuroimaging research that has been done in autism during the past 10 years and especially during the past 5 years. We review head circumference findings that have provided important clues about brain volume in autism. We

* Color representations are provided at the end of this chapter
# E-mail: janet.lainhart@hsc.utah.edu

do not attempt to duplicate recently published in-depth reviews about structural and functional imaging in autism. [1]– [6] Rather, we take a developmental approach and discuss imaging findings across modalities. A special discussion of diffusion tensor imaging is included because of the enormous opportunity it now provides to learn about white matter in autism.

Brain Size and Structure

Head Circumference

Increased head size in children with autism was first observed 60 years ago by Dr. Leo Kanner, Professor of Child Psychiatry at the Johns Hopkins Hospital. He was the first professional to describe autism and notice that some of the children had large heads. [7] During the next 20 years, medical research about the relationship between head size, brain size, and brain weight progressed. By the 1970s, it was well known in pediatrics that, in the absence of hydrocephalus and gross abnormalities of head shape, head circumference was a good index of brain size particularly during early childhood. Even more importantly, change in head circumference during early childhood was closely related to brain growth. Significant disturbances in whole brain growth during early childhood were accompanied by abnormal changes in head circumference. Aberrations of brain growth during early childhood sometimes persisted as macrocephaly or microcephaly in later childhood and adulthood.

Figure 1 shows the close relationship between head circumference, brain volume, and total intracranial volume during the first two years of life. They increase rapidly and at similar rates. About eighty-five percent of postnatal brain growth occurs by 5 years of age. Ninety-five percent of postnatal brain growth has occurred by 9 years of age. Brain volume is the first to reach its maximum and then it plateaus. Intracranial volume reaches its maximum at a slightly older age, followed by head circumference. Head circumference continues to increase for several years after brain volume plateaus because of changes in skull and scalp thickness. When brain volume gradually decreases in adulthood, head circumference and intracranial volume remain relatively constant, as persistent indices of maximal brain volume in development.

Evidence of the biological origin of autism [8] stimulated a search for physical phenomena that might give clues about what had gone wrong in brain development in children with autism. [9], [10] At first, head circumference did not appear to differ in autism. [11] Subsequent studies using new methods to reliably diagnose autism and identify and exclude medical causes consistently found increased head size in idiopathic autism. Increased mean head circumference and rates of macrocephaly were found in children and adults with autism, singletons and twins, and in both children with the full autism syndrome and children with milder forms of the disorder. [12]– [19] Overall, about 20 % of individuals with autism have macrocephaly compared to about 3 % in reference samples from the general population.

A number of factors other than autism however may have contributed to differences in head circumference between autism and reference samples. Head size in the general population and in children with autism may have increased since the reference sample data were collected. Autism and reference data samples may have differed on variables known to influence head and brain size, such as SES which is related to early childhood nutrition and maternal factors. Therefore, it is important to examine the findings of studies that compare individuals with autism to control samples.

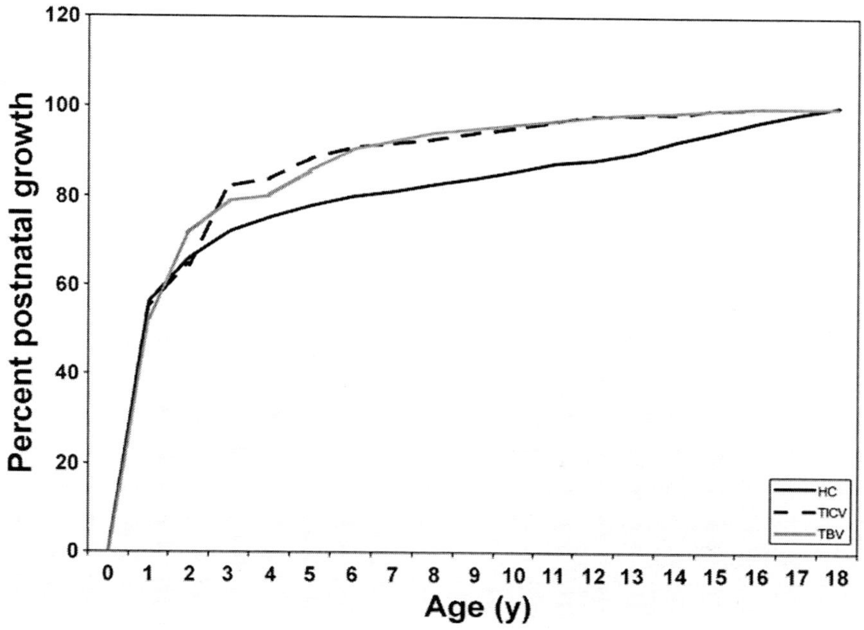

Figure 1 Percent of total postnatal growth of head circumference (HC), total intracranial volume (TICV), and total brain volume (TBV) by age in typically developing individuals.

Table 1 Mean head circumference and rates of macrocephaly and large head size in autism and comparison samples

		Mean HC (cm)	Rate of Macrocephaly (%)	Rate of HC > 90th percentile (%)
Twins [12]– [15]	autism		39.9	
	typically developing		9.0	
Singletons [12]– [15]	autism		29.7	48.7
	language disorder		9.0	13.6
	other psychiatric disorder		17.0	23.5
Children [12]– [15]	autism		12.2	
	non-autistic tuberous sclerosis or seizure disorder		9.5	
Adults [12]– [15]	autism	58.9		
	normal controls	57.4		
Adolescents and adults [12]– [15]	autism	56.9		
	typically developing	55.9		

Five head circumference studies of autism used contemporaneous control groups. All five of these studies found evidence that autism itself has an effect on head size. Table 1 shows that in all of these case-control studies, mean head circumference or rate of macrocephaly was increased in the autism samples. British male twins with autism had a higher rate of macrocephaly than 120 typically developing twins. [15] Rates of macrocephaly and head circumference above the 90th percentile were increased in 37 singletons with autism compared to children without autism who had a language disorder or another Axis I psychiatric disorder. [12] The rate of macrocephaly was higher in a different sample of 41 children with autism compared to 21 children without autism who had either tuberous sclerosis or a nonspecific seizure disorder. [18] The mean head circumference of 27 adult males with autism was greater than the grand mean of 93 typically developing adult males from other studies. [13] Mean head circumference in a sample of 67 high-functioning children and adults with autism was more than 83 age- and sex-matched typically developing individuals. [20] Thus, increased mean head circumference and rate of macrocephaly in autism appear to be sound findings. They predict increased brain volume at some time during postnatal brain development in autism.

MRI Studies of Brain Volume

Initially, two MRI studies found increased mean brain volume in children and adults with autism and neuropathologic studies found increased brain weight and megalencephaly in some cases. [21]– [25] More recent imaging studies have consistently found increased brain volume in young children with autism but not older children and adults. [20], [26]– [30]

Two MRI studies of children with autism 2 to 5 years of age have found that by this young age mean brain volume is increased in autism. [27], [28] In one of the studies, 37 % of twenty 2 and 3 year olds with autism had mean brain volumes two standard deviations or more above the mean of eight typical children. [28] As exciting as these results have been, the autism and control sample sizes have been relatively small because great effort is required to scan such young children. Nevertheless, there is a tremendous need for replication in larger samples by different laboratories. Examination of head circumference in 26 children with autism 2 to 4 years of age found macrocephaly in only 15.5 % relative to reference data. [31] Thus, the true rates of macrocephaly and megalencephaly and the relationship between head circumference and brain volume in young children with autism may not yet be known.

Whether or not mean brain volume remains increased during later childhood, adolescence, and adulthood in autism is not yet clear. Although head circumference studies have consistently found increased mean standardized head circumference in older children and adults with autism, [13], [14], [20] only one of eight MRI studies found statistically significant increases in mean brain volume in individuals with autism ranging in age from 6 years to adulthood. [20], [25], [26], [28]– [30], [32], [33]

One possible reason for the discrepancy between the results of head circumference and brain volume studies of older individuals with autism is the issue of sample size, and related to that power. Sample sizes in autism head circumference studies have generally been around 100, 5 to 7 times larger than the samples in MRI studies. To quantify case-control differences in a standardize manner and compare the results of brain volume and head circumference studies, we calculated the standardized *z* scores and effect sizes (ES) [34] of the studies that published means and standard deviations. The unit of a *z* score is the standard deviation of the control group. The unit of an effect size is the pooled standard deviation of the autism and control groups. The *z* scores and effect sizes of the MRI studies are shown in figure 2 in order of the mean age or estimated mean age of the autism samples. *z* scores and effect sizes of head circumference studies, which have predominantly been carried out in older children, adolescents, and young adults, are moderate (z = 0.52 [13] and 0.61 [16] for mean HC percentile; z = 0.45 [20] for mean HC; ES = 0.56 [16] for mean HC percentile). For MRI studies of total brain volume in autism, *z* scores and effect sizes are relatively large for young children, moderate for older children, small to moderate for adolescents, and very small for adults in, conventional terms [34] (average ES: 1.24 for 2 to 4 years of age, 0.62 for 6 to12 years of age, 0.43 for 13 to 18 years of age, 0.14 for 19 years and older). Head circumference studies predict that autism has an overall moderate effect on brain volume and this seems to be the case. Importantly, the increase in effect size from early childhood to adulthood suggests an age effect on case-control brain volume differences in autism. Power analysis shows that for brain volume studies to detect a moderate effect size of 0.50 with 80 % power at the a_2 = 0.5 significance level, imaging studies need 50 autism and 50 control subjects for a one-sided test and 64 subjects in each group for a two-sided test. [34] Few autism imaging studies have had samples this large.

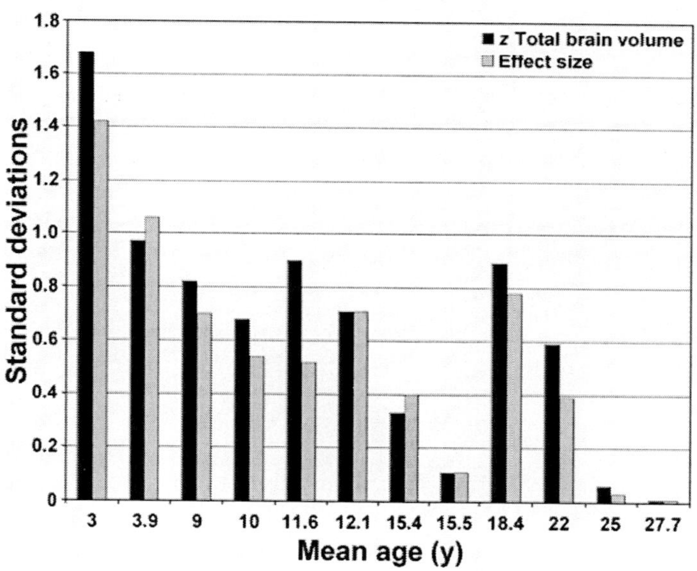

Figure 2 Standardized total brain volumes and effect sizes by mean age of sample in autism. The mean TBVs and standard deviations of the normal controls in each study were used to calculate *z* scores, $z = (\text{meanTBV}_{\text{autism}} - \text{meanTBV}_{\text{control}})$ / standard $\text{deviation}_{\text{control}}$. Effects sizes were calculated as $\text{ES} = (\text{meanTBV}_{\text{autism}} - \text{meanTBV}_{\text{control}})$ / pooled standard $\text{deviation}_{\text{autism,control}}$. Mean age of the autism sample was used when given; otherwise average age or approximate age was used. (Age 3: Courchesne et al. [28]; Age 3.9: Sparks et al. [27]; Age 9: Herbert et al. [29]; Age 10: Aylward et al. [20]; Age 11.6: low-functioning autism, Lotspeich et al. [30]; Age 12.1: high-functioning autism, Lotspeich et al. [30]; Age 15.4: Waiter et al. [33]; Age 15.5: Aylward et al. [20]; Age 18.4: Piven et al. [25]; Age 22: Hardan et al. [26]; Age est. 25: Aylward et al. [20]; Age 27.7: Haznedar et al. [32])

Sample size becomes even more important when the distribution of head circumference (and likely brain volume) in autism is considered. Data from the Collaborative Programs of Excellence in Autism suggests that the distribution ranges from microcephaly to macrocephaly, does not significantly deviate from normal, has a mean that is shifted to the right and an extended right tail reflecting the increased rate of macrocephaly. [31] This wide distribution decreases the likelihood that any given small random sample of individuals with autism will be representative of the autism population in mean head circumference and brain volume and rate of macrocephaly and megalencephaly. Figure 3 shows an autism-control simulation study of total brain volume from one of our datasets. When sample sizes are small, 16 to 20 subjects in each group, and the rate of macrocephaly in the control group is held at 6 %, an increasing rate of macrocephaly in the autism group affects the resulting *p*-value.

If there are age effects on case-control differences of brain volume in autism, the age range of the autism sample studied may also affect the results. Age effects may cancel out autism-control differences in studies that include a wide age range of subjects. Different case-control results may be expected in studies that focus on young versus older individuals with autism.

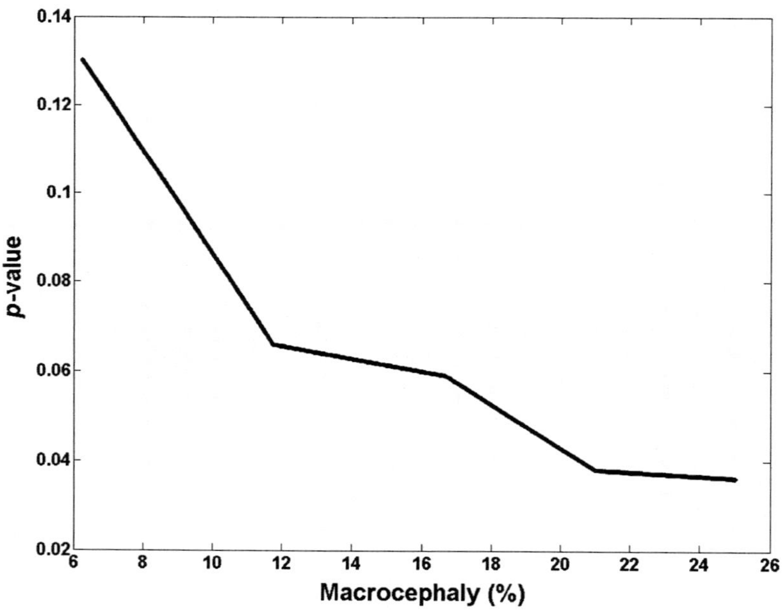

Figure 3 The effect of increasing rates of macrocephaly in the autism sample on case-control comparisons of total brain volume.

Brain Size at Birth

Because autism cannot be diagnosed at birth, information about brain size at birth in autism is indirect and comes from retrospective head circumference studies. At birth, brain volumes of children who are later diagnosed with autism appear to be similar to or smaller than "normal", depending on the reference data used. The mean birth head circumference of

37 males born at term and later diagnosed with autism in the Johns Hopkins study was similar ($z = -0.12$) to the mean of reference data. [13], [35] In a study that used different reference data, mean birth circumference of 15 children later diagnosed with autism or PDD-NOS was significantly smaller ($z = -0.66$) than the reference data mean. [36], [37] When we used the latter reference data [36] to recalculate the birth head circumference z score for the 37 subjects from the Johns Hopkins study, it was more than one standard deviation below the mean ($z = -1.30$) and suggested that birth head circumference is decreased in autism. Strong evidence, however, that birth head circumference in autism and the general population do not significantly differ comes from a Swedish epidemiologic study. [38] Birth head circumferences were similar in 398 children later diagnosed with autism and 2040 children from the general population. [38] The control children were in the same cohort as the autism children and were individually matched to the autism children by sex, birth year, and hospital of birth. Although the selection criteria of the cohort study may have resulted in an overrepresentation of more severely affected children with autism, the findings are noteworthy.

Brain Growth in Early Childhood

Similar to brain size at birth, there is little information about brain growth between birth and later childhood in autism. A major reason for this gap in our knowledge is that autism cannot be reliably diagnosed until 2 to 3 years of age. Children with high-functioning autism may not come to clinical attention until even later.

The period of brain development between birth and early childhood is extremely important. It is also the time when the clinical signs of autism appear. Neuronal proliferation and migration and proliferation of radial glial cells are completed in almost all areas of the brain during fetal development. During early postnatal life, there is an explosive increase in the number of synaptic connections, myelination increases, non-radial glial cells proliferate, and thalamocortical connections come "on-line" followed later in childhood by intrahemispheric and interhemispheric cortico-cortical connections. [39], [40] In typically developing children, brain growth during infancy and early childhood is more important than brain growth during fetal life in predicting IQ at 9 years of age. [41]

The brain seems to grow at an abnormally rapid rate during early childhood in at least some children with autism. Increased rate of brain growth in autism was first suggested by head circumference findings in macrocephalic children and adults. In most cases, the macrocephaly in autism was not present at birth but seemed to develop during childhood. [13] This original observation was quickly replicated, [42] and it was recently replicated again. [37], [43]

An increased rate of brain growth during childhood in autism is also suggested by comparison of the distributions of head circumference at birth and later childhood and adulthood and by growth curves. Figure 4 show that the distribution of head circumference of 91 individuals with autism during childhood and adulthood is nearly the mirror image of the distribution of 51 of these individuals at birth. [13] Childhood growth curves of these individuals suggest a variety of patterns of early head and brain growth in autism, as shown in Table 2. Some of the children had increased rates of head growth and others had normal or decreased rates of head growth. A small minority had decreased rate of head growth followed by an increased rate or the opposite pattern. [13] Another study examined retrospective growth data from birth and very early childhood in 22 children with autism or PDD-NOS and control children from a different cohort. Rates of head and brain growth were increased in some of the autism children during the first 1 to 1 ½ years of life. [37] The findings of these two studies are relative to reference data, and therefore need to be replicated in large autism samples with well-matched controls from the same cohort. Additional support for increased rate of brain growth during early childhood in autism comes from the two MRI studies that found increased mean brain volume by 2 to 4 years of age. [27], [28]

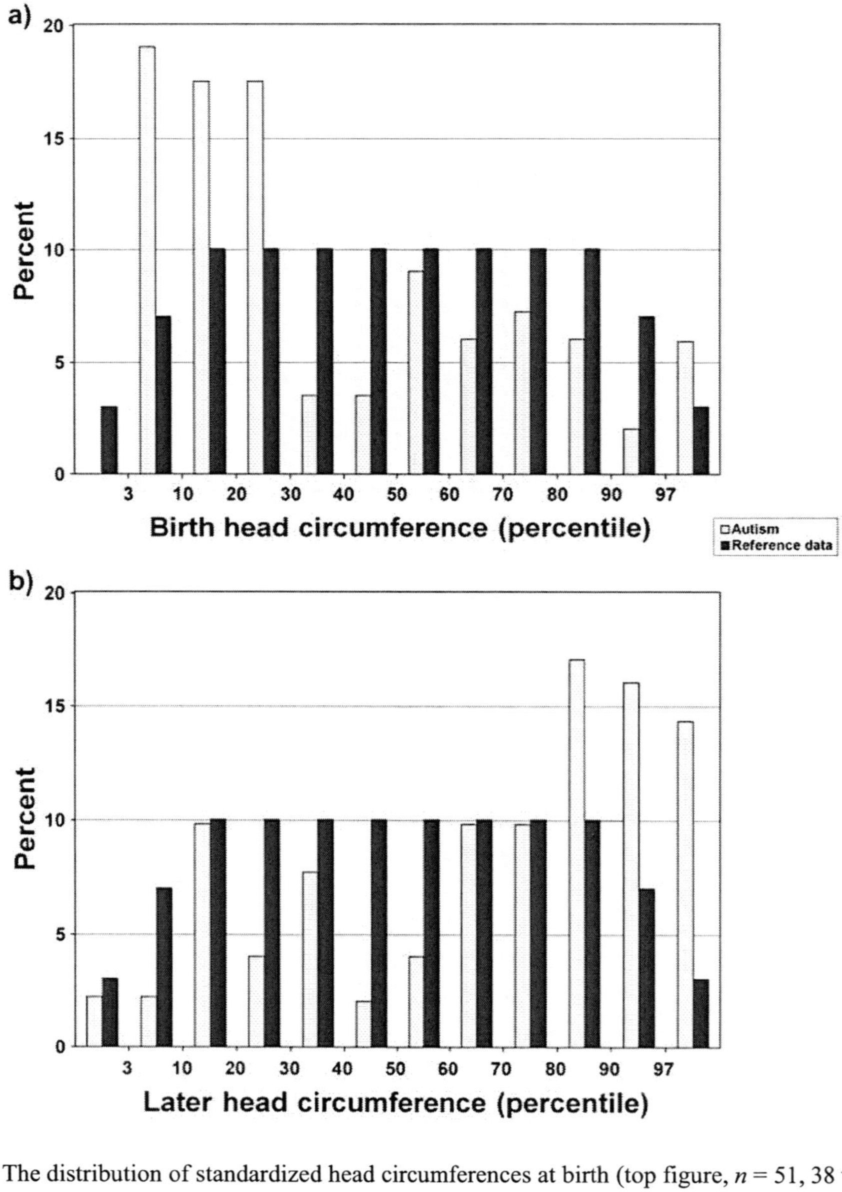

Figure 4 The distribution of standardized head circumferences at birth (top figure, $n = 51$, 38 to 42 weeks gestation) versus during later childhood and adulthood (bottom figure, $n = 91$, 3 to 38 years of age) in subjects with idiopathic autism. [13]

Table 2 Rate of head growth during childhood in autism

		Decreased Rate	Normal Rate	Increased Rate
Lainhart et al. [13]	*Autism: birth to 3 years (n=11)*	9.1 %	54.5 %	36.4 %
	Autism: 2 to 12 years (n=35)	37.1 % 2.8 %[1]	54.3 %	5.7 %
Courchesne et al. [37]	*Controls: birth to 6-14 months (n=31)*			71 %
	Autism: birth to 6-14 months (n=17)			9 %

Changes in Brain Volume in Later Childhood, Adolescence, and Adulthood

Although several longitudinal studies are in progress, all current information about changes in brain volume with age in autism comes from cross-sectional studies. [20], [28] Longitudinal changes can only be inferred from cross-sectional studies. [44], [45] Age-related findings in cross-sectional studies may be quite different from longitudinal changes observed in the same individuals over time. [44], [45]

Cross-sectional MRI studies of brain volume in autism suggest that the overall more rapid than normal increase in head and brain growth during early childhood is followed by a decrease in rate of growth below normal. By late childhood or adolescence, mean brain volumes in autism and normal controls samples do not differ even though mean head circumference remains increased in the autism groups. [20], [26], [28]

If "normalization" of brain volume truly occurs with age in autism, it may not be related to normal brain maturation. In typically developing individuals, dynamic changes in brain morphometry and circuitry occur during later childhood, adolescence, and young adulthood despite little change in total brain volume. [46]– [48] The changes in circuitry involve maturation of widely distributed neural networks. [49] Brain maturation in typically developing individuals sets the stage for peak cognitive functioning. In contrast, adolescence and young adulthood in autism are often times when cognitive and overall functioning plateau or deteriorate. In addition, seizures may develop. Individuals with autism who do not deteriorate during adolescence and young adulthood for the most part remain significantly impaired. Therefore, the brain changes associated with "normalization" of brain volume in autism may be pathologic. Longitudinal MRI studies of autism are needed during these later stages of development as well as during early life. There is essentially no imaging data about the aging brain in autism. Understanding aging in autism will become increasingly important as the disorder is more frequently recognized and diagnosed in older individuals.

[1] One child with autism had decreased rate between 2 and 4 years of age followed by an increased rate of head growth.

Head Circumference and Brain Volume in Autism Twins

Studies of head size and brain volume in twins with autism show different results. In a British epidemiologic study of male twins, 38.9 % of twins with idiopathic autism 16 years of age or younger had macrocephaly compared to 9% of 120 typically developing twins. [15] Macrocephaly was only found in twins who had the full autism syndrome. Macrocephaly was found in none of the children who had milder phenotypes including social and language features of the broader autism phenotype and milder autism spectrum disorders. These findings suggest that brain volume is increased in autism twins and larger brain volume is associated with autism versus milder forms of the disorder. Increased brain volume in autism twins was however not found in a neuroimaging study. [50] Mean total brain tissue volume was smaller ($z = -0.49$) in 9 MZ twin pairs discordant for autism relative to normal control singletons, 5 to 13 years of age, with mean IQ above average. The more severely affected group with autism had a smaller mean brain volume than twins without autism, many of whom had features of the broader phenotype of autism. The disparate findings of these two studies need to be resolved. Investigations that measure both head circumference and brain volume, stringently exclude autism twins with possibly causal medical conditions, and use typically developing twins as controls are needed. Clarification of head size and brain volume in twins with autism is important because it will advance our understanding of the relationship between genetic factors, severity of the autism phenotype, and head and brain size in autism.

Microcephaly

Neurobiologic theories of autism must wrestle with the fact that autism occurs in individuals who are microcephalic as well as those who are normocephalic and macrocephalic. Developmental brain mechanisms leading to microcephaly are different than those leading to normocephaly and macrocephaly associated with developmental disorder. [51] Neuroimaging has not yet been used to study microcephaly in autism. Head circumference studies suggest that although macrocephaly is a variable phenotypic feature of idiopathic autism in general, [13], [16], [17] microcephaly may identify distinct subtypes. Microcephaly, a head circumference 1.88 or more standard deviations below the mean for age and sex (< 3rd percentile), occurs in 3 % to 7 % of cases of idiopathic autism. [13], [16] It occurs at higher rates in children with autism who have causal medical disorders with mental retardation. [17] In idiopathic autism, microcephaly may be associated with increased rates of dysmorphology, mental retardation, and seizures, a lower male:female ratio, and a lower recurrence risk in families, compared to normocephalic and macrocephalic autism. [13], [16]

Lobar Volume

Several studies have tried to determine if brain enlargement in autism is associated with uniform enlargement of all lobes of the brain. Most sample sizes have been small. Interestingly, the findings have varied with mean age of the autism subjects studied. [52], [53] In 2 and 3 year old children with autism, an anterior-posterior gradient of enlargement was observed relative to 10 control children. The anterior lobes of the brain were most enlarged.

The occipital lobes were not enlarged. [28] In a study of older children, 9 high-functioning and 13 low-functioning children with autism, 6 to 10 years of age were compared to typically developing children. The autism children had increased mean volume in pericallosal, but not precallosal or retrocallosal regions of the two hemispheres. [24] In adolescents and adults with autism, 13 to 29 years of age, brain enlargement involved more posterior regions, the temporal, parietal, and occipital lobes. [52] Frontal lobe volume in the autism subjects was decreased relative to total brain volume. The results of these cross-sectional studies suggest an interaction between age and lobar volume in autism, with a frontal to posterior shift in lobar enlargement with age. Longitudinal data are needed to confirm these findings.

Gray and White Matter Volume

Investigations have also been carried out to determine if the increase in mean total brain volume in autism is due to an increase in gray matter, white matter, or both [24], [28], [29], [54] Once again, the cross-sectional data suggest an age-related effect. In 2 and 3 year old children with autism, total gray and white matter were increased. [28] In high- and low-functioning children with autism 6 to 10 years of age, gray matter was somewhat increased but the increase in white matter was more pronounced. [24] Some of the investigators of that study did a later analysis of 17 high-functioning autism and 15 control males, 7 to 11 years of age. Volume of the cerebral cortex was increased in the autism subjects but less than expected for total brain volume. Total white matter was increased in the autism subjects more than expected for total brain volume. [29] A different group of investigators studied 18 high-functioning and 13 low-functioning children with autism 7 to 17 years of age. This autism sample had an increase in cerebral gray rather than white matter volume compared to 21 normal controls. [30] Taken together these studies suggest that gray and white matter are increased in young children, white matter in older children, and gray but not white matter in adolescents and adults with autism.

The authors of the study of the 7 to 11 year olds also tried to determine if all white matter compartments are uniformly increased in autism. Using an automatic white matter parcellation technique they had previously developed, [55], [56] they localized the increase in white matter in 13 male autism children. White matter volume of the superficial radiate compartment was increased by 27 %. White matter volume of the combined sagittal and bridging compartments was not increased compared to 13 control males. [54] The radiate compartment of prefrontal areas was most increased (36 %). This compartment mainly contains intra-hemispheric cortico-cortical fibers. Because these exciting findings are from a small sample and one laboratory, replication is needed.

Scaling of Gray and White Matter to Brain Volume in the Enlarged Brain

In typical development, scaling of white matter to gray matter and each to total brain volume may be different in large versus small brains. Comparative anatomic studies show that as the brain enlarges across species and within primates, white matter of the neocortex increases disproportionately more than gray matter. [57] As the brain enlarges, white matter regions, which contain axons needed to communicate between more distant brain regions, increase more than gray matter regions that contain components for local processing. [58] In the human brain, the correlation between brain size and gray matter volume is negative, i.e., larger brains have smaller proportions of gray matter. [59] To complicate matters further, gray-white matter scaling may differ in different regions of the brain such as the neocortex and the cerebellum. [57] Therefore, it is not yet clear if the scaling of white matter to gray matter and each to total brain volume in autism is related to enlarged brain size in general, unique to autism, or both.

Changes in gray and white matter with age need to be further investigated in autism. The application of new methods, such as cortical pattern-matching and tensor-based morphometry, will allow detailed study of the anatomic underpinnings of increased brain volume in autism and changes across development. [60]– [63] Even when changes in total brain volume are subtle or no longer occurring, dynamic changes in regional and subregional volumes occur in typical development. [60], [62] Localized changes in the cortex may be more pronounced from later childhood into adulthood than during early childhood. [60], [61]

Regions of the Brain in Autism

Different approaches have been used to learn about the size and shape of regions of the brain in autism. Topographic patterns created by gyri and sulci and structural asymmetry of the brain have been examined. Voxel-based methods have been used to examine the entire brain for localized differences in gray and white matter. The volumes of multiple brain regions have been simultaneously examined and compared. Most autism studies have focused on the morphology of one or two regions of interests.

Structural Brain Lateralization and Asymmetry

Study of structural asymmetry provides information about how the autism brain is organized. In typical development, there is asymmetry of perisylvian language regions, Broca's and Wernicke's areas, [64] which are present at birth and stable throughout life. Children and adolescents with autism were found to have normal lateralization of the Sylvian fissure itself compared to 20 normal control children. [65] In 16 high-functioning boys with autism 7 to 11 years of age, the normal asymmetry of the inferior frontal gyrus (Broca's area) was reversed compared to 15 age- and handedness-matched normal controls. [66] In normal controls, this area was 17 % larger on the left. In the autism subjects, it was 27 % larger on the right. Normal asymmetry of the superior temporal gyrus (Wernicke's area) was present in the autism group. Volume of the posterior temporal fusiform gyrus, involved in face processing, was increased more on the left rather than the right in the autism children. The adjacent fusiform gyrus and inferior temporal gyrus showed trends toward left-ward enlargement in the autism group. Another study found decreased rather than the expected increase in gray matter volume in the left planum temporale in autism. [67] These findings suggest that normal structural asymmetry is disrupted in some of the areas involved in language and social functioning in autism.

Gyri and Sulci

Neuroimaging methods that examine the topography of the brain provide a window into the development and maturation of the cortex. Sulci and gyri form in utero as the cortex develops and expands. Changes in gyral and sulcal complexity continue during childhood and adolescence. [68] These changes are thought to be due to myelination and synaptic remodeling including elimination of synapses. Cortical complexity is believed to be associated with increased cortical surface area and hemispheric connectivity. [69] Deviation from the typical degree of gyral complexity may be a gross anatomic manifestation of underlying aberrations in microscopic cortical anatomy. [70] Thus, abnormal gyrification may provide lingering evidence of early or late disruptions of neurdevelopmental processes. [71]

In a cross-sectional study of cortical sulci in 21 children and adolescents with autism, widespread differences were found. The autism group had anterior shifting of superior frontal sulci, the right Sylvian fissure, right superior temporal sulcus, and left inferior frontal sulcus, and shifting of the olfactory sulci compared to 20 normal control children. [65] Less pronounced changes were found in the collateral and intraparietal sulci. The differences may be related to delayed cortical development in autism, particularly in the frontal lobes. [65]

In addition to suggesting brain mechanism involved in autism, study of gyri may add to our understanding of the effects of genes, epigenetic mechanisms, and environmental factors, including experience, on the brain in autism. In typically developing individuals, inter-individual variation in gyral volume is large. Scaling of the volumes of individual gyri to brain size is much different than the scaling of lobar volumes to brain size. Variance in gyral volumes appears to be strongly affected by interactive effects particular to individuals. [72]

Whole-Brain Voxel-Based Approach

In whole-brain voxel-based studies, the entire brain is examined for statistically significant case-control difference. A voxel-based study of children with autism accompanied by mental retardation and significant language impairment showed decreased gray matter in right and left superior temporal sulcal regions and decreased white matter in the right temporal pole and left cerebellum. [73] Adolescents with high-functioning autism had increased gray matter, relative to total brain volume, in frontal and temporal areas. [33] In early adulthood, high-functioning subjects with autism had gray matter differences, increases in some areas and decreases in other areas, in frontal, medial and lateral temporal, and cerebellar regions. [74]

Multiple Regions of Interest Approach

Three reports describe the volumes of multiple regions of interests and their relationship to total brain volume in autism. In 3 and 4 year old children with autism with increased mean total brain volume, cerebellar and right and left hippocampal and amygdalar volumes were increased but not significantly so when total cerebral volume was used as a covariate. [27] In 9 high-functioning and 13 low-functioning children with autism, 6 to 10 years of age, with increased mean total brain volume, volumes of the cerebral cortex, vermal lobules I–V, caudate, putamen, pallidum, diencephalons, left amygdala, cerebellum, and brainstem were increased. [24] Volumes of the hippocampus, right amygdala, ventricles, operculum, left insula, and vermal lobules VI–II were not increased. [24] In another analysis by some of the same investigators, regional brain volumes were classified relative to total brain volume in 17 high-functioning males with autism and 15 controls. [29] Volumes of the globus pallidus, putamen, caudate, diencephalons, cerebellum, and brainstem were increased in proportion to the increase in total brain volume in the autism subjects. Volumes of the cerebral cortex and hippocampus-amygdala complex were decreased in the autism group relative to total brain volume (effect sizes for adjusted volumes: cerebral cortex −0.74, amygdala-hippocampus −0.68). [29] These cross-sectional data suggest dynamic changes in scaling of the amygdala and hippocampus to total brain volume with age in autism.

C Single Region of Interest Approach

Amygdala and Hippocampus

Volumetric results of studies of the amygdala and hippampus in autism have been mixed and not consistent. Table 3 summarizes published results in order of mean age of the autism samples studied. Some of the inconsistency in the results may be due to different rates of macrocephaly in the autism samples studied, lack of systematic control for brain volume, and possible developmental effects on case-control differences and on the scaling of amygdala, hippocampus, and total brain volumes. The results of one study not included in Table 2, suggests that lack of consistent results across studies may reflect lack of consistent morphometric abnormality. Using a single subject voxel-based analysis, only 7 of 14 older children and adolescents with high-functioning autism had differences in gray matter density in either the amygdala and hippocampus: 6 children had differences in both structures, 1 child in the amygdala only, another child in the hippocampus only, compared to 18 controls. [75]

Table 3 Autism-normal control comparison of volumes of the amygdala and hippocampus

	Developmental Period Containing Mean Age of Autism Sample				
	Early childhood 2 to 4 years	Later childhood 7 to 12 years	Adolescence 13 to 18 years	Young adulthood 19 to 25 years	Older adulthood over 25 years
Amygdala	+ [27]	+ [253] − [29]	ns [253] ns [76]	− [254] + [255]	+ [74] − [93] ns [32]
Hippocampus	− [256] ns [27]	+ [253] − [29]	+ [253] ns [76] ns [257]	− [254]	Ns [32]

27 Sparks et al., 2002, $n = 29$ autism, 26 controls; mean age 3.9 y, range 3.2 y to 4.5 y.
29 Herbert et al., 2003, $n = 17$ autism, 15 controls; age range 7 y to 11 y.
32 Hazender et al., 2000, $n = 17$ autism/Asperger's, 17 controls; mean age 27.2 y.
74 Abell et al., 1999, gray matter, $n = 15$ autism, 15 controls; mean age 28.9 y.
76 Bigler et al., 2003, $n = 38$ autism, 27 controls; mean age 13.7 y, range 7 y to 31 y.
93 Pierce et al., 2001, $n = 7$ autism, 8 controls; mean age 29.5 y, range 21 y to 41 y.
253 Schumann et al., 2004, $n = 19$ autism, 11 controls; age range 7.5 y to 12.5 y.
253 Schumann et al., 2004, $n = 20$ autism, 11 controls; age range 12.75 y to 18.5 y.
254 Aylward et al., 1999, $n = 14$ autism, 14 controls; mean age 20.5 y, range 11 y to 37 y.
255 Howard et al., 2000, $n = 10$ autism/Asperger's, 10 controls; age range 15.8 y to 40.3 y.
256 Saitoh et al., 2001, cross-sectional area Area Dentata, $n = 11$ autism, 8 controls; age range 2.4 y to 4 y.
257 Piven et al., 1998, $n = 35$ autism, 36 controls; mean age 18 y, range 12 y to 29 y.

+: Autism mean volume (area) significantly increased above control mean. −: Autism mean volume (area) significantly decreased below control mean. ns: No significant difference between autism and control means.

We found that autism subjects with macrocephaly had larger hippocampi and amygdalae than normocephalic autism subjects 7 to 32 years of age. [76] When differences in brain volume were controlled for, mean volumes of the structures did not differ from controls. When we explored the relationship between amygdala volume and age in the cross-sectional sample, no age effect was observed in the autism or control group. [76] A different study found age-related changes in amygdala volume in controls but not autism subjects 7 to 18 years of age. Clearly, longitudinal studies following large numbers of individual autism and control subjects over time are needed to determine how amygdala and hippocampal volumes change relative to total brain volume with age in autism. In addition, the possibility of dynamic local increases and decreases in parts of these structures with little or no change in overall volume needs to be investigated.

Basal Ganglia

Dysfunction of the basal ganglia and frontostriatal system has long been suspected in autism. [77] Children with autism have a variety of unusual stereotyped, repetitive behaviors. In addition, they frequently have features of attention deficit hyperactivity disorder and obsessive compulsive disorder and less commonly tics. A finding in idiopathic autism, that has now been replicated four times by 3 different groups of investigators, is increased mean basal ganglia volume in autism, proportional to the increase in total brain volume. [24], [29], [78], [79] A PET study of 18 children with tuberous sclerosis (TS) and intractable epilepsy found that the TS children with autism had increased uptake of alpha-methyl-L-tryptophan in the caudate nuclei compared to TS children without autism. This finding suggests functional imbalance in circuits involving subcortical structures in at least in autism associated with TS. [80]

Cerebellum

The cerebellum has been of interest in autism because of neuropathological and early MRI findings, [22], [81] and PET findings of serotonin abnormality in the dentate nucleus. [82] The cerebellum plays a role in attention, language development, motor functioning, possibly stereotyped behaviors, in affective processing, and the processing of other higher cognitive functions. [83] Development of the cerebellum is protracted, beginning early in gestation and continuing the first year of life. [84] Brain structures with protracted periods of development are more vulnerable to factors that may perturb development. In older children and adults, males in particular, morphology of cerebellum including volume appears to be significantly affected by postnatal experience such as long-term motor skill activities and cognitive demands. [85]

A number of recent studies have examined size of the cerebellum in autism In traditional volumetric studies of 3 to 4 year olds, 7 to 11 year olds, and older adolescents and adults with autism, mean total cerebellar volume (and mid-sagittal area) were enlarged but no more than expected given the increase in mean total brain volume. [26], [27], [86] In children and adults with autism who are intellectually high- or low-functioning, significant case-control differences are lost when total brain volume is used as a covariate. These findings do not mean that the cerebellum is normal in autism. Rather, they may suggest that the process causing increased whole brain volume in autism is affecting the cerebellum in a manner that preserves their usual size relationship.

The wide distribution of head sizes and likely brain volumes in autism and the relationship between total brain and cerebellar volumes predicts a wide distribution of cerebellar volumes. By chance alone, small samples such as those used in most imaging studies of autism [87] may have had varying proportions of autism subjects with relatively large or small cerebellar and total brain volumes.

Gray and white matter of the cerebellum have been examined in voxel-based studies. In a voxel-based study comparing individual children with high-functioning autism to controls, 11 of the 14 autism children had differences in gray matter density. [75] None of the children with autism had changes in gray matter density in a "control" area of the brain, the visual cortex (V1). In low-functioning children with autism, cerebellar white matter was decreased. [73] In two studies of high-functioning adults with autism, increased gray matter in some regions of the cerebellum was found in one study [74] but not in another study that used total brain volume as a covariate. [33]

Our group has carried out a comprehensive examination of the cerebellum and its lobules in male children and adults with autism not accompanied by mental retardation. We did not find any significant case-control volumetric or area differences. We and other investigators recently examining the cross-sectional area of vermal lobules VI–VII find no autism-control differences, particularly when head and brain size are controlled for. [86], [88] Functionally, the oculomotor precision function of the cerebellar vermal lobules VI–VII was found to be normal in high-functioning adults with autism. [89] The cross-sectional area of vermis lobules VIII–X was smaller in a sample of children with autism and the finding was related to the lower IQ in the autism versus control sample. [90] When autism and control samples are matched on IQ and brain size, we find no case-control differences in these lobules. Functionally, the vestibulo-ocular reflex subserved by vermal lobules IX and X appears normal in high functioning children with autism. [91]

Although abnormalities of the cerebellum in autism may not be manifested in isolated size differences, studies of the relationships of cerebellar volume to other brain regions and to function have identified abnormalities. In children with autism 3 to 9 years of age, mid-sagittal area of cerebellar vermal lobules VI–VII was negatively related to volume of frontal lobe gray matter and rate of stereotyped behaviors. [92], [93] In young children with autism, cerebellar size at 2 to 6 years of age was related to speed of orienting to visual cues. [94 Deficits in procedural learning, subserved by cerebellar-frontal neural circuitry has been found in children and adolescents with autism. [95] Impaired fronto-cerebellar circuitry was also found in a study of attention-related event-related potential response in autism. [96] Combined neuropsychological, neurophysiological, and MRI studies of the cerebellum are needed to more clearly describe the cerebellar phenotype of autism.

Corpus Callosum

Neuroimaging study of the corpus callosum is important in autism because of increasing evidence that a key cognitive deficit in autism is in the processing of complex information. [97] It is believed that more complex tasks in any domain of functioning require more intra-hemispheric and inter-hemispheric neuronal communication than simple tasks.

The corpus callosum (CC) develops between 8 and 20 weeks of gestation and regional growth continues at different rates up to birth. [98] Approaching fibers are encouraged to properly turn and are guided across the CC midline by glial cells, pioneering cingulate axons, and a variety of chemo-repulsive and chemo-attractant molecules. [99], [100] All callosal axons are produced before birth and they are produced in excess. [101] At birth, there are over three times as many callosal axons than in adulthood, and the topography of the CC in relation to cortical areas is well established. [101] Callosal axons are rapidly eliminated after birth, particularly in the first 4 months of life. [101] Initially in infancy, callosal axons form exuberant connections with terminal fields. The connections are soon refined. [102] After birth, the splenium grows more rapidly than other regions and continues to increase in size until young adulthood. [103] On T1 weighted images, the corpus callosum appears to rapidly myelinate during the first year of life, achieving an adult-like myelinated appearance by 8 months of age. [104] Growth of the CC and decrease in signal intensity in later childhood and adolescence are thought to be due to increased axonal size and ongoing axonal cytoskeleton maturation. [105] In typically developing young individuals, there is large inter-subject variation in CC morphology. Most of the variability in mid-sagittal CC area appears to be related to genes; the heritability index is 94 %. [106] Known correlates of CC mid-sagittal area include handedness, cerebral lateralization pattern, and various cognitive abilities. [106], [107]

Table 4 Corpus callosum finding of neuroimaging studies of autism

	CC total	Anterior		Body			Posterior	
		1 rostrum	2 genu	3 rostral body	4 anterior midbody	5 posterior midbody	6 isthmus	7 splenium
MRI [24]		–		–			–	
MRI [112]	–							
MRI [111]								
MRI [86]	–							
MRI [113]								
MRI [114]	ns							
MRI [54]	ns							
MRI [110]	ns							
VBM [63]		–	–					–
VBM [108]			–					–
DTIa [116]			–	–				
DTIb [109]	ns		–					ns

–: decreased; +: increased; ns: not significant. MRI: quantitative MRI of midsagittal area; VBM: 2D voxel-based morphometry using white matter density index; DTI: diffusion tensor imaging using fractional anisotropy metric, a = whole brain using statistical parametric mapping, b = region of interest approach. Shaded cells: entire region measured (i.e. anterior CC); Witelson division not specified.

Table 4 summarizes corpus callosum findings in autism studied by quantitative measure of the midsagittal area and more recently by diffusion tensor imaging (DT-MRI) and voxel-based morphometry. [29], [54], [86], [108]– [116] What is striking about the findings is that 5 of 8 studies using traditional MRI quantitative methods and 4 of 4 studies using new methods to measure white matter metrics find abnormalities in the corpus callosum in autism. When midsagittal area or white matter differ from controls, they are always decreased in the autism group. The two DT-MRI studies examining the corpus callosum in high-functioning individuals with autism using different approaches both found decreased fractional anisotropy (FA). [109], [116] Both of the studies found decreased FA in the genu, the region of the corpus callosum where fibers from the prefrontal cortices cross the midline. Tensor-based morphometric analysis of the corpus callosum in high-functioning individual with autism shows decreased white matter in the genu and splenium in 2 of 2 studies, the rostrum in 1 of the studies, [63] and the midbody in the other study. [108] In one of the studies, there was evidence that the decrease in regional size of the CC was due to undergrowth rather than atropy. Myelination appeared to increase normally with age in the autism group, as found in an earlier study. [115], [117] Taken together, the findings suggest disordered development of the corpus callosum in autism.

Temporal Lobe

MRI examination of the brain of individuals with macrocephaly is at an early stage of development. We performed a comprehensive examination of all major components of the temporal lobe in autism subjects with and without macrocephaly. We compared them to typically developing subjects with and without macrocephaly and to individuals with dyslexia. Some of the results are shown in Figure 5. These comparisons are beginning to allow us to determine if scaling of regional to total brain volume is different when the brain enlarges across individuals in autism versus in typical development. [76]

Increased rates of macrocephaly may complicate the study of other regional brain volumes in autism. Even in typically developing individuals, all brain regions do not increase uniformly when brain volume increases across individuals. As mentioned above, when total brain volume increases, white matter increases proportionately more and gray matter proportionately less. [59] Change in regional brain volume expected in larger brains needs to be distinguished from pathologic change related to autism.

Thalamus

The thalamus is important in intra-hemispheric connectivity via connections between the cortex and thalamic nuclei and cortico-cortical connections through the thalamus. Thalamocortical afferents, transferring auditory information from the brainstem to the cortex of the temporal lobe, myelinate and come "on-line" between 4.5 months and 1 year of age. As a result, cortical processing of auditory information begins. [40] The thalamic-auditory cortex system continues to develop and mature up until 5 years of life. Maturation of the thalamo-cortical system during this period is associated with the development of auditory perception and discrimination of speech sounds. It is during this period in early childhood that signs of autism appear and language fails to develop normally.

Several studies using different imaging methods have found abnormalities of the thalamus in autism. In young children with autism, 2 to 7 years of age, perfusion of the thalami on SPECT was qualitatively decreased in 19 of 23 cases. [118] Quantitative decrease in blood perfusion of the thalami was found in a SPECT study of individuals with autism accompanied by moderate to severe mental retardation compared to mental age matched controls. [119] A volumetric study of 12 high-functioning males with autism, 11 to 37 years of age found decreased thalamic volume relative to total brain volume compared to controls. [120] In controls, thalamic volume significantly correlated with total brain volume ($r = 0.82$,

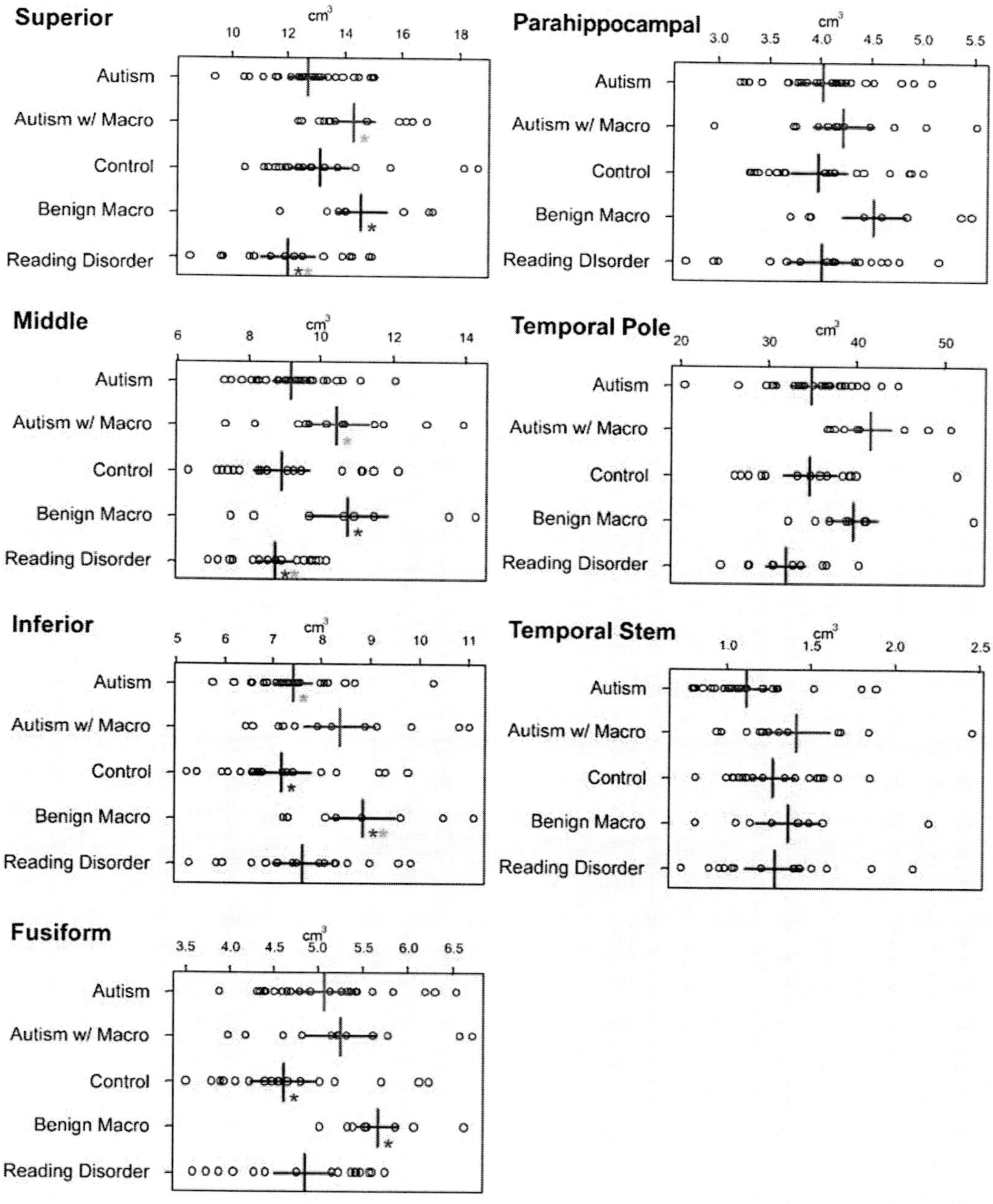

Figure 5 The effect of macrocephaly in autism and typically developing individuals on regional temporal lobe volumes.

$p = 0.001$). There was no significant correlation in the autism sample ($r = -0.15$, $p = 0.65$). [120] The atypical relationship between total brain volume and thalamic volume in the autism group appeared driven by the autism subjects with large brains. In a different study, the white matter sagittal compartment, containing thalamo-cortical as well as other fibers, was not increased relative to total brain white matter volume in high-functioning children with autism 5 to 11 years of age. [54]

Increased volumetric and neurochemical asymmetry of the thalamus has been found. Volumes of the right and left thalami were more strongly correlated in typically developing individuals ($r = 0.95$, $p = 0.001$) than in autism subjects ($r = 0.51$, $p = 0.09$). [120] In this study, the left thalamus tended to be larger than the right in the autism subjects. Using PET, serotonin synthesis was found to be asymmetrically decreased in 7 boys with autism. [82] It was decreased in the left thalamus in 5 boys and in the right thalamus in the other 2 boys. Serotonin synthesis was also abnormal in other regions of the dento-thalamo-cortical pathway. A PET study of adult men with autism has shown impaired language activation in this pathway. [121] In unusual cases autism caused by axonal dystrophy, spheroids which are characteristic of the disorder are found in numerous regions of the brain including the thalamus. [122]

Diffusion Tensor Imaging

Biological Basis

In biological tissues, properties of microstructural organization and architecture can be detected and characterized using measurements of water diffusion with MRI. In the white matter (WM) of the central nervous system, the diffusion parallel to axonal fiber orientation is relatively unhindered, whereas perpendicular to the fibers the diffusion appears to be more restricted. Thus the diffusion behavior is anisotropic, i.e., predominantly in one direction as shown in Figure 6a, rather than isotropic, i.e., identical in all directions. Anisotropic diffusion in WM was first reported in 1990. [123]

Water diffusion properties of brain tissues are highly sensitive to differences or changes in the microstructural features of the tissue, such as cellular membranes, the myelin sheath, cytoplasmic structures, and the spatial scales of these structures, i.e., cellular density, swelling, degeneration or hyperplasia. Many recent studies have demonstrated that diffusion measurements with MRI, diffusion-tensor MRI in particular, are sensitive to cellular and microstructural changes associated with a wide variety of neuropathologic and psychopathologic conditions and even normal brain development and aging.

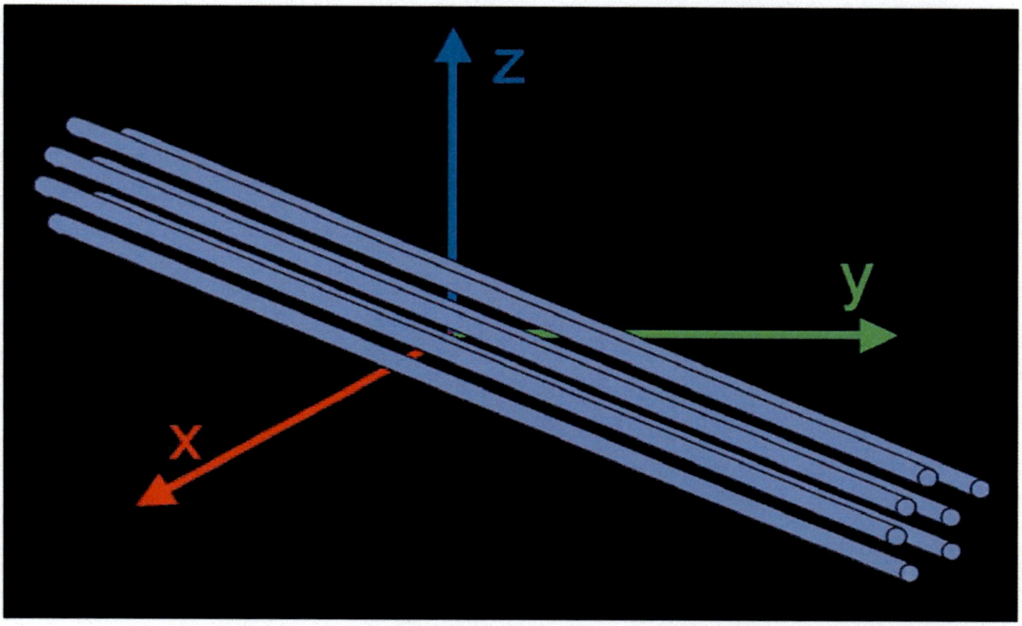

Figure 6a Bundle of axons. Water diffusion in white matter is directionally anisotropic. In white matter tracts, water diffusion perpendicular to the tracts is more "hindered." Water diffusion parallel to the tracts is unrestricted.

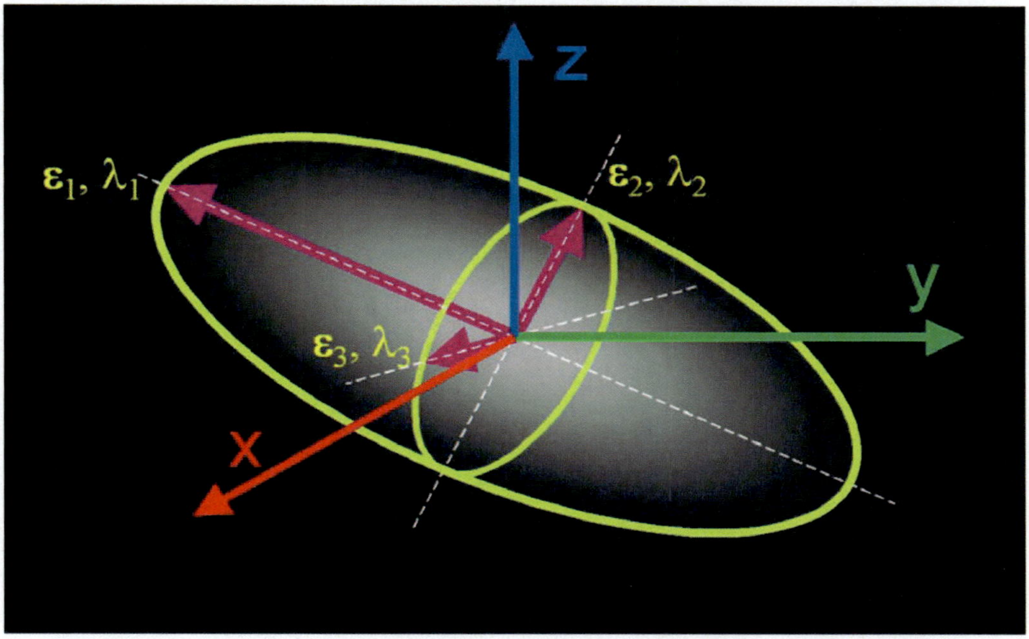

Figure 6b Directional probability of diffusion represented by an ellipse. Small changes in the density, spacing, or myelination of white matter fibers can significantly alter white matter diffusion properties, which can be measured with diffusion tensor imaging.

Diffusion Tensor MRI (DT-MRI)

In 1994, Basser et al. [124] developed an elegant tensor model to describe the anisotropic diffusion behavior of the water signal in biological tissues. (A tensor is a generalized mathematical form of a vector involving a number of indices.) The diffusion tensor D is a 3×3 matrix (with elements D_{ij}) which describes the relative diffusion in a 3 dimensional (3D) coordinate system. [124]– [127] Since this matrix is symmetric, the diffusion tensor comprises six independent variables.

It is an interesting challenge to represent the six-dimensional data in a meaningful way for interpretation. A convenient graphical way to represent the diffusion tensor is by a 3D ellipsoid as shown in Figure 6b. The axis lengths of the ellipsoid are equal to the major, medium and minor eigenvalues of the diffusion tensor. The orientation of the ellipsoid is represented by the major, medium and minor eigenvectors.

There are three important measures of the diffusion tensor. The trace of the tensor, a measure of the magnitude of diffusion, is equal to the sum of all 3 eigenvalues. Anisotropy is the measure of the degree to which diffusivity is a function of the encoding direction. [127]–[131] Currently, the most widely measure of anisotropy is probably fractional anisotropy (FA). [127] A third important measure of the diffusion tensor is tensor orientation described by the major eigenvector direction. For diffusion tensors with high anisotropy, the major eigenvector direction is generally assumed to be parallel to the direction of WM tracts which are often represented using red-green-blue color map to indicate the eigenvector orientations. [132], [133] An FA map is shown in Figure 7.

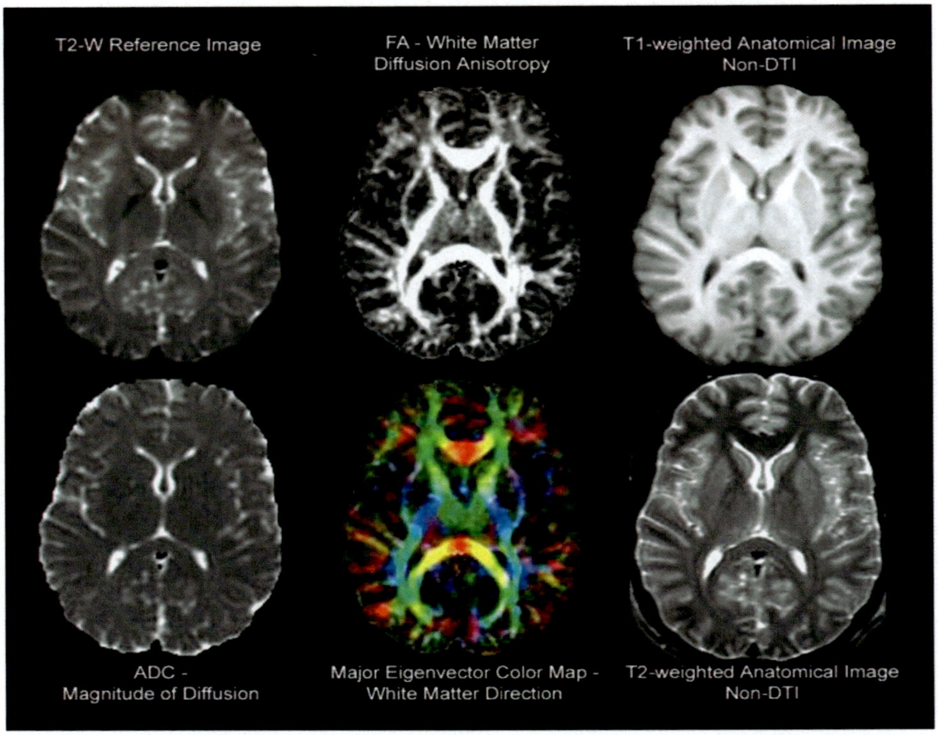

Figure 7 Fractional anisotropy map (middle brains) compared to T2- and T1-weighted anatomic images.

The diffusion tensor is based upon a 3D multivariate Gaussian model of diffusion, which appears to be a reasonable approximation in many homogeneous brain tissue regions. However, the simple Gaussian diffusion assumption may be violated in regions with complex white matter organization, or when significant partial volume averaging is present. [134], [135] New and exciting methods for measuring and characterizing complex diffusion behavior are under development, [135]– [138] but are beyond the scope of discussion here.

Measurements of DT-MRI

The apparent diffusivities of water in specific directions are estimated by measuring the signal attenuation in images with the diffusion-weighting gradients applied in the direction of interest. A minimum of six non-collinear encoding directions of diffusion-weighting are necessary to estimate the full diffusion tensor. [139], [140] A wide variety of diffusion-tensor encoding strategies with six or more encoding directions have been proposed, [140]– [143] although the encoding schemes with the most uniform angular distributions tend to provide the most accurate results. [144] There is also mounting evidence that more encoding directions diminish the variable variances of DT-MRI measures as a function of tensor orientation. [145], [146]

Diffusion-weighted, single-shot, spin-echo EPI is the most common method for diffusion-tensor measurements in the human brain. Most MRI manufacturers now offer pulse sequences (typically EPI-based) and semi-automated analysis software for DT-MRI. Single-shot EPI is well-suited for DT-MRI because it is rapid, highly efficient (2-4 images per second), and relatively insensitive to small head movements, which is problematic with many multi-shot imaging methods. However, the spatial resolution of single-shot EPI tends to be rather coarse, which is worsened by T2 blurring in the phase-encoding direction. Single-shot methods also demonstrate significant image distortions. Eddy currents induced by the strong diffusion-weighting gradients can cause DW images to be distorted and misregistered relative to one another, which leads to errors in the calculated DT-MRI images. [147] The eddy currents can be reduced using bipolar diffusion-weighting schemes. [148], [149] The distortions can also be corrected using image registration methods. [147], [150], [151] Distortions from static magnetic field (B_o) in-homogeneities cause the brain to be warped nonlinearly in the phase-encoding direction. EPI distortion can be corrected by measuring maps of the B_o field and correcting the images retrospectively. [152], [153] EPI distortions can also be reduced by using parallel imaging methods (e.g., SENSE [154], [155]).

DT-MRI Measurements in the Human Brain

Detailed diffusion tensor measurements of normal brain tissues [129], [141] demonstrate that measures of tensor anisotropy display the greatest differences between regions of GM and WM. Diffusion anisotropy is quite variable across both WM and GM structures in the brain. [128], [129], [141] By comparison, the trace is relatively homogenous for all regions of GM and WM ($\sim 2100\times10^{-6}$ mm2/s). Generally, DT changes in WM with age are characterized by increase in DT anisotropy and decrease in the trace during childhood, [156]– [159] followed by a gradual decrease in anisotropy in adulthood. [160], [161] Thus, it is absolutely critical to control for the effects of age in quantitative diffusion tensor imaging studies. Several recent studies have also shown a relationship between regional diffusion tensor measurements and cognitive ability. [162]

DT-MRI Measurements in Developmental Disorders Including Autism

It is possible that many developmental disorders such as autism have abnormalities in brain white matter that contribute to cognitive deficits, behavioral aberrations, and complex emotional and social disturbances. Generally, these white matter abnormalities are difficult to detect and characterize using conventional imaging methods.

Recently, several investigators have started to use DT-MRI as a tool to probe white matter differences in groups of patients with developmental disorders such as developmental delay, [163] leukodystrophies, [164], [165] Fragile X, [166] and velocardiofacial syndrome. [167] A number of recent studies have also used DT-MRI to study white matter abnormalities in schizophrenia. [168]– [171] To date, only one published study [116] has applied DT-MRI to investigate white matter abnormalities in autism. In that study, a voxel-based SPM analysis was performed to compare the FA maps from seven boys with autism and nine age- and IQ-matched control subjects. In this preliminary report, reduced FA was observed in white matter adjacent to the ventromedial prefrontal cortices and in the anterior cingulate gyri in the autism group. Reduced FA was also found at the junction of temporal and parietial areas, adjacent to the superior temporal sulci, in the temporal lobes near the amygdala, and in areas where tracts connect temporal and occipital lobes. FA was also reduced in corpus callosum.

Our research group is also using DT-MRI to study subjects with autism. In a preliminary investigation of our data, we examined FA measurements in the mid-sagittal plane of the corpus callosum of age- and IQ-matched males with autism (n = 16, mean age = 16.9 years) and controls (n = 11, mean age = 15.3 years). The results did not show any significant differences in FA for the full corpus callosum midsection. However, signficant differences (p = 0.026) were observed in the genu region of the corpus callosum, which contains interhemispheric connections to prefrontal brain areas. Further studies are necessary to verify this observation.

Advanced DT-MRI Analysis Methods

The complexity and richness of diffusion tensor image data offer unique opportunities for advanced image analysis, which may ultimately improve the characterization of white matter in autism and other developmental disorders. We will discuss two approaches—voxel-based statistical parametric mapping (SPM) analysis and white matter tractography.

Voxel-Based SPM Analysis of DT-MRI Data

Recently, statistical parametric mapping (SPM) methods have become quite popular for analyzing DT-MRI data either within or between groups. These approaches have been applied most commonly to FA maps and occasionally to trace maps. The general approach is similar to voxel-based morphometry (VBM).172 FA maps or some other diffusion parametric image of all the subjects are registered to a brain template and then a local smoothing kernel applied. Then, a voxel-by-voxel ANOVA is performed to estimate which brain regions exhibit consistent differences in the FA maps across subjects. The approach is attractive because the analysis is automated and doesn't require hours of tedious ROI drawing. It is performed over the entire brain, such that significant differences in areas not anticipated *a priori* can be detected. Moreover, tools exist to do the analysis (e.g., SPM, by Friston and colleagues at the University College of London; http://www.fil.ion.ucl.ac.uk/spm/) and the statistical methods for this approach have already been developed for the analysis of fMRI and morphometry data. Voxel-based SPM analysis of DT-MRI data has been applied to a broad spectrum of neuropsychiatric disorders, [116], [166]– [168], [173]– [175] to children with poor reading ability, [162] and to brain development in typically developing children. [176]

Voxel-based SPM methods are an exciting and important tool for exploratory analyses of group-wise DT-MRI data but they have some limitations. A potential confound in the SPM approach is that if the registration between data sets is not perfect, differences in brain morphology could manifest as apparent regional differences in FA between subjects. Improvements in image registration algorithms will improve the confidence in SPM studies of DT-MRI data. A challenge with this approach is that the orientation of the diffusion tensor must be rotated to the same orientation as the target image or template space. [134] Several investigators have recently reported approaches to the registration of DT-MRI images with tensor transformation. [134], [177]– [179] Another current limitation of the SPM approach is that the case-control analyses have considered only a single scalar parameter, FA, whereas the diffusion tensor is a multidimensional entity. The use of multivariate statistical models could potentially improve the detection of group differences and increase the flexibility in developing models to describe the interactions between variables. Finally, the large numbers of voxels in DT images lead to multiple comparisons which increase the likelihood of false positives. Few, if any DT-MRI SPM studies have corrected their results for multiple comparisons.

White Matter Tractography

White matter tractography (WMT) methods offer a unique opportunity to segment white matter pathways in the brain as well as within specific white matter structures, such as the corpus callosum and corona radiate, as shown in figures 8, 9, and 10. There are currently no other non-invasive methods that are capable of structural parcellation of the white matter based upon apparent connectivity patterns.

Recently, several investigators have developed WMT algorithms to estimate WM connectivity using the anisotropic and directional information of the diffusion tensor. Most of these algorithms use the major eigenvector to estimate the tangent of the trajectory for a WM fiber bundle. [180]– [182] Tracing methods based upon the full diffusion tensor field have also been developed. [183]– [186] The latter methods show promise for resolving pathways in regions with intersecting oblique WM fibers. Other investigators have developed more continuous methods for estimating connectivity between a single location and multiple terminal points. These approaches include variations of probabilistic Monte Carlo methods to perturb estimated tract pathways, [187], [188] wavefront propagation methods, [189] and solutions to the diffusion equation in the diffusion tensor field. WMT methods have been used to generate anatomically plausible tract reconstructions of major WM pathways in the human brain. [181], [190]– [194] DT-MRI measurements (including the eigenvector directions) are highly sensitive to measurement noise which influences the accuracy of WMT. Several studies have simulated noise effects on the estimated tract accuracy, [195]– [198] and have generally found the errors to be small over large distances in homogeneous white matter pathways. However, in regions of complex white matter geometry (e.g., small and/or intersecting white matter structures), current WMT methods have difficulty in resolving the correct pathways.

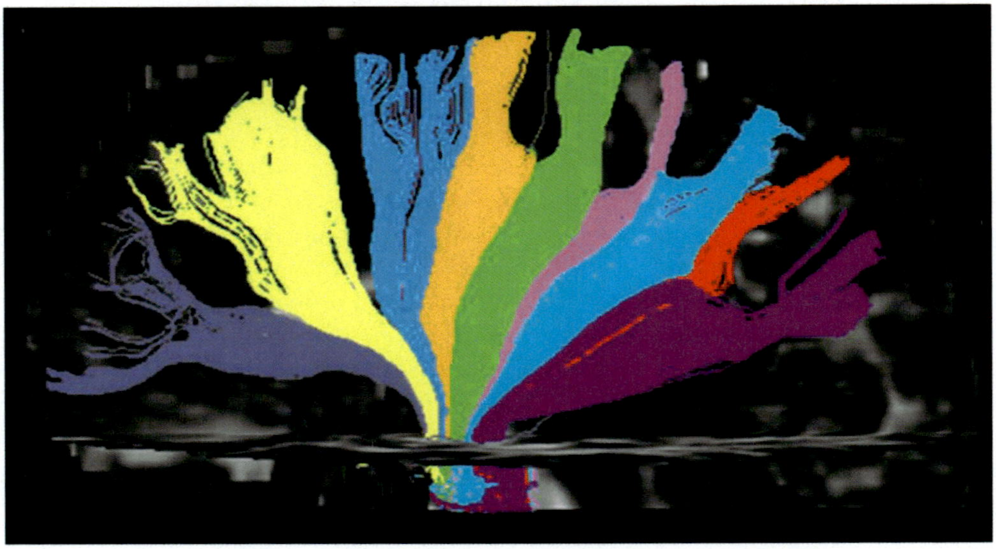

Figure 8 White matter tractography images of the main projection pathways between the brainstem and cortex through the cerebral peduncles, internal capsule, and corona radiate.

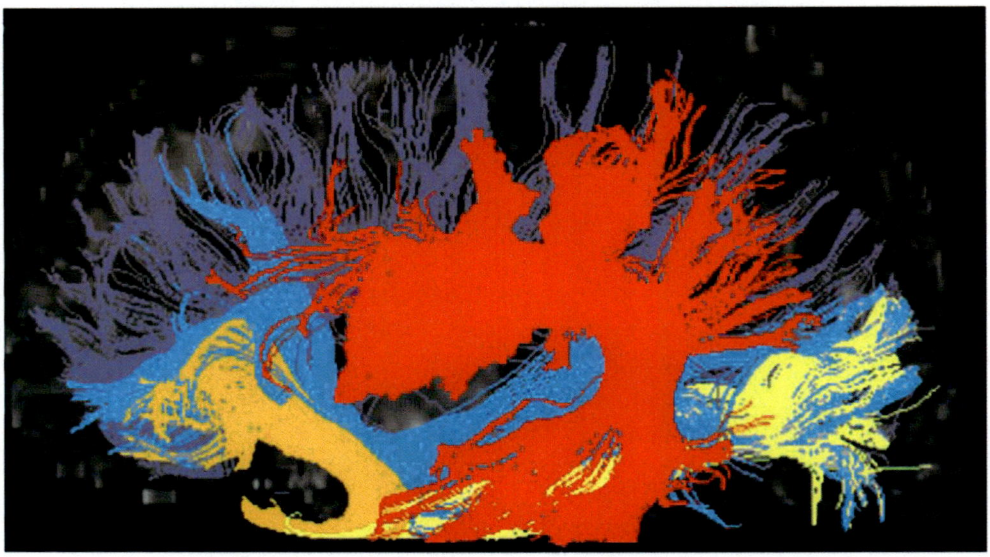

Figure 9 White matter tractography images of intra-hemispheric cortico-cortical major association pathways: uncinate fasciculus (left-side of image, second lightest tract); inferior longitudinal fasciculus (right-side of image, lightest tract); superior longitudinal fasciculus (darkest tract); occipitofrontal fasciculus (lower medium bright, posterior to anterior tract); corpus callosum (diffuse upper medium-shaded fibers).

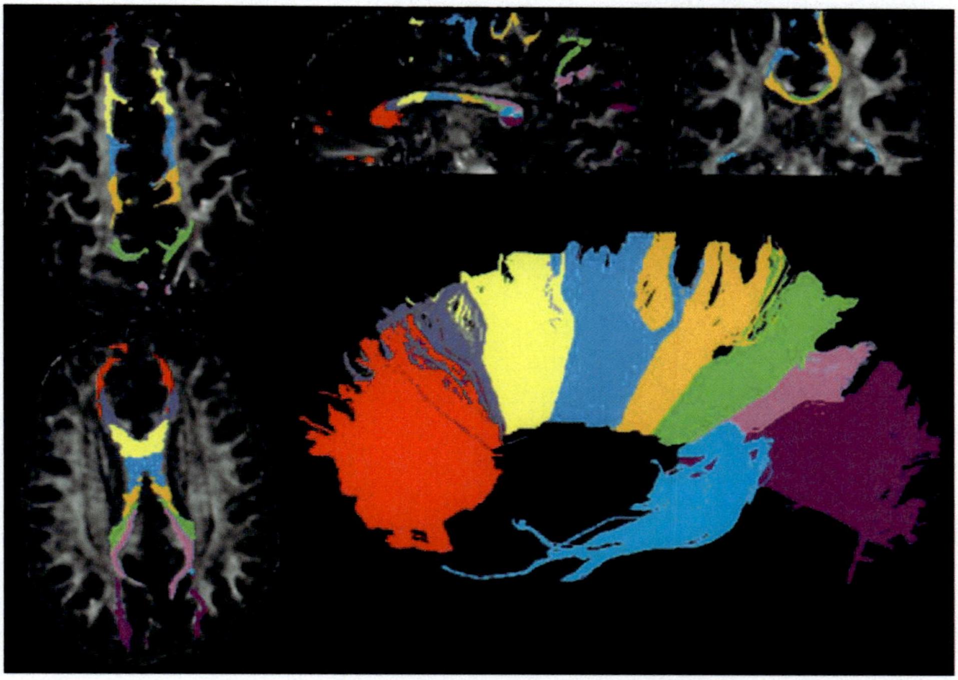

Figure 10 White matter tractography segmentation of the corpus callosum. In the figure, the corpus callosum (CC) has been parcellated according to specific cortical regions of connectivity. This parcellation approach allows for unique cortical specific labeling of parts of a structure for further analysis.

Brain Function

Functional neuroimaging has begun to help us understand how differences in brain function in autism are related to the unusual forms of thought and behavior that characterize the disorder. Most functional brain studies in autism have been performed on relatively small samples of specific subgroups of individuals with autism, specifically selected so the sample is as homogeneous in intellectual functioning, gender, and age as possible. Much work still needs to be done to determine if the findings in one subgroup of autism generalize to the population of individuals with idiopathic autism, including the large group with mental retardation. Also extremely important is work to determine if the fMRI findings of abnormal patterns and amounts of activation are the "chicken or the egg," i.e., primary deficits or the downstream results of other primary deficits and the resulting atypical life experience.

Perfusion in the Non-Activated Brain

A number of investigators have quantitatively examined regional cerebral blood flow (rCBF) in the brains of children with autism in a variety of unstimulated states, i.e. when they are not performing some task. Examination of the brain at "rest" is important because even when not activated by a task the brain is very active producing ongoing energy for homeostasis and cycling of neurotransmitters. [199]

Unactivated states studied in autism have included those just before or during sedation-induced sleep. The size of the autism samples studied have ranged from 5 to 23. Five of these studies used SPECT, [118], [200]– [202] one used PET,203 and two used voxel-based whole-brain analysis methods. [203], [204] One of the studies was the first longitudinal imaging study of autism. [200] Taken together the studies suggest distributed abnormalities of regional cerebral blood flow involving frontal and temporal areas in the unactivated brain in autism.

All five SPECT studies found hypoperfusion in one or both frontal lobes in individuals with autism at various ages. One PET study of autistic children 5 to13 years of age did not. [203] Five young children with autism had hypoperfusion of the frontal lobes when they were 3 to 4 years of age but not when they were 6 to 7 years of age. [200] A cross-sectional study examining the relationship of age to rCBF found prefrontal hypoperfusion followed by increasingly prominent frontal and temporal hypoperfusion with age in autism. [201]

Five of six studies found hypoperfusion in the temporal lobes. The longitudinal SPECT study did not find temporal hypoperfusion in 5 autism children with they were 3 to 4 or 6 to 7 years old. Using PET, the same investigators later found significant temporal hypoperfusion, centered in the auditory associative and adjacent multimodal cortices. [203] Temporal hypoperfusion was present in 76 % of 21 children with autism 5 to 13 years of age and in a replication sample of 12 children with autism. [203] Single studies have found evidence of relationships between the amount of frontal and temporal perfusion and IQ, [202] decreased perfusion of prefrontal and anterior cingulate areas and social and communication impairment, and decreased medial temporal rCBF and stereotyped, repetitive tendencies in autism. [204] One of the 6 studies found decreased perfusion in the parietal lobe. [205]

Functional Neuroimaging and Mental Processes in Autism

Functional neuroimaging using fMRI or PET has permitted an unprecedented opportunity to learn about how the brains of the individuals with autism work when the individuals are presented with a stimulus or asked to perform a particular cognitive task. Small samples (n = 6, 8, 11, etc.) have been used in fMRI studies of autism because of the need for higher-functioning and verbal subjects who can understand the tasks and cooperate, the difficulty of finding homogeneous groups of such subjects, and because processing and analyzing functional imaging data is labor-intensive.

Motor Functioning

The motor domain is important in autism because many affected children and adults have some degree of impairment in fine and gross motor functioning. The motor impairment often leads to an avoidance of physical games, sports, health-promoting physical activities, and thus to a lack of social opportunities. fMRI studies of simple motor tasks, visually-driven motor tasks, and simple motor versus attentional tasks have suggested that brain functioning, in terms of the areas of the brain involved and degree of involvement, may be different in autism than in typical development. These studies suggest that patterns of brain functioning during motor tasks in autism are idiosyncratic, varying from individual to individual. [206]– [208]

Exceptional Skills

Dr. Leo Kanner observed that some individuals with autism had "islets of ability" in the midst of otherwise pervasive disability. fMRI study of the Embedded Figures Task suggests that adults with autism or Asperger's disorder use different cognitive strategies and brain areas, specifically less working memory and prefrontal areas and more visual processing and ventral occipito-temporal areas, than typical adults. [209] A child with autism and hyperlexia was found to have "hyperactivation" of phonological systems of the left superior temporal and inferior frontal cortices and visual form recognition systems adjacent to the right inferior temporal sulcus compared to age- or reading level-matched controls. [210]

Higher Order Working Memory

Instead of examining fMRI-derived activation in one or two regions of interest, some studies have performed whole-brain imaging to examine multiple areas of the brain known to be parts of a distributed neural network involved in performance of a task. As task complexity increases, it is believed that more regions of the brain must "communicate" with each other for successful task performance. Examination of distributed neural networks is particularly important in autism because autism is thought to be a disorder of complex information processing involving multiple developmental and neurological domains. fMRI was used to examine the functioning of component parts of the distributed neural network involved in spatial working memory. Subjects with autism showed differences in the bilateral dorsolateral prefrontal cortex and right posterior cingulate cortex. [211] There were no differences detected by fMRI in other components of the network which includes widespread cortical and subcortical regions and the cerebellum. The findings suggest frontal cortex dysfunction in high-functioning autism.

Mentalizing

An advance in cognitive neuroscience that has had a major impact on imaging research in autism was conceptualization and operationalization of the difficulty children and adults with autism have "reading" the minds of others. [212]– [214] Mentalizing, also referred to as "theory of mind," describes thinking about such things as what the another person knows versus does not know about a situation, how the other person is feeling, what he might be thinking and intending, and what he might do next. The ability to infer the mental states of other people begins at about 18 months of age. This ability rapidly increases in complexity during childhood. [215] Recognition that "theory of mind" was impaired in autism stimulated research about social cognition and the "social brain."

Exploration of the brain-basis of mentalizing in autism began with a study of recognition of mental state words by children and a SPECT study of regional cerebral blood flow in normal adults during the word recognition task. [216] Since that investigation, imaging studies of autism have examined a variety of the cognitive components of mentalizing. Most of these studies have been in combined samples of individuals with autism and Asperger's disorder, which we refer to as autism spectrum disorders (ASD).

When individuals with high-functioning ASDs were asked to judge, from looking at a person's eyes, what they might be thinking, fMRI evidence of amygdala dysfunction was found. [217] When individuals with ASDs had to perceptually discriminate between faces and objects, the fusiform face area of the right fusiform gyrus appeared dysfunctional on fMRI. [218] Dysfunction of right fusiform gyrus, left amydgala, and left cerebellum were suggests during an fMRI study of ASD subjects explicitly and implicitly processing facial expressions of emotion. [219] Further evidence of fusiform and amygdala dysfunction in autism came from an fMRI study of face versus shape perception. [93] A PET study of regional cerebral blood flow suggested fusiform dysfunction along with other areas of dysfunction in individuals with autism even when emotional voice sounds increased the salience of facial expressions of emotion. [220] Amygdala function appeared particularly important in processing complex facial stimuli, such as those involved in emotions that have complex social significance, compared to than the facial stimuli of simple emotions. [221] It was proposed that all of these regions may be parts of more widespread dysfunction affecting social and emotional cognition. [222] The dysfunction seen with fMRI in adolescents and adults with autism may be related to the abnormal experience of the social world that begins very early in childhood. [223]

One fMRI study followed fascinating neuropsychological work that investigated the impaired tendency of children and adults with autism to give social meaning to stimuli, i.e., social attribution. [224] The fMRI findings suggested that impaired social attribution in autism was related to dysfunction in the medial prefrontal cortex, the cortex adjacent to the superior temporal sulcus, and the basal temporal area. [225] In addition, the findings suggested abnormal connectivity in autism between anterior and posterior parts of the brain network involved in mentalizing, specifically between the cortex adjacent to the superior temporal sulcus and the extrastriate cortex. [225]

More recent fMRI studies have further investigated what happens in the brain when people with autism look at faces. Recent evidence suggests that there may be some, but not severe dysfunction of the fusiform gyrus in children with autism but not in adults when they process basic facial expressions of emotions. [226]– [229] The fusiform gyrus was activated normally in 2 studies of adults with ASD. [227], [229] It was activated, but not as much as in typically developing peers, in 2 studies of children and adolescents with ASDs. [226], [228] Prefrontal function may be adequate. [226], [228], [229] Findings in the amygdala are mixed. [226], [228] Together these most recent studies suggest that individuals with autism may use some brain areas not used in typically developing individuals to process facial expressions of emotion. [226] In addition there is further evidence that components, other than the fusiform gyrus, of widely distributed networks involved in processing faces and facial expressions of emotions may be impaired in autism. [226], [227], [229] Suspected neural networks are those that processes complex social and emotional information, [230] including networks involved in motivation, salience, and attention.

Language

Children and adults with autism have a variety of abnormalities of language which are severely impairing. Age at onset of meaningful single words and phrases is usually delayed. Many children with autism never develop functional language. Apparently normal onset of language can be followed by a plateau in language development or complete loss of language skills. Early receptive language and attention to the talk of others is often so impaired that young children with autism may seem like they are deaf. When language does develop, it is often peculiar in forms with structural and pragmatic abnormalities. Understanding of other than simple or literal language is usually impaired.

Windows of functioning of the brain when children and adults with autism hear and speak language are beginning to open. Information about auditory and language processing in autism comes from event-related potential (ERP), functional magnetic resonance (fMRI), and positron emission tomographic (PET) studies. Most studies examining aspects of auditory and language processing in autism have been performed on small samples of high-functioning children and adults with autism (IQ > 70 or 80) and have not yet been replicated.

An exploratory study using [^{15}O]-water positron emission tomography was carried out in 4 high-functioning adults with autism during receptive and expressive language tasks. Less activation, suggestive of atypical specialization, was found in 3 ROIs, the dentate nucleus of the cerebellum, the thalamus, and the dorsolateral prefrontal cortex. [121], [231] The three regions are components of the widely distributed dentato-thalamo-cortical pathway that is important in involving the cerebellum in some complex cognitive and motor functions, including language.

A variety of intriguing abnormalities have been found more recently. Several studies have tapped automatic aspects of the brain's response to sounds and speech. When a subject intentionally focuses on a stimulus of his choice, his brains "hears" and discriminates between background sounds and involuntarily orients to the sounds whether he realizes it or not. When 8 high-functioning male children, 6 to 12 years of age, were watching a video they liked, simple tones, complex tones, and vowel sounds were presented as background sounds. Resulting ERPs showed that involuntary perception (P1, N2, N4) and discrimination (MMN [mismatch negativity]) of all 3 sounds were similar in the autism and typically developing children. Both groups of children also showed evidence of involuntary orientation to the simple and complex tones (P3a). The typically developing children showed P3a evidence of involuntary orientation to the vowel speech-like sounds. The children with autism did not. This suggests that high-functioning children with autism have normal, or near-normal automatic perception and discrimination of vowel and non-speech sounds, and automatic orienting to non-speech but not vowel speech-like sounds. Automatic perception and discrimination of sounds are believed to require cortico-cortical neuronal communication in primary and secondary auditory cortices. Involuntary orienting to sound appears to involve neuronal communication in a more widely-distributed neural network, involving auditory cortex, multi-modal sensory areas in the parietal lobe, and the dorsolateral prefrontal cortex.

Evidence of abnormally distributed brain processing of auditory stimuli in autism has also been shown by a H_2 [15]O PET study. [232] Regional cerebral blood flow while listening to complex speech-like sounds was compared in 5 adolescent and young adults with autism (mean IQ of 65, standard deviation 5, including one non-verbal subject) and 8 University students. Activation in the autism and control groups showed some differences. The autism sample had a larger volume of activation in the right, rather than left, superior temporal gyrus. Peak activation in the autism subjects occurred in several areas outside of the auditory cortex that were not activated in the controls. [232] Although the effects of a large difference in mean IQ between the autism and control samples on the results of this study are uncertain, the results suggest differences in regions activated by complex sounds in autism. The same voice versus non-vocal sound paradigm was tested in 5 male adults with autism (4 with IQs >80, 1 with an IQ of 50). The autism adults did not activate the voice-selective part of the auditory cortex that is activated in the normal controls. [233]

Voices, in the auditory realm, appear to play a similar role to faces in the visual realm. [234] Characteristics of voice help identify a person and how the person is feeling. The development of voice recognition begins very early. Newborn babies are able to perceive basic differences between sounds in their environment and recognize the voice of their mothers. [235] Cortical development allows perception and processing of more complex aspects of voice. The area sensitive to voice in adults lies outside of the primary auditory cortex along the anterior and central, upper part of the superior temporal sulcus. The activation is believed to respond to the combination of high- and low-frequency sounds in speech. The voice-sensitive area appears bilateral but predominantly right-sided and it appears to be part of a neural network involved in high-level analysis of complex sounds. [236], [237] Thus, the findings in autism suggest impairment in cortical processing required for high-level analysis of the complex sound of voice, including speech.

Comprehension of everyday language requires not only processing of voice sounds but also an understanding of words, syntax (how words are put together in sentences), and semantics (the meaning of language). Even the highest-functioning adults with autism, who have full scale and verbal IQs >80 and good understanding of single words, are impaired in comprehension of every-day language, especially non-literal language.

In an elegant experiment in 17 individuals with this specific subtype of autism, comprehension of active and passive sentences was tested. [230] Activation in 35 cortical regions likely to show activation during sentence comprehension was examined. The study particularly focused on the left superior and middle temporal gyri (Wernicke's area) which are involved in the processing of individual words, and the left inferior frontal gyrus (Broca's area) which is involved in the analysis of syntax, semantics, and working memory, all important in sentence comprehension. There were a number of extremely important findings. First, the adults with autism activated over twice as many voxels in Wernicke's area and five times fewer voxels in Broca's area than the normal controls. This finding suggests that high-functioning adults with autism do more local processing of the individual words in a sentence and less distributed processing of the more complex aspects of a sentence. [230] Processing the complex aspects of a sentence is critical to understanding meaning. [230]

The nature of the underlying brain abnormality in autism was suggested by the second part of the experiment. This part involved examination of the correlations of the patterns of increases and decreases in activation over time as the experimental tasks were administered. Correlations of the time activation series were analyzed in 10 sets of brain areas which showed significant case-control differences. The strength of the correlation of the time activation series of different brain regions over time as experimental tasks are administered is believed to be a quite precise measure of even subtle differences in functional connectivity between regions. In the autism group, the differences from controls in correlations of the time activation series were not subtle. For each of the 10 sets of brain regions, this measure of functional connectivity was substantially less in the autism group than in the normal control adults. [230] The 10 sets of brain regions included cortical areas that are connected intra-hemispherically and others that are connected across the two hemispheres and included connections between frontal, temporal, parietal, and occipital lobe areas. Across the 10 sets of brain regions, the differences in standardized functional connectivity between autism and control groups were similar in magnitude. In addition, the pattern of standardized connectivity was similar across the 10 area sets; the sets of areas with the strongest functional connectivity in the control group were the same areas with the strongest albeit less connectivity in the autism group.

Contingent on replication by other laboratories, the findings suggest that the relative connectivity of different sets of brain areas is similar in autism and typical controls. (For example, the connectivity between brain areas A and B is greater than between areas C and D in both autism and controls.) In all cases, however, the functional connectivity between two areas is less in the autism group. (Example continued, the connectivity between areas A and B is less in autism than controls; the connectivity between areas C and D is also less in autism.) The similarity of the findings across sets of brain areas suggests that some mechanism, involving white matter, cortical grey matter, or both, is decreasing non-local cortico-cortico intra- and inter-hemispheric functional connectivity in autism in a fairly uniform and diffuse fashion.

The investigators of this language comprehension study report similar differences in functional connectivity in autism when experimental tasks focus on other cognitive domains affected in autism, such as social cognition and problem-solving. [238] The authors propose that the "underconnectivity" demonstrated by their findings involves all, or nearly all, cortically-mediated functions impaired in autism. [230] Given the increased mean brain volume in autism, studies are needed to determine if normal and abnormal brain enlargement affect indices of brain connectivity.

New Information Relevant to fMRI and PET Studies of Brain Function

Neither fMRI or PET directly measure the activity of neurons or how neurons respond to a stimulus or during a task. fMRI and PET measure changes (increments) in blood flow and in the consumption of glucose and oxygen that are used to produce energy. Elegant experiments and decades of work are resulting in major inroads to the understanding of the complex relationship between the activity of neurons in response to a stimulus or during a cognitive task and changes in regional cerebral blood flow and glucose and oxygen consumption. [239]

These experiments show that total energy consumption, not just the increment measured in functional imaging studies, is the biologic link between stimulus and neural activity. When the brain is at rest, it is incredibly active and consuming a lot of energy. This high level of energy consumption by the un-stimulated brain is referred to as "REST." [240] Neuronal activity in response to a stimulus is measured by the sum of the activity at REST + any incremental activity during stimulation. [199], [239] This new finding may allow additional interpretations of functional neuroimaging studies of autism that measured only the location and magnitude of the increment in cerebral blood flow or glucose or oxygen consumption during a task or stimulus. Past interpretations that may need further thought include: 1) that regions showing a significant increment in metabolic activity during an activity or task (i.e., the regions activated) are all the brain areas involved in performance of the task; 2) decreased or absent increment in metabolic activity (i.e., "decreased activation" or "not activated") in an area during a task, in cases vs. controls or in a given task with practice, means that the area is not importantly involved and active during the task; 3) the magnitude of the increment in metabolic activity reflects the amount of neural activity involved in performance of the task.

Brain Chemistry

Serotonin

One of the major advances in neuroimaging that has been little applied to the study of autism is the ability to study levels of neurotransmitters and their receptors in the brain. One center has done most of this work in autism to date and has focused on serotonin. Elevated mean blood serotonin is one of the most replicated biological findings in autism. [241] Depletion of brain tryptophan, the precursor of brain serotonin, is associated with worsening of symptoms in individuals with autism. [242] Treatment with serotonin re-uptake inhibitor medications may be associated with some improvement in social interaction, language, stereotyped and compulsive behaviors, and other psychiatric symptoms in children and adults with autism. [243] In addition, serotonin is known to be important in brain development, including the development of brain connectivity. [244]

PET studies are beginning to elucidate differences in the synthesis of serotonin in the brain in autism. The conversion of radio-labeled tryptophan to serotonin in the brain allows serotonin synthesis to be quantitatively visualized. Altered levels of serotonin synthesis were found in the components of a pathway important in language functioning that connects the dentate nucleus of the cerebellum, the thalamus, and the frontal cortex. In 7 boys with autism, serotonin synthesis was asymmetric in the frontal cortex, thalamus, and dentate nucleus, decreased in either the right or left frontal cortex and thalamus, and increased in the contralateral dentate nucleus. [82] The authors then studied the relationship between global serotonin synthesis and age in an enlarged, cross-sectional sample of 30 children with autism and controls. [245] In the controls, serotonin synthesis was increased above adult level in early childhood until age 5 years and then it declined. In the autism children, serotonin synthesis continued to increase from very early childhood until 15 years of age at which time it reached 150 % of adult value.

Chemical Markers of Neuronal Integrity, Cell Energy, and Cell Membranes

Magnetic resonance spectroscopy (MRS) allows study of the concentrations of chemical markers of neuronal integrity and homeostasis, cell membrane and myelin turnover, and cell energy metabolism including energy-producing compounds in the brain. Advances in MRS now allow study of these chemicals in multiple whole slices of the brain and the brain regions included in these slices in contrast to isolated, smaller volumes.

N-acetyl aspartate (NAA), a sensitive marker of the integrity of neurons and their homeostatic interactions with neuroglia, has been studied from early childhood into adulthood in autism. Changes in NAA appear related to the density and metabolic health of neurons, including myelination. In typical development, levels of NAA increase dramatically in the brain during the first 2 years of life and then plateau, reach adult levels in the late teenage years, and decline during adulthood. Decreases in NAA are seen in disease states and traumatic injury of the brain. Increased NAA is believed to be related to increase neuron cell packing density or metabolism.

When a change in NAA has been found in autism, it has always been decreased. But the findings of where it is decreased are mixed, perhaps due to different age ranges and regions studied, whether NAA in grey or white matter was measured, and possible developmental effects. Decreased NAA was found in the frontal lobe, [246]– [248] and the cingulate gyrus in one of three studies, [247]– [249] and in the parietal lobe in one of two studies. [247], [248] NAA was decreased in two of three studies in the medial temporal lobe [248], [250], [251] and lateral temporal lobe [246]– [248] and in two of two studies in the cerebellum. [250], [251] The most comprehensive and largest study to date was carried out in 45 three and four year old children with either autism or PDD-NOS. Their mean cognitive level was in the intellectually handicapped range. In this group of children, NAA was decreased in left frontal white matter, both cingulated gyri, right superior temporal gyrus, right parietal lobe white matter, and right thalamus. [248] NAA in the autism spectrum disorder and 13 typically developing children did not differ in the medial temporal lobe, insula, corpus callosum, caudate, putamen, or occipital lobe. [248] Interestingly, a study of adults with Asperger's disorder, who by definition are verbal and cognitively high-functioning, NAA was increased in the prefrontal, but not the parietal, regions and prefrontal NAA significantly correlated with obsessional behavior. [252]

MRS studies of autism have examined the spectral peak of creatinine concentration (Cr), which included creatinine and phosphocreatine, the "fuels" for oxidative metabolism in the brain. In typical development, these biochemicals increase during the first 2 years of life, remain at high levels during childhood, and decrease to adult levels in adolescence. Like NAA, theses biochemical usually decrease in brain regions affected by disease or trauma.

Studies of Cr in autism spectrum disorders present mixed finding that suggest developmental and IQ (or other disorder severity) effects. In 3 and 4 year old children with ASDs, Cr concentration was decreased in left hemisphere frontal white matter, insula, parietal white matter, and in the anterior corpus callosum. [248] No change from typically developing children was found the right hemisphere of the above regions or in the cingulated gyrus, caudate, putamen, superior temporal gyrus, medial temporal lobe and oc/cipital lobe of either hemisphere. [248] In 22 children with autism 5 to 16 years of age, Cr was increased in the head of the right caudate, and decreased in the body of the left caudate and in the right occipital cortex. [249] In the 14 adults with Asperger's disorder, Cr was increased in the prefrontal but not parietal lobe. [252]

The choline concentration (Cho) measured by MRS includes a number of different biochemicals that are indicators of turnover of cell membranes in the brain. They are found in highest concentration in myelin and neuroglia cells. In typical development, the net concentration of choline compounds increases during the first year of life as myelination increases, is high during childhood, and decreases to adult levels by the latter part of adolescence. The concentration of choline in the brain increases when neurons are injured and cell membranes and myelin breakdown. In autism, MRS findings of choline in the brain are mixed, with very young impaired children with ASD showing different results than older children with autism and adults with Asperger's disorder. In the 3 and 4 years olds with ASD, Cho was decreased in the right medial temporal lobe and superior temporal gyrus and left thalamus. [248] Cho concentration was no different from typically developing children in the frontal, parietal, and occipital lobes including the cingulate gyri and insula, corpus callosum, caudate and putamen. [248] In older children with autism, Cho was decreased in the anterior cingulate gyrus and increased in the head of the caudate on the right. [249] In adults with Asperger's disorder, choline was increased in prefrontal but not parietal lobes. [252]

Two other biochemicals have been examined in autism. Myo-inositol, which is involved in maintaining the correct balance of water inside and outside of cells and in the transmission of chemical messages across cell membranes in the brain, was decreased in the 3 to 4 year old children with ASD. Brain lactate can increase when metabolism in the brain is increased (e.g., seizures) or disordered (e.g. inborn errors of metabolism) or when blood and oxygen supply to the brain are decreased (e.g. hyperventilation, hypoxia, vascular compromise). Brain lactate was increased in 1 of 9 children with autism in one study, [246] but mean brain lactate was not decreased in the 45 young children with ASD. [248] To date there are no published studies of brain glutamate, glutamine, or GABA, important neurotransmitters, in autism.

Ethical Considerations

Autism is a very impairing lifelong disorder which drastically alters the course of development of multiple cognitive and neurological domains. From early in life, autism also alters experience. Autism stands as barrier to the achievement of basic and more complex skills that allow effective communication with others and appropriate functioning in many different social situations. It impairs the ability to solve the myriad of little and big problems that are part of everyday life, cope adaptively with the never-ending changes of daily life, and live independently as adults.

We do not know if the findings of imaging studies, the majority of which have been done with older, high-functioning children and adults with autism, generalize to younger children and those who also have mental retardation or seizures. Although the majority of imaging research has been done in high-functioning older individuals with autism who do not have seizures, the majority of individuals with autism have mental retardation and a sizeable minority (about 30 % to 35 %) has seizures by young adulthood.

Autism needs to be understood in all of these subgroups and other subgroups that exist. What the review of the autism imaging research for this chapter showed us very clearly, is that although the field has substantially progressed in recent years, there are many, many crucial important questions that remain unanswered. Therefore, the key question may not be whether or not imaging research in autism is ethical, but rather how can what must be done to understand autism be done as safely and effectively as possible. This appears to be as true for low-functioning and very young children with autism, the majority of whom require sedation for scanning, as for high-functioning older children and adults. The key questions may not be whether autism should be studied in young and low-functioning children, but rather how can sedation be administered so these children can be scanned as safely and as effectively as possible. As much as is possible needs to be learned from the data that result from the child's time in the scanner and the family's effort. With research come knowledge, hope, and progress.

Conclusion

In this chapter we discuss numerous advances in neuroimaging in autism. These include convergent evidence of increased mean brain volume particularly during early childhood in autism, preliminary findings of the anatomic basis of brain enlargement, investigations of scaling between total and regional brain and the effects of age on brain structure, function, and chemistry. Advances also include the application of relatively new neuroimaging methods such as diffusion tensor imaging, functional imaging, comprehensive spectroscopy, and new measures of functional connectivity. Challenges for future autism imaging research include the need to elucidate 1) how the brain grows, develops, and changes across the lifespan in autism, and how these changes are related to clinical manifestations and impairment; 2) how brain enlargement in autism affects regional morphometry, spectroscopic and functional characteristics, white matter organization, and connectivity; 3) how heterogeneity and comorbidity in autism affect neuroimaging findings. Finally, large gaps between macroscopic and microscopic brain research need to be bridged so that neuroimaging research can be used to help determine the cellular and molecular basis of autism.

Acknowledgments

This work was supported by the NICHD/NICDC Collaborative Programs of Excellence in Autism: 2 U19 HD35476 to the University of Utah, Neuroimaging Component (Drs. Lainhart, Bigler, Alexander, and Lazar). Additional support came from the Utah Autism Foundation, Valley Mental Health, the Ira B. Fulton Foundation, and the National Alliance for Research on Schizophrenia and Depression (Dr. Lazar). We thank Mr. Craig Vickers for his technical assistance in the preparation of this chapter. We also thank the children and adults who have participated in our research studies, and our families.

References

[1] Sokol DK, Edwards-Brown M. Neuroimaging in autistic spectrum disorder (ASD). *Journal of Neuroimaging.* 2004;14:8-15.

[2] Brambilla P, Hardan A, di Nemi SU, Perez J, Soares JC, Barale F. Brain anatomy and development in autism: Review of structural MRI studies. *Brain Research Bulletin.* 2003;61:557-569.

[3] Palmen SJ, Van Engeland H. Review on structural neuroimaging findings in autism. *Journal of Neural Transmission.* 2004;111:903-929.

[4] Frith C. What do imaging studies tell us about the neural basis of autism? *Novartis Foundation Symposium.* 2003;251:149-166.

[5] Courchesne E, Redcay E, Kennedy DP. The autistic brain: Birth through adulthood. *Current Opinion in Neurology.* 2004;17:489-496.

[6] Boddaert N, Zilbovicius M. Functional neuroimaging and childhood autism. *Pediatric Radiology.* 2002;32:1-7.

[7] Kanner L. Autistic disturbances of affective contact. *Nervous Child.* 1943;2:217-250.

[8] Folstein S, Rutter M. Genetic influences and infantile autism. *Nature.* 1977;265:726-728.

[9] Walker HA. Incidence of minor physical anomaly in autism. *Journal of Autism and Childhood Schizophrenia.* 1977;7:165-176.

[10]Steg JP, Rapoport JL. Minor physical anomalies in normal, neurotic, learning disabled, and severely disturbed children. *Journal of Autism and Childhood Schizophrenia.* 1975;5:299-307.

[11]Tuchman RF, Rapin I, Shinnar S. Autistic and dysphasic children. I: Clinical characteristics. *Pediatrics.* 1991;88:1211-1218.

[12]Woodhouse W, Bailey A, Rutter M, Bolton P, Baird G, Le Couteur A. Head circumference in autism and other pervasive developmental disorders. *Journal of Child Psychology and Psychiatry.* 1996;37:665-671.

[13]Lainhart JE, Piven J, Wzorek M, et al. Macrocephaly in children and adults with autism. *Journal of the American Academy of Child and Adolescent Psychiatry.* 1997;36:282-290.

[14]Bolton P, Macdonald H, Pickles A, et al. A case-control family history study of autism. *Journal of Child Psychology and Psychiatry.* 1994;35:877-900.

[15]Bailey A, Le Couteur A, Gottesman I, et al. Autism as a strongly genetic disorder: Evidence from a British twin study. *Psychological Medicine.* 1995;25:63-77.

[16]Miles JH, Hadden LL, Takahashi TN, Hillman RE. Head circumference is an independent clinical finding associated with autism. *American Journal of Medical Genetics.* 2000;95:339-350.

[17]Fombonne E, Roge B, Claverie J, Courty S, Fremolle J. Microcephaly and macrocephaly in autism. *Journal of Autism and Developmental Disorders.* 1999;29:113-119.

[18]Fidler DJ, Bailey JN, Smalley SL. Macrocephaly in autism and other pervasive developmental disorders. *Developmental Medicine Child Neurology.* 2000;42:737-740.

[19]Davidovitch M, Patterson B, Gartside P. Head circumference measurements in children with autism. *Journal of Child Neurology.* 1996;11:389-393.

[20]Aylward EH, Minshew NJ, Field K, Sparks BF, Singh N. Effects of age on brain volume and head circumference in autism. *Neurology.* 2002;59:175-183.

[21]Bailey A, Luthert P, Dean A, et al. A clinicopathological study of autism. *Brain.* 1998;121:889-905.

[22]Bauman ML, Kemper TL. *Neurobiology of Autism.* Baltimore, MD: Johns Hopkins University Press; 1994.

[23]Bailey A, Luthert P, Bolton P, Le Couteur A, Rutter M, Harding B. Autism and megalencephaly. *Lancet.* 1993;341:1225-1226.

[24]Filipek PA, Richelme C, Kennedy DN, et al. Morphometric analysis of the brain in developmental language disorder and autism (abstract). *Annals of Neurology.* 1992;32:475.

[25]Piven J, Arndt S, Bailey J, Havercamp S, Andreasen NC, Palmer P. An MRI study of brain size in autism. *American Journal of Psychiatry.* 1995;152:1145-1149.

[26]Hardan AY, Minshew NJ, Mallikarjuhn M, Keshavan MS. Brain volume in autism. *Journal of Child Neurology.* 2001;16:421-424.

[27]Sparks BF, Friedman SD, Shaw DW, et al. Brain structural abnormalities in young children with autism spectrum disorder. *Neurology.* 2002;59:184-192.

[28]Courchesne E, Karns CM, Davis HR, et al. Unusual brain growth patterns in early life in patients with autistic disorder: An MRI study. *Neurology.* 2001;57:245-254.

[29]Herbert MR, Ziegler DA, Deutsch CK, et al. Dissociations of cerebral cortex, subcortical and cerebral white matter volumes in autistic boys. *Brain.* 2003;126:1182-1192.

[30]Lotspeich LJ, Kwon H, Schumann CM, et al. Investigation of neuroanatomical differences between autism and Asperger syndrome. *Archives of General Psychiatry.* 2004;61:291-298.

[31]Lainhart J. Head and brain growth in autism: Advances and implications for neuroimaging research. Paper presented at: NIH CPEA/STAART Network Meeting; May 18-19, 2004; Bethesda, MD.

[32]Haznedar MM, Buchsbaum MS, Wei TC, et al. Limbic circuitry in patients with autism spectrum disorders studied with positron emission tomography and magnetic resonance imaging. *American Journal of Psychiatry.* 2000;157:1994-2001.

[33]Waiter GD, Williams JH, Murray AD, Gilchrist A, Perrett DI, Whiten A. A voxel-based investigation of brain structure in male adolescents with autistic spectrum disorder. *Neuroimage.* 2004;22:619-625.

[34]Cohen J. *Statistical power analysis for the behavioral sciences.* Second ed. Hillsdale, New Jersey: Lawrence Erlbaum Associates; 1988.

[35]Roche AF, Mukherjee D, Guo SM, Moore WM. Head circumference reference data: Birth to 18 years. *Pediatrics.* 1987;79:706-712.

[36]Center for Disease Control. CDC Growth Charts: United States. *National Center for Health Statistics.* Available at: www.cdc.gov/growthcharts.

[37]Courchesne E, Carper R, Akshoomoff N. Evidence of brain overgrowth in the first year of life in autism. *Journal of the American Medical Association.* 2003;290:337-344.

[38]Hultman CM, Sparen P, Cnattingius S. Perinatal risk factors for infantile autism. *Epidemiology.* 2002;13:417-423.

[39]Levitt P. Structural and functional maturation of the developing primate brain. *Journal of Pediatrics.* 2003;143:S35-S45.

[40]Moore JK. Maturation of human auditory cortex: Implications for speech perception. *Annals of Otology, Rhinology and Laryngology: Supplement.* 2002;189:7-10.

[41]Gale CR, O'Callaghan FJ, Godfrey KM, Law CM, Martyn CN. Critical periods of brain growth and cognitive function in children. *Brain.* 2004;127:321-329.

[42]Stevenson RE, Schroer RJ, Skinner C, Fender D, Simensen RJ. Autism and macrocephaly. *Lancet.* 1997;349:1744-1745.

[43]Lainhart JE. Increased rate of head growth during infancy in autism. *Journal of the American Medical Association.* 2003;290:393-394.

[44]Kraemer HC, Yesavage JA, Taylor JL, Kupfer D. How can we learn about developmental processes from cross-sectional studies, or can we? *American Journal of Psychiatry.* 2000;157:163-171.

[45]Giedd JN, Blumental J, Jeffries NO, et al. Brain development during childhood and adolescence: A longitudinal MRI study. *Nature Neuroscience.* 1999;2:861-863.

[46]Giedd JN. Structural magnetic resonance imaging of the adolescent brain. *Annals of the New York Academy of Science.* 2004;1021:77-85.

[47]Sowell ER, Trauner DA, Gamst A, Jernigan TL. Development of cortical and subcortical brain structures in childhood and adolescence: A structural MRI study. *Develomental Medicine Child Neurology.* 2002;44:4-16.

[48]Caviness VS, Jr., Kennedy DN, Richelme C, Rademacher J, Filipek PA. The human brain age 7-11 years: A volumetric analysis based on magnetic resonance images. *Cerebral Cortex.* 1996;6:726-736.

[49]Luna B, Thulborn KR, Munoz DP, et al. Maturation of widely distributed brain function subserves cognitive development. *Neuroimage.* 2001;13:786-793.

[50]Kates WR, Burnette CP, Eliez S, et al. Neuroanatomic variation in monozygotic twin pairs discordant for the narrow phenotype for autism. *American Journal of Psychiatry.* 2004;161:539-546.

[51]Woods CG. Human microcephaly. *Current Opinion in Neurobiology.* 2004;14:112-117.

[52]Piven J, Arndt S, Bailey J, Andreasen N. Regional brain enlargement in autism: A magnetic resonance imaging study. *Journal of the American Academy of Child and Adolescent Psychiatry.* 1996;35:530-536.

[53]Carper RA, Moses P, Tigue ZD, Courchesne E. Cerebral lobes in autism: Early hyperplasia and abnormal age effects. *Neuroimage.* 2002;16:1038-1051.

[54]Herbert MR, Ziegler DA, Makris N, et al. Localization of white matter volume increase in autism and developmental language disorder. *Annals of Neurology.* 2004;55:530-540.

[55]Meyer JW, Makris N, Bates JF, Caviness VS, Kennedy DN. MRI-Based topographic parcellation of human cerebral white matter. *Neuroimage.* 1999;9:1-17.

[56]Makris N, Meyer JW, Bates JF, Yeterian EH, Kennedy DN, Caviness VS. MRI-Based topographic parcellation of human cerebral white matter and nuclei II. Rationale and applications with systematics of cerebral connectivity. *Neuroimage.* 1999;9:18-45.

[57]Bush EC, Allman JM. The scaling of white matter to gray matter in cerebellum and neocortex. *Brain Behavior and Evolution.* 2003;61:1-5.

[58]Zhang K, Sejnowski TJ. A universal scaling law between gray matter and white matter of cerebral cortex. *Proceedings of the National Academy of Science U S A.* 2000;97:5621-5626.

[59]Luders E, Steinmetz H, Jancke L. Brain size and grey matter volume in the healthy human brain. *Neuroreport.* 2002;13:2371-2374.

[60]Sowell ER, Thompson PM, Toga AW. Mapping changes in the human cortex throughout the span of life. *Neuroscientist.* 2004;10:372-392.

[61]Gogtay N, Giedd JN, Lusk L, et al. Dynamic mapping of human cortical development during childhood through early adulthood. *Proceedings of the National Academy of Science U S A.* 2004;101:8174-8179.

[62]Chung MK, Worsley KJ, Robbins S, et al. Deformation-based surface morphometry applied to gray matter deformation. *Neuroimage.* 2003;18:198-213.

[63]Chung MK, Dalton KM, Alexander AL, Davidson RJ. Less white matter concentration in autism: 2D voxel-based morphometry. *Neuroimage.* 2004;23:242-251.

[64]Geschwind DH, Miller BL, DeCarli C, Carmelli D. Heritability of lobar brain volumes in twins supports genetic models of cerebral laterality and handedness. *Proceedings of the National Academy of Science U S A.* 2002;99:3176-3181.

[65]Levitt JG, Blanton RE, Smalley S, et al. Cortical sulcal maps in autism. *Cerebral Cortex.* 2003;13:728-735.

[66]Herbert MR, Harris GJ, Adrien KT, et al. Abnormal asymmetry in language association cortex in autism. *Annals of Neurology.* 2002;52:588-596.

[67]Rojas DC, Bawn SD, Benkers TL, Reite ML, Rogers SJ. Smaller left hemisphere planum temporale in adults with autistic disorder. *Neuroscience Letter.* 2002;328:237-240.

[68]Blanton RE, Levitt JG, Thompson PM, et al. Mapping cortical asymmetry and complexity patterns in normal children. *Psychiatry Research.* 2001;107:29-43.

[69]Luders E, Narr KL, Thompson PM, et al. Gender differences in cortical complexity. *Nature Neuroscience.* 2004;7:799-800.

[70]Casanova MF, Araque J, Giedd J, Rumsey JM. Reduced brain size and gyrification in the brains of dyslexic patients. *Journal of Child Neurology.* 2004;19:275-281.

[71]Narr KL, Bilder RM, Kim S, et al. Abnormal gyral complexity in first-episode schizophrenia. *Biological Psychiatry.* 2004;55:859-867.

[72]Kennedy DN, Lange N, Makris N, Bates J, Meyer J, Caviness VS, Jr. Gyri of the human neocortex: an MRI-based analysis of volume and variance. *Cerebral Cortex.* 1998;8:372-384.

[73]Boddaert N, Chabane N, Gervais H, et al. Superior temporal sulcus anatomical abnormalities in childhood autism: A voxel-based morphometry MRI study. *Neuroimage.* 2004;23:364-369.

[74]Abell F, Krams M, Ashburner J, et al. The neuroanatomy of autism: A voxel-based whole brain analysis of structural scans. *Neuroreport.* 1999;10:1647-1651.

[75]Salmond CH, de Haan M, Friston KJ, Gadian DG, Vargha-Khadem F. Investigating individual differences in brain abnormalities in autism. *Philosophical Transactions of theRoyal Society of London B Biological Sciences.* 2003;358:405-413.

[76]Bigler ED, Tate DF, Neeley ES, et al. Temporal lobe, autism, and macrocephaly. *American Journal of Neuroradiology.* 2003;24:2066-2076.

[77]Maurer RG, Damasio AR. Childhood autism from the point of view of behavioral neurology. *Journal of Autism and Developmental Disorders.* 1982;12:195-205.

[78]Sears LL, Vest C, Mohamed S, Bailey J, Ranson BJ, Piven J. An MRI study of the basal ganglia in autism. *Progress in Neuropsychopharmacology and Biological Psychiatry.* 1999;23:613-624.

[79]Hardan AY, Kilpatrick M, Keshavan MS, Minshew NJ. Motor performance and anatomic magnetic resonance imaging (MRI) of the basal ganglia in autism. *Journal of Child Neurology.* 2003;18:317-324.

[80]Asano E, Chugani DC, Muzik O, et al. Autism in tuberous sclerosis complex is related to both cortical and subcortical dysfunction. *Neurology.* 2001;57:1269-1277.

[81]Courchesne E, Yeung-Courchesne R, Press GA, Hesselink JR, Jernigan TL. Hypoplasia of cerebellar vermal lobules VI and VII in autism. *New England Journal of Medicine.* 1988;318:1349-1354.

[82]Chugani DC, Muzik O, Rothermel R, et al. Altered serotonin synthesis in the dentatothalamocortical pathway in autistic boys. *Annals of Neurology.* 1997;42:666-669.

[83]Riva D, Giorgi C. The cerebellum contributes to higher functions during development: evidence from a series of children surgically treated for posterior fossa tumours. *Brain.* 2000;123 (Pt 5):1051-1061.

[84]ten Donkelaar HJ, Lammens M, Wesseling P, Thijssen HO, Renier WO. Development and developmental disorders of the human cerebellum. *Journal of Neurology.* 2003;250:1025-1036.

[85]Hutchinson S, Lee LH, Gaab N, Schlaug G. Cerebellar volume of musicians. *Cerebral Cortex.* 2003;13:943-949.

[86]Manes F, Piven J, Vrancic D, Nanclares V, Plebst C, Starkstein SE. An MRI study of the corpus callosum and cerebellum in mentally retarded autistic individuals. *Journal of Neuropsychiatry and Clinical Neuroscience.* 1999;11:470-474.

[87]Kaufmann WE, Cooper KL, Mostofsky SH, et al. Specificity of cerebellar vermian abnormalities in autism: A quantitative magnetic resonance imaging study. *Journal of Child Neurology.* 2003;18:463-470.

[88]Hardan AY, Minshew NJ, Harenski K, Keshavan MS. Posterior fossa magnetic resonance imaging in autism. *Journal of the American Academy of Child and Adolescent Psychiatry.* 2001;40:666-672.

[89]Minshew N, Luna B, Sweeney JA. Oculomotor evidence for neocortical systems but not cerebellar dysfunction in autism. *Neurology.* 1999;52:917.

[90]Levitt JG, Blanton R, Capetillo-Cunliffe L, Guthrie D, Toga A, McCracken JT. Cerebellar vermis lobules VIII-X in autism. *Progress in Neuropsychopharmacology and Biological Psychiatry.* 1999;23:625-633.

[91]Goldberg MC, Landa R, Lasker A, Cooper L, Zee DS. Evidence of normal cerebellar control of the vestibulo-ocular reflex (VOR) in children with high-functioning autism. *Journal of Autism and Developmental Disorders.* 2000;30:519-524.

[92]Carper RA, Courchesne E. Inverse correlation between frontal lobe and cerebellum sizes in children with autism. *Brain.* 2000;123 (Pt 4):836-844.

[93]Pierce K, Muller RA, Ambrose J, Allen G, Courchesne E. Face processing occurs outside the fusiform 'face area' in autism: evidence from functional MRI. *Brain.* 2001;124:2059-2073.

[94]Harris NS, Courchesne E, Townsend J, Carper RA, Lord C. Neuroanatomic contributions to slowed orienting of attention in children with autism. *Brain Research Cognitive Brain Research.* 1999;8:61-71.

[95]Mostofsky SH, Goldberg MC, Landa RJ, Denckla MB. Evidence for a deficit in procedural learning in children and adolescents with autism: implications for cerebellar contribution. *Journal of the International Neuropsychological Society.* 2000;6:752-759.

[96]Townsend J, Westerfield M, Leaver E, et al. Event-related brain response abnormalities in autism: evidence for impaired cerebello-frontal spatial attention networks. *Brain Research Cognitive Brain Research.* 2001;11:127-145.

[97]Minshew NJ, Goldstein G, Siegel DJ. Neuropsychologic functioning in autism: profile of a complex information processing disorder. *Journal of International Neuropsychological Society.* 1997;3:303-316.

[98]Probst FP. Congenital defects of the corpus callosum. Morphology and encephalographic appearances. *Acta Radiologica Supplement.* 1973;331:1-152.

[99]Richards LJ. Axonal pathfinding mechanisms at the cortical midline and in the development of the corpus callosum. *Brazilian Journal of Medical Biological Research.* 2002;35:1431-1439.

[100]Shu T, Puche AC, Richards LJ. Development of midline glial populations at the corticoseptal boundary. *Journal of Neurobiology.* 2003;57:81-94.

[101]LaMantia AS, Rakic P. Axon overproduction and elimination in the corpus callosum of the developing rhesus monkey. *Journal of Neuroscience.* 1990;10:2156-2175.

[102]Rochefort N, Quenech'du N, Watroba L, Mallat M, Giaume C, Milleret C. Microglia and astrocytes may participate in the shaping of visual callosal projections during postnatal development. *Journal of Physiology Paris.* 2002;96:183-192.

[103]Giedd JN, Blumenthal J, Jeffries NO, et al. Development of the human corpus callosum during childhood and adolescence: A longitudinal MRI study. *Progress in Neuropsychopharmacology and Biological Psychiatry.* 1999;23:571-588.

[104]Paus T, Collins DL, Evans AC, Leonard G, Pike B, Zijdenbos A. Maturation of white matter in the human brain: A review of magnetic resonance studies. *Brain Research Bulletin.* 2001;54:255-266.

[105]Keshavan MS, Diwadkar VA, DeBellis M, et al. Development of the corpus callosum in childhood, adolescence and early adulthood. *Life Sciences.* 2002;70:1909-1922.

[106]Scamvougeras A, Kigar DL, Jones D, Weinberger DR, Witelson SF. Size of the human corpus callosum is genetically determined: An MRI study in mono and dizygotic twins. *Neuroscience Letter.* 2003;338:91-94.

[107]Witelson SF. Hand and sex differences in the isthmus and genu of the human corpus callosum. A postmortem morphological study. *Brain.* 1989;112:799-835.

[108]Vidal CN, DeVito TJ, Hayashi KM, Drost DJ, Williamson PC, Craven-Thuss B, Herman D, Sui Y, Toga AW. Detection and visualization of corpus callosum deficits in autisitc children using novel anatomical mapping algorithms. Proceedings of the International Society for Magnetic Resonance in Medicine. http://www.loni.ucla.edu/_thompson/ISMRM2003/cvISMRM2003.html.

[109]Alexander AL, Lazar M, Bigler ED, et al. Diffusion tensor imaging of white matter in autism [abstract]. Paper presented at: Proceedings of CPEA/STAART Annual Meeting; May 17-20, 2004; Bethesda, MD.

[110]Rice S, Bigler ED, Cleavinger H, Tate DF, Sayer J. Macocephaly, corupus callosum morphology and autism. *Journal of Child Neurology.* in press.

[111]Piven J, Bailey J, Ranson BJ, Arndt S. An MRI study of the corpus callosum in autism. *American Journal of Psychiatry.* 1997;154:1051-1056.

[112]Egaas B, Courchesne E, Saitoh O. Reduced size of corpus callosum in autism. *Archives of Neurology.* 1995;52:794-801.

[113]Hardan AY, Minshew NJ, Keshavan MS. Corpus callosum size in autism. *Neurology.* 2000;55:1033-1036.

[114]Elia M, Ferri R, Musumeci SA, Panerai S, Bottitta M, Scuderi C. Clinical correlates of brain morphometric features of subjects with low-functioning autistic disorder. *Journal of Child Neurology.* 2000;15:504-508.

[115]Chung MK, Dalton KM, Alexander AL, Davidson RJ. Less white matter concentration in autism: 2D voxel-based morphometry. *Neuroimage.* in press.

[116]Barnea-Goraly N, Kwon H, Menon V, Eliez S, Lotspeich L, Reiss AL. White matter structure in autism: Preliminary evidence from diffusion tensor imaging. *Biological Psychiatry.* 2004;55:323-326.

[117]Belmonte M, Egaas B, Townsend J, Courchesne E. NMR intensity of corpus callosum differs with age but not with diagnosis of autism. *Neuroreport.* 1995;6:1253-1256.

[118]Ryu YH, Lee JD, Yoon PH, Kim DI, Lee HB, Shin YJ. Perfusion impairments in infantile autism on technetium-99m ethyl cysteinate dimer brain single-photon emission tomography: Comparison with findings on magnetic resonance imaging. *Europearn Journal of Nuclear Medicine.* 1999;26:253-259.

[119]Starkstein SE, Vazquez S, Vrancic D, et al. SPECT findings in mentally retarded autistic individuals. *Journal of Neuropsychiatry Clinical Neuroscience.* 2000;12:370-375.

[120]Tsatsanis KD, Rourke BP, Klin A, Volkmar FR, Cicchetti D, Schultz RT. Reduced thalamic volume in high-functioning individuals with autism. *Biological Psychiatry.* 2003;53:121-129.

[121] Muller RA, Chugani DC, Behen ME, et al. Impairment of dentato-thalamo-cortical pathway in autistic men: Language activation data from positron emission tomography. *Neuroscience Letters.* 1998;245:1-4.

[122] Weidenheim KM, Goodman L, Dickson DW, Gillberg C, Rastam M, Rapin I. Etiology and pathophysiology of autistic behavior: Clues from two cases with an unusual variant of neuroaxonal dystrophy. *Journal of Child Neurology.* 2001;16:809-819.

[123] Moseley ME, Cohen Y, Kucharczyk J, et al. Diffusion-weighted MR imaging of anisotropic water diffusion in cat central nervous system. *Radiology.* 1990;176:439-445.

[124] Basser PJ, Mattiello J, LeBihan D. MR diffusion tensor spectroscopy and imaging. *Biophysics Journal.* 1994;66:259-267.

[125] Basser PJ, Mattiello J, LeBihan D. Estimation of the effective self-diffusion tensor from the NMR spin echo. *Journal of Magnetic Resonance.* 1994;103:247-254.

[126] Basser PJ. Inferring microstructural features and the physiological state of tissues from diffusion-weighted images. *NMR in Biomedicine.* 1995;8:333-344.

[127] Basser PJ, Pierpaoli C. Microstructural and physiological features of tissues elucidated by quantitative-diffusion-tensor MRI. *Journal of Magnetic Resonance.* 1996;111:209-219.

[128] Alexander AL, Hasan K, Kindlmann G, Parker DL, Tsuruda JS. A geometric analysis of diffusion tensor measurements of the human brain. *Magnetic Resonance Medicine.* 2000;44:283-291.

[129] Pierpaoli C, Basser PJ. Toward a quantitative assessment of diffusion anisotropy. *Magnetic Resonance Medicine.* 1996;36:893-906.

[130] Conturo TE, McKinstry RC, Akbudak E, Robinson BH. Encoding of anisotropic diffusion with tetrahedral gradients: A general mathematical diffusion formalism and experimental results. *Magnetic Resonance Imaging.* 1996;35:399-412.

[131] Ulug AM, van Zijl PC. Orientation-independent diffusion imaging without tensor diagonalization: anisotropy definitions based on physical attributes of the diffusion ellipsoid. *Journal of Magnetic Resonance Imaging.* 1999;9:804-813.

[132] Makris N, Worth AJ, Sorensen AG, et al. Morphometry of in vivo human white matter association pathways with diffusion-weighted magnetic resonance imaging. *Annals of Neurology.* 1997;42:951-962.

[133] Pajevic S, Pierpaoli C. Color schemes to represent the orientation of anisotropic tissues from diffusion tensor data: Application to white matter fiber tract mapping in the human brain. *Magnetic Resonance in Medicine.* 1999;42:526-540.

[134] Alexander DC, Pierpaoli C, Basser PJ, Gee JC. Spatial transformations of diffusion tensor magnetic resonance images. *IEEE Transactions on Medical Imaging.* 2001;20:1131-1139.

[135] Tuch DS, Reese TG, Wiegell MR, Makris N, Belliveau JW, Wedeen VJ. High angular resolution diffusion imaging reveals intravoxel white matter fiber heterogeneity. *Magnetic Resonance in Medicine.* 2002;48:577-582.

[136] Mulkern RV, Gudbjartsson H, Westin CF, et al. Multi-component apparent diffusion coefficients in human brain. *NMR in Biomedicine.* 1999;12:51-62.

[137] Frank LR. Characterization of anisotropy in high angular resolution diffusion-weighted MRI. *Magnetic Resonance in Medicine.* 2002;47:1083-1099.

[138] Ozarslan E, Mareci TH. Generalized diffusion tensor imaging and analytical relationships between diffusion tensor imaging and high angular resolution diffusion imaging. *Magnetic Resonance in Medicine.* 2003;50:955-965.

[139] Shrager RI, Basser PJ. Anisotropically weighted MRI. *Magnetic Resonance in Medicine.* 1998;40:160-165.

[140] Papadakis NG, Xing D, Huang CL, Hall LD, Carpenter TA. A comparative study of acquisition schemes for diffusion tensor imaging using MRI. *Journal of Magnetic Resonance.* 1999;137:67-82.

[141] Shimony JS, McKinstry RC, Akbudak E, et al. Quantitative diffusion-tensor anisotropy brain MR imaging: Normative human data and anatomic analysis. *Radiology.* 1999;212:770-784.

[142] Jones DK, Horsfield MA, Simmons A. Optimal strategies for measuring diffusion in anisotropic systems by magnetic resonance imaging. *Magnetic Resonance Medicine.* 1999;42:515-525.

[143] Basser PJ, Pierpaoli C. A simplified method to measure the diffusion tensor from seven MR images. *Magnetic Resonance Imaging.* 1998;39:928-934.

[144] Hasan KM, Parker DL, Alexander AL. Comparison of gradient encoding schemes for diffusion-tensor MRI. *Journal of Magnetic Resonance Imaging.* 2001;13:769-780.

[145] Batchelor PG, Atkinson D, Hill DL, Calamante F, Connelly A. Anisotropic noise propagation in diffusion tensor MRI sampling schemes. *Magnetic Resonance Imaging.* 2003;49:1143-1151.

[146] Jones DK. The effect of gradient sampling schemes on measures derived from diffusion tensor MRI: A Monte Carlo study. *Magnetic Resonance in Medicine.* 2004;51:807-815.

[147] Haselgrove JC, Moore JR. Correction for distortion of echo-planar images used to calculate the apparent diffusion coefficient. *Magnetic Resonance in Medicine.* 1996;36:960-964.

[148] Alexander AL, Tsuruda JS, Parker DL. Elimination of eddy current artifacts in diffusion-weighted echo-planar images: the use of bipolar gradients. *Magnetic Resonance in Medicine.* 1997;38:1016-1021.

[149] Reese TG, Heid O, Weisskoff RM, Wedeen VJ. Reduction of eddy-current-induced distortion in diffusion MRI using a twice-refocused spin echo. *Magnetic Resonance in Medicine.* 2003;49:177-182.

[150] Andersson JL, Skare S. A model-based method for retrospective correction of geometric distortions in diffusion-weighted EPI. *Neuroimage.* 2002;16:177-199.

[151] Kindlmann G, Whitacer R, Jones G. Diffusion tensor imaging. Paper presented at: Science and Industry and Mathematics, 2004; Salt Lake City, Utah.

[152] Jezzard P, Balaban RS. Correction for geometric distortion in echo planar images from B0 field variations. *Magnetic Resonance in Medicine.* 1995;34:65-73.

[153] Lee KJ, Papadakis NG, Barber DC, Wilkinson ID, Griffiths PD, Paley MN. A method of generalized projections (MGP) ghost correction algorithm for interleaved EPI. *IEEE Transactions on Medical Imaging.* 2004;23:839-848.

[154] Pruessmann KP, Weiger M, Scheidegger MB, Boesiger P. SENSE: Sensitivity encoding for fast MRI. *Magnetic Resonance in Medicine.* 1999;42:952-962.

[155] Bammer R, Auer M, Keeling SL, et al. Diffusion tensor imaging using single-shot SENSE-EPI. *Magnetic Resonance Imaging.* 2002;48:128-136.

[156] Huppi PS, Maier SE, Peled S, et al. Microstructural development of human newborn cerebral white matter assessed in vivo by diffusion tensor magnetic resonance imaging. *Pediatric Research.* 1998;44:584-590.
[157] Schmithorst VJ, Dardzinski BJ, Holland SK. Simultaneous correction of ghost and geometric distortion artifacts in EPI using a multiecho reference scan. *IEEE Transactions of Medical Imaging.* 2001;20:535-539.
[158] O'Sullivan M, Jones DK, Summers PE, Morris RG, Williams SC, Markus HS. Evidence for cortical "disconnection" as a mechanism of age-related cognitive decline. *Neurology.* 2001;57:632-638.
[159] Mukherjee P, Miller JH, Shimony JS, et al. Normal brain maturation during childhood: Developmental trends characterized with diffusion-tensor MR imaging. *Radiology.* 2001;221:349-358.
[160] Pfefferbaum A, Sullivan EV, Hedehus M, Lim KO, Adalsteinsson E, Moseley M. Age-related decline in brain white matter anisotropy measured with spatially corrected echo-planar diffusion tensor imaging. *Magnetic Resonance in Medicine.* 2000;44:259-268.
[161] Abe O, Aoki S, Hayashi N, et al. Normal aging in the central nervous system: Quantitative MR diffusion-tensor analysis. *Neurobiology of Aging.* 2002;23:433-441.
[162] Klingberg T, Vaidya CJ, Gabrieli JD, Moseley ME, Hedehus M. Myelination and organization of the frontal white matter in children: A diffusion tensor MRI study. *Neuroreport.* 1999;10:2817-2821.
[163] Filippi CG, Lin DD, Tsiouris AJ, et al. Diffusion-tensor MR imaging in children with developmental delay: Preliminary findings. *Radiology.* 2003;229:44-50.
[164] Guo AC, Petrella JR, Kurtzberg J, Provenzale JM. Evaluation of white matter anisotropy in Krabbe disease with diffusion tensor MR imaging: Initial experience. *Radiology.* 2001;218:809-815.
[165] Schneider JF, Il'yasov KA, Boltshauser E, Hennig J, Martin E. Diffusion tensor imaging in cases of adrenoleukodystrophy: preliminary experience as a marker for early demyelination? *American Journal of Neuroradiology.* 2003;24:819-824.
[166] Barnea-Goraly N, Eliez S, Hedeus M, et al. White matter tract alterations in fragile X syndrome: Preliminary evidence from diffusion tensor imaging. *American Journal of Medical Genetics.* 2003;118B:81-88.
[167] Barnea-Goraly N, Menon V, Krasnow B, Ko A, Reiss A, Eliez S. Investigation of white matter structure in velocardiofacial syndrome: A diffusion tensor imaging study. *American Journal of Psychiatry.* 2003;160:1863-1869.
[168] Buchsbaum MS, Tang CY, Peled S, et al. MRI white matter diffusion anisotropy and PET metabolic rate in schizophrenia. *Neuroreport.* 1998;9:425-430.
[169] Foong J, Symms MR, Barker GJ, Maier M, Miller DH, Ron MA. Investigating regional white matter in schizophrenia using diffusion tensor imaging. *Neuroreport.* 2002;13:333-336.
[170] Kubicki M, Westin CF, Nestor PG, et al. Cingulate fasciculus integrity disruption in schizophrenia: a magnetic resonance diffusion tensor imaging study. *Biological Psychiatry.* 2003;54:1171-1180.
[171] Lim KO, Hedehus M, Moseley M, de Crespigny A, Sullivan EV, Pfefferbaum A. Compromised white matter tract integrity in schizophrenia inferred from diffusion tensor imaging. *Archives of General Psychiatry.* 1999;56:367-374.

[172]Ashburner J, Friston KJ. Voxel-based morphometry--the methods. *Neuroimage.* 2000;11:805-821.

[173]Agartz I, Andersson JL, Skare S. Abnormal brain white matter in schizophrenia: A diffusion tensor imaging study. *Neuroreport.* 2001;12:2251-2254.

[174]Ardekani BA, Nierenberg J, Hoptman MJ, Javitt DC, Lim KO. MRI study of white matter diffusion anisotropy in schizophrenia. *Neuroreport.* 2003;14:2025-2029.

[175]Foong J, Maier M, Barker GJ, Brocklehurst S, Miller DH, Ron MA. In vivo investigation of white matter pathology in schizophrenia with magnetisation transfer imaging. *Journal of Neurology Neurosurgery and Psychiatry.* 2000;68:70-74.

[176]Schmithorst VJ, Wilke M, Dardzinski BJ, Holland SK. Correlation of white matter diffusivity and anisotropy with age during childhood and adolescence: A cross-sectional diffusion-tensor MR imaging study. *Radiology.* 2002;222:212-218.

[177]Jones DK, Griffin LD, Alexander DC, et al. Spatial normalization and averaging of diffusion tensor MRI data sets. *Neuroimage.* 2002;17:592-617.

[178]Park HJ, Kubicki M, Shenton ME, et al. Spatial normalization of diffusion tensor MRI using multiple channels. *Neuroimage.* 2003;20:1995-2009.

[179]Xu D, Mori S, Shen D, van Zijl PC, Davatzikos C. Spatial normalization of diffusion tensor fields. *Magnetic Resonance in Medicine.* 2003;50:175-182.

[180]Conturo TE, Lori NF, Cull TS, et al. Tracking neuronal fiber pathways in the living human brain. *Proceedings of the National Academy of Sciences U S A.* 1999;96:10422-10427.

[181]Basser PJ, Pajevic S, Pierpaoli C, Duda J, Aldroubi A. In vivo fiber tractography using DT-MRI data. *Magnetic Resonance in Medicine.* 2000;44:625-632.

[182]Mori S, Crain BJ, Chacko VP, van Zijl PC. Three-dimensional tracking of axonal projections in the brain by magnetic resonance imaging. *Annals of Neurology.* 1999;45:265-269.

[183]Westin CF, Maier SE, Mamata H, Nabavi A, Jolesz FA, Kikinis R. Processing and visualization for diffusion tensor MRI. *Medical Image Analysis.* 2002;6:93-108.

[184]Weinstein DM, Kindlmann GL, Lundberg EC. Tensorlines: Advection-diffusion based propagation through diffusion tensor fields. *IEEE Visualization Proceedings*. San Francisco; 1999:249-253.

[185]Lazar M, Weinstein DM, Hasan KM, Alexander AL. Axon tractography with tensorlines. *Proceeding of the 8th Scientific Meeting of International Society Magnetic Resonance Medicine*. Denver; 2000:482.

[186]Lazar M, Weinstein DM, Tsuruda JS, et al. White matter tractography using diffusion tensor deflection. *Human Brain Mapping.* 2003;18:306-321.

[187]Koch MA, Norris DG, Hund-Georgiadis M. An investigation of functional and anatomical connectivity using magnetic resonance imaging. *Neuroimage.* 2002;16:241-250.

[188]Behrens TE, Johansen-Berg H, Woolrich MW, et al. Non-invasive mapping of connections between human thalamus and cortex using diffusion imaging. *Nature Neuroscience.* 2003;6:750-757.

[189]Tournier JD, Calamante F, Gadian DG, Connelly A. Diffusion-weighted magnetic resonance imaging fibre tracking using a front evolution algorithm. *Neuroimage.* 2003;20:276-288.

[190] Stieltjes B, Kaufmann WE, van Zijl PC, et al. Diffusion tensor imaging and axonal tracking in the human brainstem. *Neuroimage.* 2001;14:723-735.

[191] Mori S, van Zijl PC. Fiber tracking: principles and strategies - a technical review. *Nuclear Magnetic Resonance in Biomedicine.* 2002;15:468-480.

[192] Xu D, Mori S, Solaiyappan M, van Zijl PC, Davatzikos C. A framework for callosal fiber distribution analysis. *Neuroimage.* 2002;17:1131-1143.

[193] Poupon C, Clark CA, Frouin V, et al. Regularization of diffusion-based direction maps for the tracking of brain white matter fascicles. *Neuroimage.* 2000;12:184-195.

[194] Catani M, Howard RJ, Pajevic S, Jones DK. Virtual in vivo interactive dissection of white matter fasciculi in the human brain. *Neuroimage.* 2002;17:77-94.

[195] Lori NF, Akbudak E, Shimony JS, et al. Diffusion tensor fiber tracking of human brain connectivity: Aquisition methods, reliability analysis and biological results. *Nuclear Magnetic Resonance in Biomedicine.* 2002;15:494-515.

[196] Anderson AW. Theoretical analysis of the effects of noise on diffusion tensor imaging. *Magnetic Resonance in Medicine.* 2001;46:1174-1188.

[197] Tournier JD, Calamante F, King MD, Gadian DG, Connelly A. Limitations and requirements of diffusion tensor fiber tracking: an assessment using simulations. *Magnetic Resonance in Medicine.* 2002;47:701-708.

[198] Lazar M, Alexander AL. An error analysis of white matter tractography methods: synthetic diffusion tensor field simulations. *Neuroimage.* 2003;20:1140-1153.

[199] Shulman RG, Rothman DL, Behar KL, Hyder F. Energetic basis of brain activity: implications for neuroimaging. *Trends Neuroscience.* 2004;27:489-495.

[200] Zilbovicius M, Garreau B, Samson Y, et al. Delayed maturation of the frontal cortex in childhood autism. *American Journal of Psychiatry.* 1995;152:248-252.

[201] Wilcox J, Tsuang MT, Ledger E, Algeo J, Schnurr T. Brain perfusion in autism varies with age. *Neuropsychobiology.* 2002;46:13-16.

[202] Hashimoto T, Sasaki M, Fukumizu M, Hanaoka S, Sugai K, Matsuda H. Single-photon emission computed tomography of the brain in autism: effect of the developmental level. *Pediatric Neurology.* 2000;23:416-420.

[203] Zilbovicius M, Boddaert N, Belin P, et al. Temporal lobe dysfunction in childhood autism: A PET study. Positron emission tomography. *American Journal of Psychiatry.* 2000;157:1988-1993.

[204] Ohnishi T, Matsuda H, Hashimoto T, et al. Abnormal regional cerebral blood flow in childhood autism. *Brain.* 2000;123 (Pt 9):1838-1844.

[205] Mountz JM, Tolbert LC, Lill DW, Katholi CR, Liu HG. Functional deficits in autistic disorder: characterization by technetium-99m-HMPAO and SPECT. *Journal of Nuclear Medicine.* 1995;36:1156-1162.

[206] Muller RA, Pierce K, Ambrose JB, Allen G, Courchesne E. Atypical patterns of cerebral motor activation in autism: a functional magnetic resonance study. *Biological Psychiatry.* 2001;49:665-676.

[207] Muller R-A, Kleinhans N, Kemmotsu N, Pierce K, Courchesne E. Abnormal variability and distribution of functional maps in autism: An fMRI study of visuomotor learning. *American Journal of Psychiatry.* 2003;160:1847-1862.

[208] Allen G, Courchesne E. Differential effects of developmental cerebellar abnormality on cognitive and motor functions in the cerebellum: An fMRI study of autism. *American Journal of Psychiatry.* 2003;160:262-273.

[209]Ring HA, Baron-Cohen S, Wheelwright S, et al. Cerebral correlates of preserved cognitive skills in autism: a functional MRI study of embedded figures task performance. *Brain.* 1999;122 (Pt 7):1305-1315.
[210]Turkeltaub PE, Flowers DL, Verbalis A, Miranda M, Gareau L, Eden GF. The neural basis of hyperlexic reading. An FMRI case study. *Neuron.* 2004;41:11-25.
[211]Luna B, Minshew NJ, Garver KE, et al. Neocortical system abnormalities in autism: An fMRI study of spatial working memory. *Neurology.* 2002;59:834-840.
[212]Baron-Cohen S, Leslie AM, Frith U. Does the autistic child have a "theory of mind"? *Cognition.* 1985;21:37-46.
[213]Baron-Cohen S. The cognitive neuroscience of autism. *Journal of Neurology Neurosurgery and Psychiatry.* 2004;75:945-948.
[214]Hill EL, Frith U. Understanding autism: insights from mind and brain. *Philosophical Transactions of the Royal Society of Lond B Biological Sciences.* 2003;358:281-289.
[215]Frith U, Frith CD. Development and neurophysiology of mentalizing. *Philosophical Transactions of the Royal Society of Lond B Biological Sciences.* 2003;358:459-473.
[216]Baron-Cohen S, Ring H, Moriarty J, Schmitz B, Costa D, Ell P. Recognition of mental state terms. Clinical findings in children with autism and a functional neuroimaging study of normal adults. *British Journal of Psychiatry.* 1994;165:640-649.
[217]Baron-Cohen S, Ring HA, Wheelwright S, et al. Social intelligence in the normal and autistic brain: an fMRI study. *European Journal of Neuroscience.* 1999;11:1891-1898.
[218]Schultz RT, Gauthier I, Klin A, et al. Abnormal ventral temporal cortical activity during face discrimination among individuals with autism and Asperger syndrome. *Archives of General Psychiatry.* 2000;57:331-340.
[219]Critchley HD, Daly EM, Bullmore ET, et al. The functional neuroanatomy of social behaviour: changes in cerebral blood flow when people with autistic disorder process facial expressions. *Brain.* 2000;123 (Pt 11):2203-2212.
[220]Hall GBC, Szechtman H, Nahmias C. Enhanced salience and emotion recognition in autism: A PET study. *American Journal of Psychiatry.* 2003;160:1439-1441.
[221]Adolphs R, Baron-Cohen S, Tranel D. Impaired recognition of social emotions following amygdala damage. *Journal of Cognitive Neuroscience.* 2002;14:1264-1274.
[222]Adolphs R, Sears L, Piven J. Abnormal processing of social information from faces in autism. *Journal of Cognitive Neuroscience.* 2001;13:232-240.
[223]Dawson G, Carver L, Meltzoff AN, Panagiotides H, McPartland J, Webb SJ. Neural correlates of face and object recognition in young children with autism spectrum disorder, developmental delay, and typical development. *Child Development.* 2002;73:700-717.
[224]Klin A. Attributing social meaning to ambiguous visual stimuli in higher-functioning autism and Asperger syndrome: The Social Attribution Task. *Journal of Child Psychology and Psychiatry.* 2000;41:831-846.
[225]Castelli F, Frith C, Happe F, Frith U. Autism, Asperger syndrome and brain mechanisms for the attribution of mental states to animated shapes. *Brain.* 2002;125:1839-1849.
[226]Wang AT, Dapretto M, Hariri AR, Sigman M, Bookheimer SY. Neural correlates of facial affect processing in children and adolescents with autism spectrum disorder. *Journal of the American Academy of Child and Adolescent Psychiatry.* 2004;43:481-490.

[227] Pierce K, Haist F, Sedaghat F, Courchesne E. The brain response to personally familiar faces in autism: findings of fusiform activity and beyond. *Brain.* 2004.

[228] Piggot J, Kwon H, Mobbs D, et al. Emotional attribution in high-functioning individuals with autistic spectrum disorder: a functional imaging study. *Journal of the American Academy of Child and Adolescent Psychiatry.* 2004;43:473-480.

[229] Hadjikhani N, Joseph RM, Snyder J, et al. Activation of the fusiform gyrus when individuals with autism spectrum disorder view faces. *Neuroimage.* 2004;22:1141-1150.

[230] Just MA, Cherkassky VL, Keller TA, Minshew NJ. Cortical activation and synchronization during sentence comprehension in high-functioning autism: Evidence of underconnectivity. *Brain.* 2004;127:1811-1821.

[231] Muller RA, Behen ME, Rothermel RD, et al. Brain mapping of language and auditory perception in high-functioning autistic adults: A PET study. *Journal of Autism and Developmental Disorders.* 1999;29:19-31.

[232] Boddaert N, Belin P, Chabane N, et al. Perception of complex sounds: Abnormal pattern of cortical activation in autism. *American Journal of Psychiatry.* 2003;160:2057-2060.

[233] Gervais H, Belin P, Boddaert N, et al. Abnormal cortical voice processing in autism. *Nature Neuroscience.* 2004;7:801-802.

[234] Belin P, Zatorre RJ, Ahad P. Human temporal-lobe response to vocal sounds. *Brain Research Cognitive Brain Research.* 2002;13:17-26.

[235] Winkler I, Kushnerenko E, Horvath J, et al. Newborn infants can organize the auditory world. *Proceedings of the National Academy of Science.* 2003;100:11812-11815.

[236] Belin P, Zatorre RJ, Lafaille P, Ahad P, Pike B. Voice-selective areas in human auditory cortex. *Nature.* 2000;403:309-312.

[237] Belin P, Zatorre RJ. Adaptation to speaker's voice in right anterior temporal lobe. *Neuroreport.* 2003;14:2105-2109.

[238] Spice B. Autism seen as problem of connections in brains. *Post Gazette.* August 15, 2004. http://www.post-gazette.com/pg/04228/361572.stm.

[239] Shulman RG. Functional imaging studies: linking mind and basic neuroscience. *American Journal of Psychiatry.* 2001;158:11-20.

[240] Andreasen NC, O'Leary DS, Cizadlo T, et al. Remembering the past: two facets of episodic memory explored with positron emission tomography. *American Journal of Psychiatry.* 1995;152:1576-1585.

[241] Anderson GM. Genetics of childhood disorders: XLV. Autism, part 4: serotonin in autism. *Journal of the American Academy of Child and Adolescent Psychiatry.* 2002;41:1513-1516.

[242] McDougle CJ, Naylor ST, Cohen DJ, Aghajanian GK, Heninger GR, Price LH. Effects of tryptophan depletion in drug-free adults with autistic disorder. *Archives of General Psychiatry.* 1996;53:993-1000.

[243] McDougle CJ, Kresch LE, Posey DJ. Repetitive thoughts and behavior in pervasive developmental disorders: treatment with serotonin reuptake inhibitors. *Journal of Autism and Developmental Disorders.* 2000;30:427-435.

[244] Chugani DC. Serotonin in autism and pediatric epilepsies. *Mental Retardation Developmental Disabilities Research Review.* 2004;10:112-116.

[245] Chugani DC, Muzik O, Behen M, et al. Developmental changes in brain serotonin synthesis capacity in autistic and nonautistic children. *Annals of Neurology.* 1999;45:287-295.

[246] Chugani DC, Sundram BS, Behen M, Lee ML, Moore GJ. Evidence of altered energy metabolism in autistic children. *Progress in Neuropsychopharmacol Biological Psychiatry.* 1999;23:635-641.

[247] Hisaoka S, Harada M, Nishitani H, Mori K. Regional magnetic resonance spectroscopy of the brain in autistic individuals. *Neuroradiology.* 2001;43:496-498.

[248] Friedman SD, Shaw DW, Artru AA, et al. Regional brain chemical alterations in young children with autism spectrum disorder. *Neurology.* 2003;60:100-107.

[249] Levitt JG, O'Neill J, Blanton RE, et al. Proton magnetic resonance spectroscopic imaging of the brain in childhood autism. *Biological Psychiatry.* 2003;54:1355-1366.

[250] Mori K, Hashimoto T, Harada M, et al. [Proton magnetic resonance spectroscopy of the autistic brain]. *No To Hattatsu.* 2001;33:329-335.

[251] Otsuka H, Harada M, Mori K, Hisaoka S, Nishitani H. Brain metabolites in the hippocampus-amygdala region and cerebellum in autism: an 1H-MR spectroscopy study. *Neuroradiology.* 1999;41:517-519.

[252] Murphy DG, Critchley HD, Schmitz N, et al. Asperger syndrome: A proton magnetic resonance spectroscopy study of brain. *Archives of General Psychiatry.* 2002;59:885-891.

[253] Schumann CM, Hamstra J, Goodlin-Jones BL, et al. The amygdala is enlarged in children but not adolescents with autism; the hippocampus is enlarged at all ages. *Journal of Neuroscience.* 2004;24:6392-6401.

[254] Aylward EH, Minshew NJ, Goldstein G, et al. MRI volumes of amygdala and hippocampus in non-mentally retarded autistic adolescents and adults. *Neurology.* 1999;53:2145-2150.

[255] Howard MA, Cowell PE, Boucher J, et al. Convergent neuroanatomical and behavioural evidence of an amygdala hypothesis of autism. *Neuroreport.* 2000;11:2931-2935.

[256] Saitoh O, Karns CM, Courchesne E. Development of the hippocampal formation from 2 to 42 years: MRI evidence of smaller area dentata in autism. *Brain.* 2001;124:1317-1324.

[257] Piven J, Bailey J, Ranson BJ, Arndt S. No difference in hippocampus volume detected on magnetic resonance imaging in autistic individuals. *Journal of Autism and Developmental Disorders.* 1998;28:105-110.

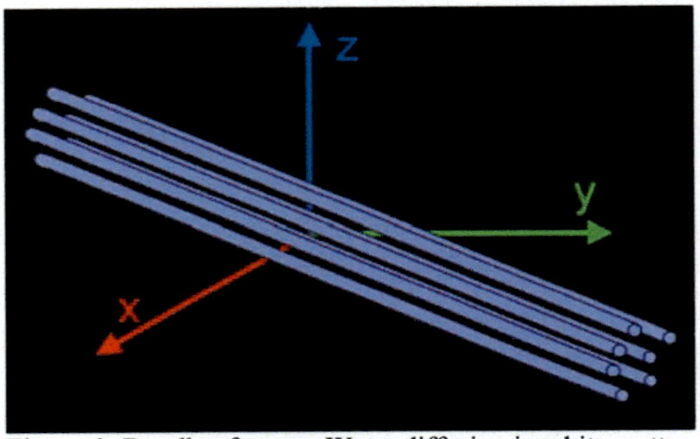

Figure 6a Bundle of axons. Water diffusion in white matter is directionally anisotropic. In white matter tracts, water diffusion perpendicular to the tracts is more "hindered." Water diffusion parallel to the tracts is unrestricted.

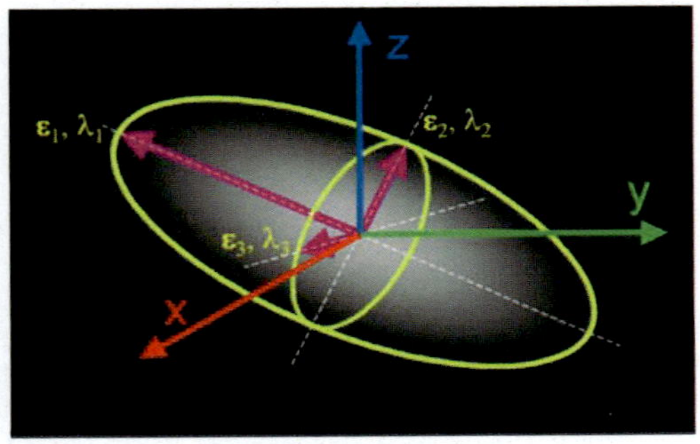

Figure 6b Directional probability of diffusion represented by an ellipse. Small changes in the density, spacing, or myelination of white matter fibers can significantly alter white matter diffusion properties, which can be measured with diffusion tensor imaging.

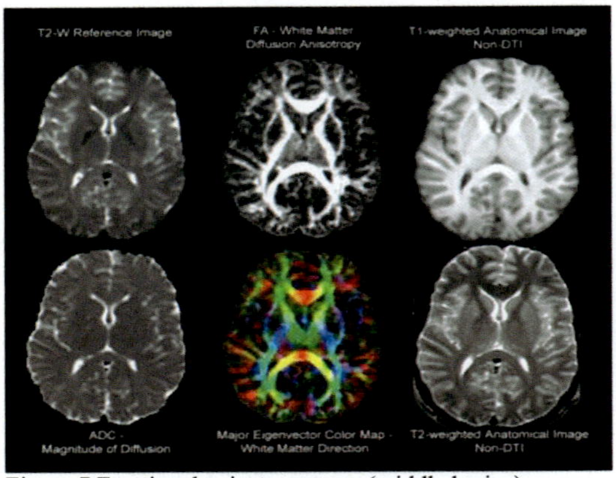

Figure 7 Fractional anisotropy map (middle brains) compared to T2- and T1-weighted anatomic images.

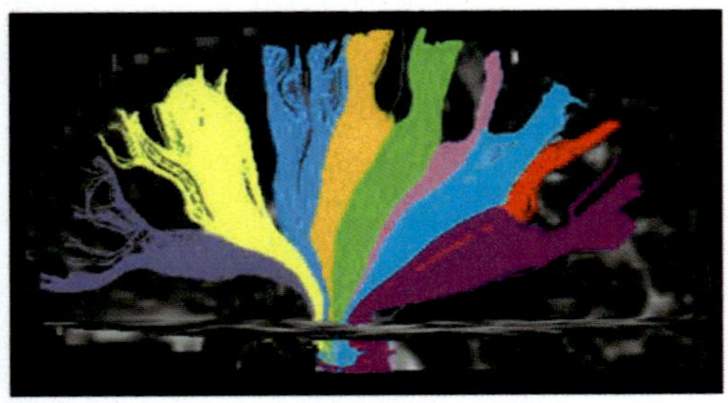

Figure 8 White matter tractography images of the main projection pathways between the brainstem and cortex through the cerebral peduncles, internal capsule, and corona radiate

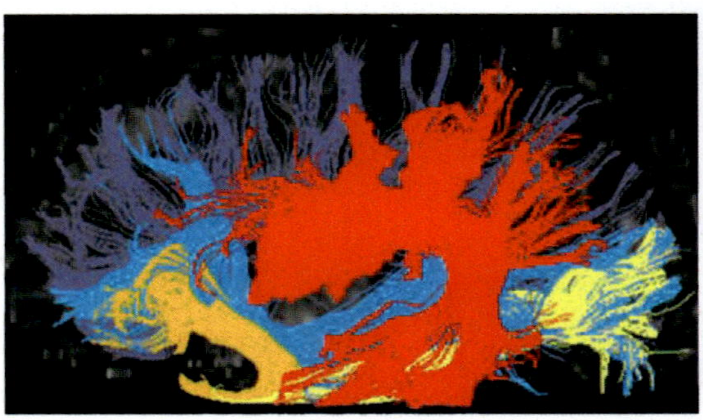

Figure 9 White matter tractography images of intra-hemispheric cortico-cortical major association pathways: uncinate fasciculus (left-side of image, second lightest tract); inferior longitudinal fasciculus (right-side of image, lightest tract); superior longitudinal fasciculus (darkest tract); occipitofrontal fasciculus (lower medium bright, posterior to anterior tract); corpus callosum (diffuse upper medium-shaded fibers).

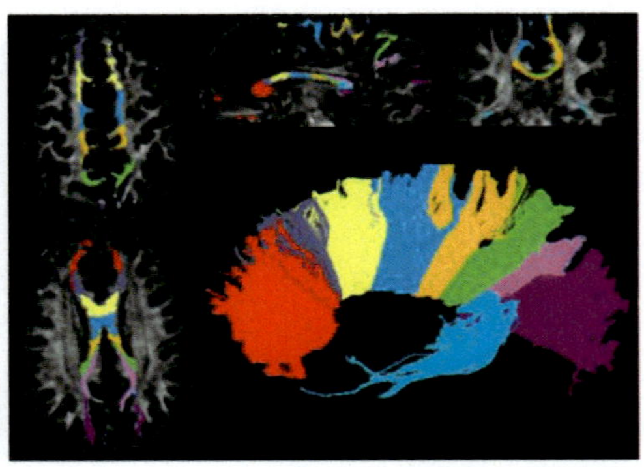

Figure 10 White matter tractography segmentation of the corpus callosum. In the figure, the corpus callosum (CC) has been parcellated according to specific cortical regions of connectivity. This parcellation approach allows for unique cortical specific labeling of parts of a structure for further analysis.

In: Recent Developments in Autism Research
Editor: Manuel F. Casanova, pp. 109-126

ISBN 1-59454-358-5
© 2005 Nova Science Publishers, Inc.

Chapter IV

EEG in Autism: Is There Just Too Much Going on in There?

Caroline Brown*
Department of Experimental Psychology University of Bristol, Bristol, UK

The Attentional Network

Early research into anomalous brain function in autism looked for differences in one or more specific brain areas. It has become clear however, that the brain works as a dynamic network, combining sensory, emotional, physical and mental information from many cells in many brain regions in an ongoing process. It is necessary to take the same wider view when trying to understand how the brain works in autism, that is when looking for function or functions that are aberrant. Conventional electroencephalographic (EEG) research indicates that there are differences in brain activity in both perception and attention in people with autism, and the processes of attention and perception are intrinsically linked *because* of the "network" structure of information processing in the brain. Table 1 lists some of the areas that contribute to the attentional network.

Briefly, incoming sensory information from the eyes and ears (and other senses too, but for simplicity we will focus on visual and auditory processes here) passes through central structures of the brain on its way to the cortical region specific to that information. Figure 1 shows a diagram of where these perceptually specific regions of cortex are in Figure 1a—visual cortex is at the back of the head, and auditory cortex in the middle at the side. Figure 1b shows some of the structures in the brain that are part of a central pathway, which is important because incoming information is also passed through these structures to other areas of the brain (both cortical and sub-cortical) thus enabling decisions regarding the allocation of attention or the instigation of automatic behaviour *before* we are even conscious of the need to do so.[1]

* caroline.brown@bris.ac.uk

[1] This serves as a very useful defence mechanism, so for instance closing the eyelid *before* the globule of hot fat hits the cornea thus protecting the eyeball from permanent and non-repairable damage.

Table 1.

	EEG measure	Attention	Perception	
			Visual	Audition
Frontal cortical lobe	#	*		
Frontal sub-cortical (anterior cingulate gyrus)		*		
Parietal lobe	#	*	*	*
Mid-brain structures (thalamus, limbic system)		*		
Cerebellum (timing of events)		*		
Occipital lobes	#		*	
Temporal lobes posterior	#		*	
Temporal lobes anterior and inside	#			*

* brain areas that contribute to the attentional network.
# we can measure activity from these areas using EEG.

EEG—How is EEG Measured, and What Does it Assess?

EEG is the measurement of electrical activity output by neurons in the outer cortex as they fire. The amount of electrical activity at the scalp is tiny, it is measured in $1/1000^{th}$s of a volt (microvolts or μV), and is recorded by metal electrodes held against the scalp forming an electrical "bridge" by means of an electrically sensitive gel or liquid. The electrical signal picked up by each electrode is then sent to a computer through an amplifier, and recorded as digital data, the data from each electrode being known as the "signal" from a "channel." The number of electrodes used can vary from one or two right up to two-hundred-and-fifty-six—the limiting factors being *computing power*, the *time* it takes to get a good recording and *sensitivity* to movement, which causes huge interference with EEG recordings.

This latter problem has been almost insurmountable until fairly recently when attempting to record EEG from babies, young children and mentally handicapped individuals.[1] This is because muscle activity produces electrical activity, which is more powerful than that measured from the brain, so any movement of the eyes (including blinks) or the head causes huge surges of electrical activity—relative to the very low power being measured by EEG. Modern methods of analysis now enable eye blinks, eye movements and other muscle related electrical activity to be removed from the recording, theoretically leaving only the brain activity for analysis.

EEG measures the electrical activity of cells in the cortex so it can tell us only about cortical processes and not what is happening in sub-cortical structures of the brain. Much of the evidence for brain processes involved in both active and passive tasks must be taken from other sources of imaging like functional Magnetic Resonance Imaging (fMRI), which looks at

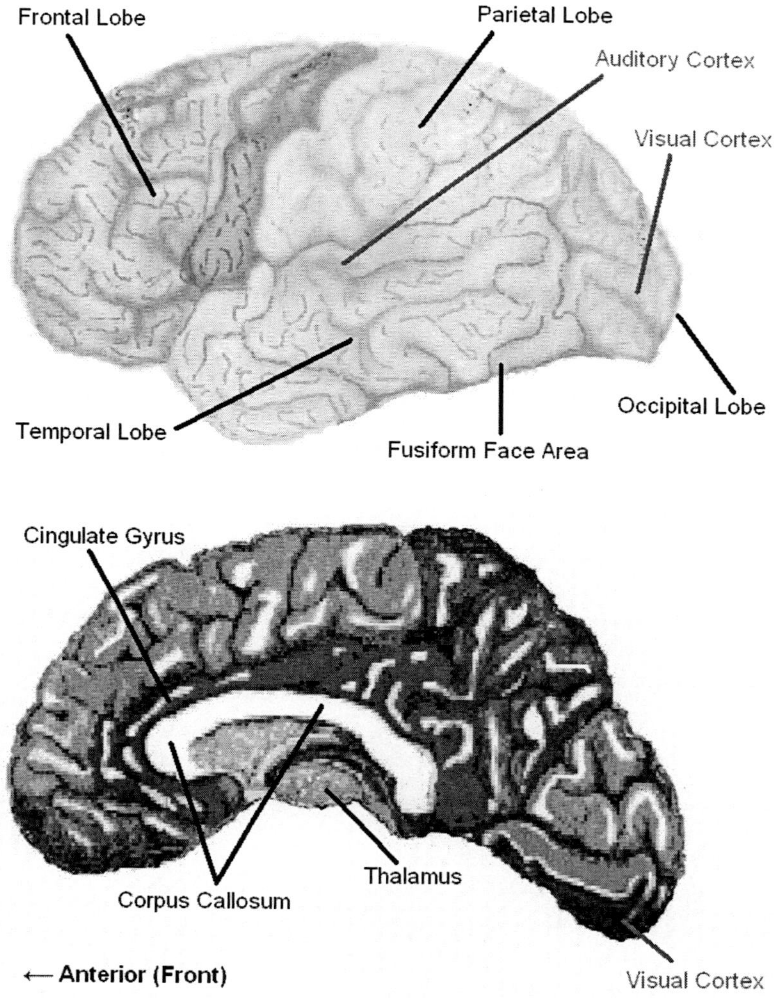

Figure 1 (A) The cortex of the human brain, showing main lobes. (B) The inside of the human brain showing the cingulate gyrus, corpus callosum, and the thalamus, structures important in passing information between areas of the brain.

the amount of blood an area uses during a particular thinking task. Such imaging tells us very well *where* something happens, but has to be measured over several seconds which is not very precise in terms of the timing. However, EEG records at a rate of between 1 and 5 milliseconds per data point and therefore gives very accurate information regarding the timing of both increases and decreases in brain activity.

There are several ways of analysing the electrical data collected, the simplest being the analysis of "background" EEG, where no sounds or pictures are used as stimuli, and the level of brain activity is recorded whilst the participant is either asleep or awake. Other types of analysis are the event-related potential (ERP), coherence and spectral analysis, and these are outlined below.

In research we want to find out *which* brain processes occur and *where* and *when* they happen. To do this EEG is averaged around "events" which are varied experimentally and then compared. Figure 2a shows how the EEG for events where the participant sees the word "dog" can be recorded and then averaged in an event-related potential (ERP). As a comparison the ERP could then be compared to the ERP created by recording EEG whilst the word "cat" is used as a stimulus. This same experimental technique can be used in visual or auditory experiments as well as those varying attention, memory or any other brain function of interest.

Figure 2b shows the typical pattern of an ERP and consists of components named either N (for negative) or P (for positive) and either order of occurrence (e.g. N1, P1, N2, P2 etc) or in terms of the time (in milliseconds) after the event (e.g. P120 or N250). These components can be compared by how big they are (that is the amplitude in microvolts [μv]) or in latency (time after the event) between conditions or between groups of participants. In this way, activity that happens earlier or uses greater brain-power in one group or one experimental condition can be identified in comparison to another group or experimental condition.

A second, and rather more complicated approach to analysing EEG data involves looking at how consistently two brain areas are working together at the same rate of firing. In this analysis, known as **coherence**, the rate of firing within a longish time period either before, during or after an event is compared for similarity between areas. This more complex analysis is often also used when "background" EEG has been measured, and often as a way of identifying changes in brain activity changes during development.

Finally, a fairly recent approach to analysing EEG information looks at the changes in the *frequency* of electrical firing in the brain. This type of analysis is called **spectral analysis** and is quite exciting because instead of comparing average activity, the relationships between areas during active processing are compared. In the dynamic network model of outlined above this is likely to be extremely important. We know that as neurons are excited they increase their firing rate, but what appears to be important is that areas working together on the same information increase their firing rate together and synchronise that activity. To give some idea of the different frequencies that are looked at in EEG research a diagram showing differences in frequency at EEG defined bandwidths is shown in Figure 3.

Behavioural and Brain Measures That Have Traditionally Been Investigated in Autism

In autism, individuals are impaired in social interaction, cognitive function often involving language and exhibit odd or stereotyped behaviours. Additionally, some individuals report perceptual abnormalities such as over-sensitivity to sounds or colours, and indeed to smells and somatosensory stimulation too. Much of the brain research in autism has focussed on particular aspects of these symptoms—for instance comparison is made between perception of non-verbal tones and verbal tones and the brain response over the auditory area is measured, which give us some indication of brain differences in language perception. Social and cognitive impairments however are likely to show as differences in activity across the attentional network because they involve the combination of perception, attention and higher cognitive functions underlying memory and emotional processing.

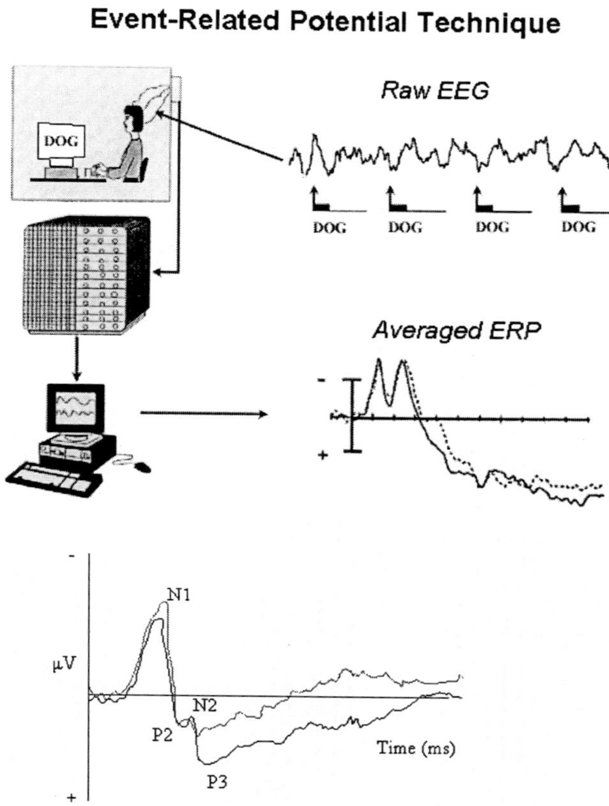

Figure 2 (A) Electrical activity is collected continuously, then segmented into portions related to "events." All the segments are then averaged to create the Event-Related Potential (ERP) for that event, which may be compared to an ERP of a different event. (B) ERPs often show specific components, named with an N if negative and P if positive, e.g. N1, N2, P2, and P3.

The Development of Attention

In typically developing infants between about 3 and 6 months the behavioural ability to shift attention from one object (thought/sound/visual item) to another develops. This is known as the "orienting system," and is thought to involve the development of communication between the parietal lobes, which encode the spatial relationship between the object in focus and the self, and areas in the centre of the brain including the thalamus.[2] As this orienting system comes on line, infants start to respond to social information from other people, known as joint-attention bids, from around 6 months onwards. For instance, if someone points to an object, the infant will turn their attention towards that object, and interestingly this ability in pre-vocal months is highly related to later language ability, which allows us to infer that it is linked to early language learning skills too.[3]–[6] This then is the "posterior" attention system developing, and involves the parietal lobe regions around cortical regions kn own to receive information from many senses.

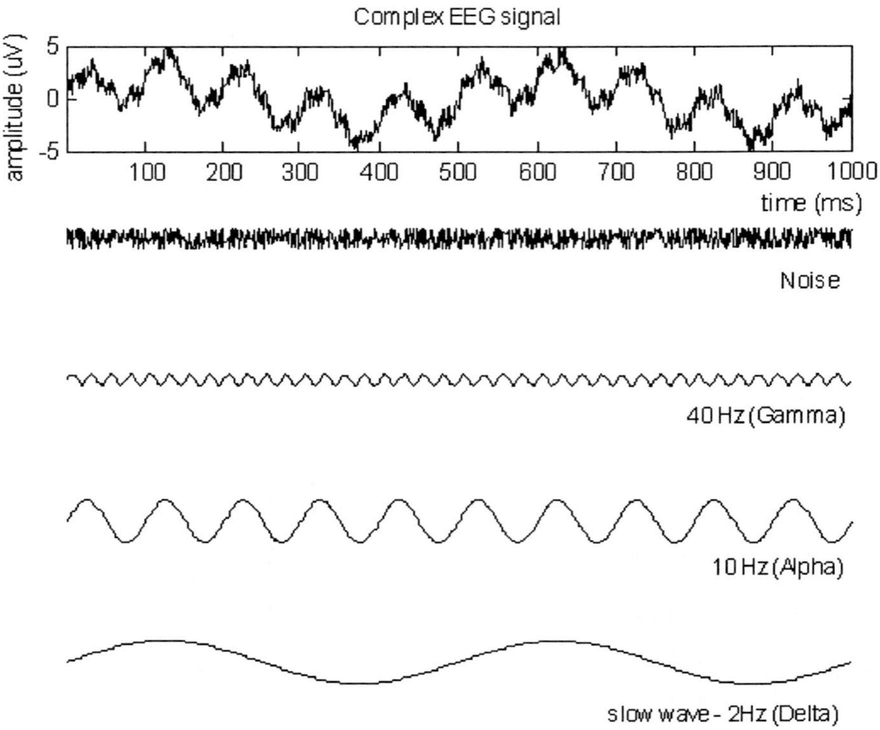

Figure 3 A complex wave from an EEG recording over the time of 1 second (1000 ms). Spectral analysis shows that it is made up of wave-forms of different frequency and a certain amount of "noise." Names and frequencies of EEG bandwidths of interest: Delta: 1–3 Hz; Theta: 4–7 Hz; Alpha: 8–13 Hz; Beta: 14–30 Hz; Gamma: 30–100 Hz; Hz = cycles per second.

Later, the "anterior" (frontal) attention system develops—this involves frontal cortical areas and frontal sub-cortical regions called the anterior cingulate gyrus, which lies just beneath the cortex at the front of the brain, and the parts of the brain that regulate both bodily function and emotions called the limbic system. The anterior attentional system regulates voluntary control of where to focus attention, and how to share it when two or more things need to be concentrated on—whether these are external or internal.[2] This type of attention is termed as the cognitive, executive and/or motivational type, and its development is seen as changes in EEG over frontal and parietal parts of the brain.[7],[8]

The development of the frontal attentional system is likely to continue right through to adulthood, with the most marked changes occurring in the frontal lobes during adolescence. What EEG recordings of typically developing children also tell us is that overall children's brains are far more active when younger, and that this activity reduces and becomes more focussed as children progress through adolescence to the point at which, as in adult EEG recordings, very precise patterns of activity at particular times are found in particular brain

[2] For instance when Mum disappears from the room baby diverts his attention to follow her and then drops the toy he has been playing with. This in turn causes baby to notice that his nappy area does not feel so very good which may well have been out of the focus of his attention previously whilst playing with the toy!

locations.[9],[10] Thatcher et al[11]–[14] (1986; 1992; 1994a; 1994b) also showed that as children developed there were 2–4 year cycles where coherence firstly increased and then reduced. It is thought that the periods of greater coherence coincide with periods when children are learning specialised behaviours, like using a spoon or reading for instance. Periods during which coherence reduces coincide with periods when children learn to differentiate between newly learnt tasks, for instance using a knife and fork compared to using a pen or pencil, and during periods when reliance on automation of well-learnt tasks such as riding a bike occurs.

With this general background we are now ready to look at what EEG recordings from both children and adults with autism tell us.

How Does EEG Vary in Autism?

Background EEG

In adults with autism measures of background EEG during sleep showed increased activity over left frontal areas whereas the control group (adults matched for gender, age and IQ) showed greater activity over right frontal and right posterior (occipital-lobe) visual areas.[15]

This difference in brain area is not apparent in young children, although in early development, the background measures of EEG activity in the lower frequency bands (theta and alpha) at 14 months old over frontal regions strongly correlate with measures of social attention at 18 months old in *typically* developing infants.[8],[16] Such activity is thought to represent the early development of the anterior attention system, and given the cognitive deficits associated with autism it is likely that frontal background EEG activity would be absent, reduced or located at substantially different scalp areas in children with autism.[3]

Perception of Sound and Attention to Sound Types

The perception of simple non-speech sounds, like clicks, gives rise to exactly the same "normal" patterns of activity in both autistic and non-autistic individuals.[17] Such sound perception is likely to utilise the parietal (or posterior) attention system since it does not require the conscious allocation of attention, since the information in a click only needs to be localised in terms of its direction *not* made sense of. The brain is particularly good at detecting differences between incoming stimuli, in any sensory mode.

There is one particular experimental method, called the "oddball task" that enables the measurement of brain activity generated in response to "difference" because brain cells actively increase their firing rate when they detect a variation from "the normal." So, if the same sound is played at differing intervals over a long time, each time it is heard the same group of cells will fire and a particular pattern will emerge in the ERP. When an occasional "target" sound is played, which may be of a slightly different tone, or for a slightly different duration, the parietal attention system is alerted by the change in activity because additional

---

[3] Of course most children would not have a formal diagnosis of autism or autistic spectrum disorder at 14 months old—especially those that are undergoing "autistic regression."

cells respond to the difference in the tone. Because participants do not have to make any behavioural action (like pressing a button) to the sounds, the brain will simply register the change by itself. The "oddball task" is therefore very useful for testing individuals who cannot make behavioural responses e.g. small infants and people with physical and mental disabilities. Using this task, Courchesne et al.[18] found that in young people with autism the attentional component at around 300 ms was smaller than that in age and gender matched controls. In Courchesne and colleagues' experiment however, the sounds the experimenters used incorporated both verbal and non-verbal components, which may account for the differences between the young people with autism and those without, but which the experimenters attributed to differences in attention.

The difference in perceiving non-speech and speech sounds in autism is quite marked, with speech sounds being associated with reduction in brain activity and non-speech sounds with increased or earlier brain activity. Autistic children aged 5–9 years when perceiving a difference in pure tone showed a very early increase in activity over left-frontal regions compared to age and gender-matched children.[19] When speech-related sounds are used however the orienting system appears not to function in the same way. In an experiment that compared orienting (the parietal attention system) to simple and complex non-speech and vowel sounds, Čeponienė et al.[20] found normal ERP patterns over right auditory brain regions to both the simple and complex non-speech sounds. In the vowel-change condition however, the children with autism showed *no* attentional component at all between 300 and 400 ms.

Visual Perception and Attention

In vision it might be expected that the social impairment evidenced in autism would manifest itself in differences in perception of social stimuli like faces. There is also evidence that suggests that some people with autism have specifically good visual abilities to pick out patterns from backgrounds which non-autistic people see as whole pictures.[21]–[24] In simple visual oddball tasks, some interesting EEG differences are found between people with autism and people without.

People with autism show a bigger and quicker early attentional component, combined with a smaller and later attentional component. Stauder and Mottron[25] compared a group with autism (children and adults ranging in age from 8 to 36) with age, IQ and gender matched controls. They found that the early attentional components were both more powerful (the P1) and quicker (N2 latency reduced) in the group with autism. The P3 component over right frontal and temporal electrodes was also significantly reduced in the group with autism, suggesting the later attentional component is impaired.

The late positive component, the P3, which occurs over posterior regions of the brain, usually over parietal lobes, has been shown to be smaller in autistic groups than in non-autistic in many other studies too.[26]–[28] This suggests that in the perception of visual information, the posterior attention system does not contribute in the same way in autism as it does in non-autistic populations. It may be that one of the functions of the posterior attention system is to gather all the information together—or to look at it another way perhaps all the information from distributed parts of the brain *focuses* onto the parietal lobe. This explanation of the P3 is at best tentative, but would account for why the P3 (or P300) is associated with many different tasks, and appears to be sensitive to multi-modal stimuli, since any difference in processing or in the signalling mechanisms from anywhere in the brain would ultimately lead to a difference in the summation of that activity.

Visual Attention Tasks

Social functioning relies on the ability to recognise and presumably process faces of other human beings. Face recognition and face processing have been identified as occurring within a wide network of brain areas using many imaging techniques. Over a wide area of brain activity, averaged event-related EEG data may not be able to give the same depth of information that other imaging techniques and other EEG analysis techniques can give. Nevertheless, it is of great interest that when even quite young children with autistic spectrum disorders (ASD) were tested for face and object recognition that they showed the same clear EEG differences to objects (familiar versus novel toys), but no EEG difference to a picture of their own mother (familiar) compared to that of someone else's mother (novel). The children, aged 3–4 were compared with two other groups of children, one a group of typically developing children of the same age, and the other a group of children with developmental delay of the same age. In both these other groups EEG differences were found for both the face and the object tasks.[29] The EEG differences found between the groups were those measured at periods of time from 400 ms to over 1500 ms after onset of stimuli, which indicates that these effects are not necessarily related to either of the attentional components described above. This is probably because face processing entails activity from a very wide network of brain areas, and it takes this extra time for all the information to come together.

Certainly there is corroborating evidence that face processing in particular is done very differently in the autistic brain than in the non-autistic brain. This can be seen from research utilising functional Magnetic Resonance imaging (fMRI), in a face processing task testing adults with autism and comparing the results with a non-impaired group of adults matched for age, gender and handedness.[30] As with previously reported research, this task used the oddball paradigm, here changed so that participants pressed a button to either female faces (as targets within the commoner pictures of males as standards) or to circles (as targets within rectangles as standards). The circles and rectangles were morphed from the faces that were used, so that the percentage of light and dark pixels on the display were exactly equivalent. In the non-impaired participants the area of the brain known as the Fusiform Face Area, which is marked on Figure 1, always showed greater activation during the face task. By contrast only one of the participants with autism showed increased activation at this site—instead each individual with autism showed a different pattern of activation using widely differing parts of their brains, despite being as accurate and as fast as the control group in the task. Because of the way that fMRI data is analysed the brain images during the shape task are used as comparisons for brain activity during the face-processing task. In the group with autism, this analysis suggests that they may have shown preferential attention to the shapes rather than to the faces.

Spectral Analysis

In the last ten years, research into the co-ordination of cognitive functions has been influenced by the finding that individual brain cells co-ordinate their activities with other neurons by increasing their firing rates to around 40 Hz (called the gamma band) and that they fire together, that is synchronously. This research was first carried out in the brains of live animals (see Singer and Gray[31] for a review) and was later tested using EEG measures in humans.[32],[33] In a system that evidently works by combining information from many areas (the network) there needs to be a mechanism that enables large groups of cells working on the same thing to connect, whilst at the same time activity from cells not involved needs to be kept separate.

In normal processing groups of cells combine their activity at around 40 Hz to signal their joint contribution to the cognitive task being undertaken. This mechanism functions as a binding system, enabling the joining or combination of processing across a network of areas in the brain. Neurons generally fire at a fairly constant rate, until they receive information from other neurons that either increases (excitation) or decreases (inhibition) their firing rate. The information they receive comes as chemicals from other neurons at points where they make contact (synapses), and the receipt of sufficient chemical information results in neurons sending an electrical impulse along their long output tails (axons), which in turn triggers increased firing in cells further along the line. For the last part of last century it was thought that the simply increasing firing rate would be a sufficiently informative signal for groups of cells working on the same object to recognise that they were part of a single assembly.[34] However, it became clear as more was discovered about what makes neurons become active, that different groups of cells working on separate objects would not be able to signal their relatedness without an alternative mechanism.[35],[36]

It is likely however, that synchronous firing is only one of several ways in which cells in a large network join their information together. Another way, which happens through learning, is that cells which frequently send information to other cells create many contact points (synapses), and probably as a consequence, those cells become attuned to respond to particular patterns. For instance, there are cells which fire most rapidly to pictures of hands,[37] but they do also increase their firing rate to pictures of forks—which suggests that there are cells which have "learnt" particular shapes or items or associations. The question of how information is shared between cells that are situated both close together within a functional region and at greater distances, between regions is still open to debate. As with most complex problems, it is unlikely that the answer will be a simple "either this or this" answer, and is more likely to be a combination of many signalling mechanisms. However, the simple hypothesis put forward by Singer and Gray[31] was that co-ordinated activity in the gamma bandwidth was the way in which cells in the same area bound information together, and that it was likely that cells in different brain areas but working on the same task would also do the same.

A binding mechanism such as synchronised gamma activity would therefore enable the brain network to identify novel input (perception) *and* the active combination of "attentional" input to perception. It would in effect enable the co-ordination of information stored across widespread parts of the brain; learnt items, procedures, emotions, language, social information and posture for instance. In autism, the lack of co-ordination evidenced in social and verbal impairments and language deficits may be a result of impairments to the binding system,[38] and this might therefore be manifested in differences in measures of gamma EEG.

In one experiment, researchers asked adults with autism and a group of gender and handedness matched adults to view pictures of upright or inverted faces whilst recording EEG. In the unimpaired adults, upright faces generated a burst of gamma activity over frontal scalp regions, which was larger than the inverted face condition. By contrast, both upright and inverted faces generated the same burst of gamma in the group with autism therefore giving no useful information in order to discriminate between upright and inverted faces.[39] This result indicates that whereas in unimpaired adults attention was greater to upright faces, in those with autism equal attention was paid to both upright and inverted faces. In the light of the recent imaging research by Pierce et al,[30] reported above, this result may have been because faces do not utilise the same network of brain areas in autism. This might account for why the frontal 40 Hz burst in the group with autism was the same whether the face was upright or upside-down because individuals with autism may not have access to specific face-processing areas, but instead a wide-spread and personally exclusive network.

However, other research testing adolescents with autism in an experiment which presented either shapes or random pictures[40] found that gamma activity in autism was significantly different in the group with autism than in an age and IQ matched group of youngsters. In this experiment, shapes are apparent but are in fact visual illusions that appear when the background shapes (inducers) all face one another (Figure 4). This experimental design has the advantage that simply changing the direction of one or more of the inducers allow a control condition where no shape appears. In perceptual tasks of this kind, gamma bursts have been reliably recorded over the posterior attention areas in unimpaired adults at both around 300 ms,[41],[42] and at the same scalp areas as an early response suggesting that attention is being paid to the incoming visual information at around 100 ms.[43] To make sure that differences in gamma EEG were not due to developmental differences or IQ differences, a group of youngsters the same age and same IQ were tested. In the UK such youngsters are described as having moderate learning difficulties (MLD), and any other developmental or neurological disorder was excluded as a reason for reduced IQ in all the children who took part in the experiment.

Behaviourally, there was no difference between the groups in either reaction time or in accuracy. Figure 5 shows the gamma activity in both groups for the shape and random conditions measured over parietal regions. Whereas both groups show almost identical activity in the Kanizsa-random condition they are very different in the Kanizsa-shape condition. When perceiving the shape, the group with autism differ from the control group in three ways: Firstly, overall gamma power is much higher than in the control group. Secondly, the group with autism show a very early burst of gamma activity at between 80 and 120 ms. Finally, the later gamma component is present in both the control group and the group with autism, but in the group with autism it is more powerful and starts much earlier.

What does this tell us about the gamma activity in the brains of children with autism? Well, developmentally babies start to show a gamma response frontally at around the same time as they start to perceive the shapes in the Kanizsa illusion, that is at around 6–9 months.[44] Children also show higher gamma power when they are younger, which reduces in power and extent as they age.[45]–[47] In normal development as networks develop and refine through learning and experience, less cells take part in signalling a cognitive event—

this is seen in the reduction in power of conventional EEG and reduction in extent to small focal areas in both conventional and gamma EEG. In autism however the increased gamma activity indicates that many cells increase their activity very soon after the start of a cognitive event, like perception, but that instead of reducing their activity until other network information can be combined, these cells remain active and indeed may continue to increase in activity.

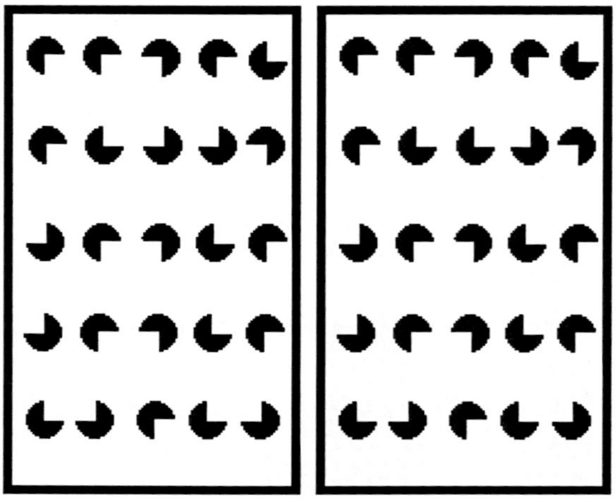

Figure 4 Kanizsa stimuli: In the picture on the left (Kanizsa-shape), a white rectangular shape can be seen, whereas in the picture on the right, although several candidates appear, none are proper rectangles (Kanizsa-random).

Logical Inferences from Gamma Data

The inability to reduce activity until required may well be a failure of inhibition—that is the cells in the autistic brain simply continue to fire and do not (can not) learn to stop. If this is the case then we would expect several consequences, firstly it would lead to the inability to decide which event requires paying attention to when there is a choice of two or more. This may be the underlying cause of an inability to direct attention either internally or externally.

Secondly in cases where perceptual gamma activity is early enough and sufficiently powerful some individuals may be able to utilise it, thus improving their perception within specific modalities. Such a response may be what underlies the better performance of people with autism at finding hidden patterns or re-creating complex patterns.

Finally, if there is a problem with not being able to inhibit gamma activity to limited brain areas there is likely to be an increased chance of epilepsy, which is manifested in uncontrolled high frequency EEG activity. Certainly, there is a far greater incidence both of epilepsy within autism (estimates ranging from 7–42 %) and an increased rate of EEG abnormalities.[48]–[50]

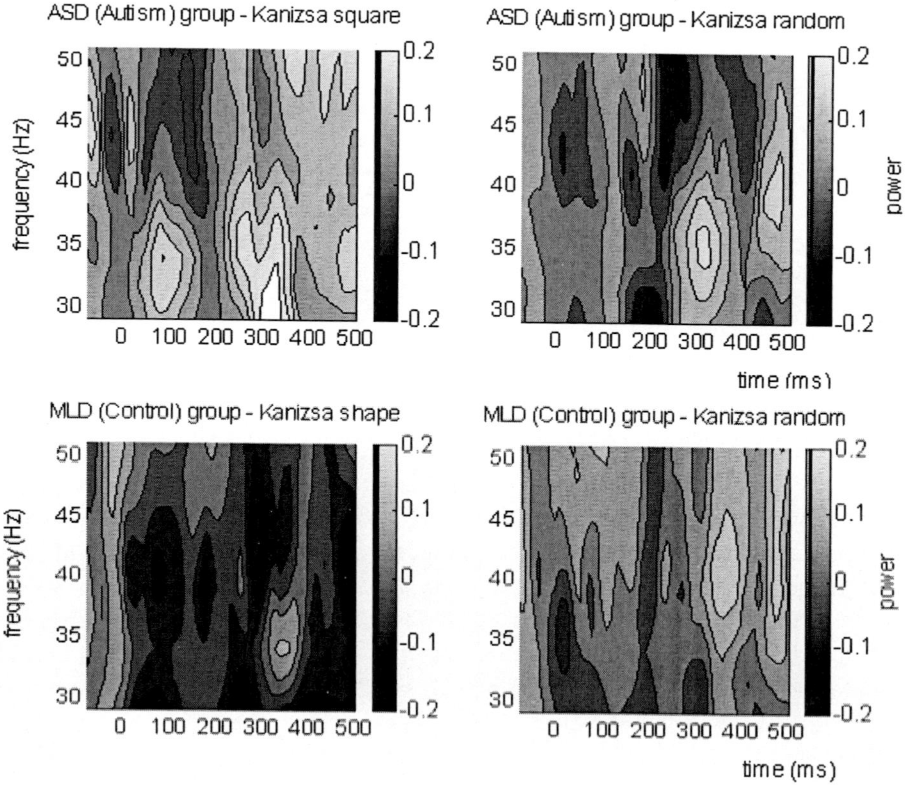

Figure 5 Spectrograms showing the increase and decrease in 30–40 Hz gamma activity in both the Kanizsa shape and random conditions for the ASD group (upper panels) and the age and IQ matched MLD group (lower panels).

Summary

Why should too much gamma activity be linked to a reduction in the ability to focus attention? In such a complex and ever-changing (dynamic) system, it is likely to be the circuits whose overall activity is sufficiently different from other co-active circuits that come to dominance.[51] In the context of neural communication, most neurons increase their firing rate as they are stimulated, but as they do so, many of the cells surrounding them reduce their firing rate. This inhibition is a result of neuro-chemical input from surrounding cells. If the arrangement of surrounding cells were altered in the brains of people with autism then we should expect to see a difference in the patterns of electrical activity measured by EEG. One hypothesis is that attention can be thought of as the focussing of the brain circuit onto the activity of a particular group or assembly of cells (which may be active in many different parts of the brain). In autism, this focussing may not happen because of an inability to "switch-off" the activity of irrelevant brain cells.

Attention however serves several purposes—in terms of vision we need to focus our eyes on what we need to pay attention to, as we see things more clearly in the centre of our visual field, and with less clarity at the outside or periphery. So, in the early part of visual processing when we are paying attention to an item, there is a bigger burst of activity over posterior visual regions. As the visual information progresses through the brain it is integrated with information from diverse brain regions regarding emotional, contextual, temporal and spatial relationships along with previously learned knowledge and automatic (well-learnt) skills. Such integration may be measurable in terms of the increased gamma burst found at between 250 and 400 ms over parietal and frontal regions.[52]–[54]

In autism, we know that both language and socialisation are impaired, both of which essentially entail the wide integration of such information, which suggests that there are either differences in the way the which the brain is put together or that there are differences in the way that relevant bits of brain communicate with one another. Our findings that there is much more powerful and uninhibited gamma activity in autism suggests that none (or few) of the circuits in the brain can come to dominance because too many are active at the same time.[40]

One way in which this inability to utilise context may benefit people with autism is that they may be able to focus on incoming perceptual information and use it more quickly if it can be tied up with an appropriate response network. There is some evidence that people with autism are better at tasks in which they do not have to use contextual information.[21],[55] In Figure 5 it is noticeable that the group with autism showed a clear early burst of gamma that was not found in the control group[4] data, which because of the way the analysis was performed indicates that this gamma activity is different from that found in the control group. This increased and earlier burst of gamma activity *might* be linked to increased ability to perform tasks where ignoring the contextual information is an advantage, as shown for instance in being able to pick out hidden objects from larger pictures.[24]

The disadvantages of such an overactive system however are twofold. In the first place, it is not possible to flexibly re-focus the brain system onto rapidly occurring events occurring in sequence. For non-autistic people it is thought that the gamma binding signal allows the rapid formation of thought networks, which can be updated very quickly from both external and internally generated information (e.g. memory or feelings).[56] The second disadvantage of an uninhibited or overactive gamma system is the increased likelihood of epilepsy or epileptic like absence that is apparent so widely in autism.[57]

A Final Comment

The spectral research reported here is in the earliest of stages, and therefore the conclusions being drawn here are at best tentative. They are currently the subject of debate between several groups of developmental scientists, and there is a great need to carry out far more research both into autism and indeed into the normal developmental sequence of brain activity, to serve as a reference for all developmental disorders.

[4] It is important to note though that this does not mean the control group do not show this component—the type of analysis that this data underwent however takes out any activity that always occurs at the same point in every trial, so such a component may be there in the control group but very regular. The autism group early component varies in both its time of starting and its duration for it to show so clearly in this type of analysis.

Acknowledgements

Grateful acknowledgement is made to Thomas Gruber (University of Leipzig) for his assistance in data analysis and programming.

References

[1] Casey BJ, de Haan M. Introduction: new methods in developmental science. *Developmental Science.* 2002; 5: 265-267.

[2] Johnson MH. Cortical maturation and the development of visual attention in early infancy. *Journal of Cognitive Neuroscience.* 1990; 2: 81-95.

[3] Butterworth G. Origins of mind in perception and action. In: Moore C, Dunham PJ, eds. *Joint Attention: Its Origins and Role in Development.* Hillsdale, NJ: Lawrence Erlbaum Associates, 1995: 29-40.

[4] Morales M, Mundy P, Rojas J. Following the direction of gaze and language development in 6-month-olds. *Infant Behavior and Development.* 1998; 21: 373-377.

[5] Baldwin DA. Infants' contribution to the achievement of joint reference. *Child Development.* 1991; 62: 875-890.

[6] Mundy P, Gomes A. Individual differences in joint attention skill development in the second year. *Infant Behavior and Development.* 1998; 21: 469-482.

[7] Rothbart M, Posner M, Rosicky J. Orienting in normal and pathological development. *Development and Psychopathology.* 1994; 6: 635-652.

[8] Mundy P, Card J, Fox N. EEG correlates of the development of infant joint attention skills. *Developmental Psychobiology.* 2000; 36: 325-338.

[9] Taylor MJ, Baldeweg T. Application of EEG, ERP and intracranial recordings to the investigation of cognitive functions in children. *Developmental Science.* 2002; 5: 318-334.

[10]Thomas KM, Nelson CA. Age-related changes in the electrophysiological response to stimulus novelty: a topographic approach. *Electroencephalography and Clinical Neurophysiology.* 1996; 98: 294-308.

[11]Thatcher RW, Krause PJ, Hrybyk M. Cortico-cortical associations and EEG coherence: a two-compartmental model. *Electroencephalography and Clinical Neurophysiology.* 1986; 64: 123-143.

[12]Thatcher RW. Cyclic cortical reorganization during early childhood. *Brain and Cognition.* 1992; 20: 24-50.

[13]Thatcher RW. Cyclic cortical reorganization: Origins of human cognitive development. In: Dawson G, Fischer K, eds. *Human Behavior and the Developing Brain.* New York, NY: Guilford Press, 1994: 232-266.

[14]Thatcher RW. Psychopathology of early frontal lobe damage: dependence on cycles of development. *Development and Psychopathology.* 1994; 6: 565-596.

[15]Bolduc C, Daoust AM, Limoges E, Mottron L, Braun CMJ, Godbout R. EEG lateralization in high functioning autism. *International Journal of Psychophysiology.* 2002; 45: 150.

[16]Henderson LM, Yoder PJ, Yale ME, McDuffie A. Getting the point: electrophysiological correlates of protodeclarative pointing. *International Journal of Developmental Neuroscience.* 2002; 20: 449-458.

[17]Courchesne E, Courchesne RY, Hicks G, Lincoln AJ. Functioning of the brain-stem auditory pathway in non-retarded autistic individuals. *Electroencephalography and Clinical Neurophysiology.* 1985; 61: 491-501.

[18]Courchesne E, Kilman BA, Galambos R, Lincoln AL. Autism: processing of novel auditory information assessed by event-related brain potentials. *Electroencephalography and Clinical Neurophysiology.* 1984; 59: 238-248.

[19]Gomot M, Giard MH, Adrien JL, et al. Auditory mismatch process in children with autism: an ERP topographic study. *International Journal of Psychophysiology.* 2001; 41: 217-218.

[20]Čeponienė R, Lepistö T, Shestakova A, et al. Speech-sound-selective auditory impairment in children with autism: they can perceive but do not attend. *Proceedings of the National Academy of Sciences of the United States of America.* 2003; 100: 5567-5572.

[21]Happé FGE. Studying weak central coherence at low levels: children with autism do not succumb to visual illusions: a research note. *Journal of Child Psychology and Psychiatry and Allied Disciplines.* 1996; 37: 873-877.

[22]Shah A, Frith U. An islet of ability in autistic children: a research note. *Journal of Child Psychology and Psychiatry and Allied Disciplines.* 1983; 24: 613-620.

[23]Shah A, Frith U. Why do autistic individuals show superior performance on the block design task? *Journal of Child Psychology and Psychiatry and Allied Disciplines.* 1993; 34: 1351-1364.

[24]Jolliffe T, Baron-Cohen S, Are people with autism and Asperger syndrome faster than normal on the embedded figures test? *Journal of Child Psychology and Psychiatry and Allied Disciplines.* 1997; 38: 527-534.

[25]Stauder JEA, Mottron L. Visual gating, -attention and -context in autism: a cognitive ERP study. *International Journal of Psychophysiology.* 2002; 45: 39.

[26]Kemner C, van der Gaag RJ, Verbaten M, van Engeland H. ERP differences among subtypes of pervasive developmental disorders. *Biological Psychiatry.* 1999; 46: 781-789.

[27]Kemner C, Verbaten MN, Cuperus JM, Camfferman G, van Engeland H. Visual and somatosensory event-related brain potentials in autistic children and three different control groups. *Electroencephalography and Clinical Neurophysiology.* 1994; 92: 225-237.

[28]Verbaten MN, Roelofs JW, van Engeland H, Kenemans JK, Slangen JL. Abnormal visual event-related potentials of autistic children. *Journal of Autism and Developmental Disorders.* 1991; 21: 449-470.

[29]Dawson G, Carver L, Meltzoff, AN, Panagiotides H, McPartland J, Webb SJ. Neural correlates of face and object recognition in young children with autism spectrum disorder, developmental delay, and typical development. *Child Development.* 2002; 73: 700-717.

[30]Pierce K, Muller RA, Ambrose J, Allen G, Courchesne E. Face processing occurs outside the fusiform "face area" in autism: evidence from functional MRI. *Brain.* 2001; 124: 2059-2073.

[31]Singer W, Gray C. Visual feature integration and the temporal correlation hypothesis. *Annual Review of Neuroscience.* 1995; 18: 555-586.

[32]Müller MM, Bosch J, Elbert T, et al. Visually induced gamma-based responses in human electroencephalographic activity: a link to animal studies. *Experimental Brain Research.* 1996; 112: 96-102.

[33]Müller MM, Junghofer M, Elbert T, Rockstroh B. Visually induced gamma-band responses to coherent and incoherent motion: a replication study. *Neuroreport.* 1997; 8: 2575-2579.

[34]Hebb DO. *The Organization of Behavior: A Neuropsychological Theory.* New York, NY: Wiley, 1949.

[35]Milner PM. A model for visual shape recognition. *Psychology Review.* 1974; 81: 521-535.

[36]von der Malsburg C, Schneider W. A neural cocktail-party processor. *Biological Cybernetics.* 1986; 54: 29-40.

[37]Tanaka K, Saito H, Fukada Y, Moriya M. Coding visual images of objects in the inferotemporal cortex of the macaque monkey. *Journal of Neurophysiology.* 1991; 66: 170-189.

[38]Brock J, Brown CC, Boucher J, Rippon G. The temporal binding deficit hypothesis of autism. *Development and Psychopathology.* 2002; 14: 209-224.

[39]Grice SJ, Spratling MW, Karmiloff-Smith A, et al. Disordered visual processing and oscillatory brain activity in autism and Williams Syndrome. *Neuroreport.* 2001; 12: 2697-2700.

[40]Brown C, Gruber T, Boucher J, et al. Gamma abnormalities during perception of illusory figures in autism. *Cortex.* 2004; in press.

[41]Tallon C, Bertrand O, Bouchet P, Pernier J. Gamma-range activity evoked by coherent visual stimuli in humans. *European Journal of Neuroscience.* 1995; 7: 1285-1291.

[42]Tallon-Baudry C, Bertrand O, Delpuech C, Pernier J. Stimulus specificity of phase-locked and non-phase-locked 40 Hz visual responses in human. *Journal of Neuroscience.* 1996; 16: 4240-4249.

[43]Herrmann CS, Mecklinger A, Pfeifer E. Gamma responses and ERPs in a visual classification task. *Clinical Neurophysiology.* 1999; 110: 636-642.

[44]Csibra G, Davis G, Spratling MW, Johnson MH. Gamma oscillations and object processing in the infant brain. *Science.* 2000; 290: 1582-1585.

[45]Yordanova J, Kolev V, Heinrich H, Woerner W, Banaschewski T, Rothenberger A. Developmental event-related gamma oscillations: effects of auditory attention. *European Journal of Neuroscience.* 2002; 16: 2214-2224.

[46]Yordanova J, Kolev V, Heinrich H, Banaschewski T, Woerner W, Rothenberger A. Gamma band response in children is related to task-stimulus processing. *Neuroreport.* 2000; 11: 2325-2330.

[47]Böttger D, Herrmann CS, von Cramon DY. Amplitude differences of evoked alpha and gamma oscillations in two different age groups. *International Journal of Psychophysiology.* 2002; 45: 245-251.

[48]Tuchman R. Treatment of seizure disorders and EEG abnormalities in children with autism spectrum disorders. *Journal of Autism and Developmental Disorders.* 2000; 30: 485-489.

[49]Tuchman RF, Rapin I. Regression in pervasive developmental disorders: seizures and epileptiform electroencephalogram correlates. *Pediatrics.* 1997; 99: 560-566.

[50]Rossi PG, Parmeggiani A, Bach V, Santucci M, Visconti P. EEG features and epilepsy in patients with autism. *Brain and Development.* 1995; 17: 169-174.

[51]Nunez PL. Toward a quantitative description of large scale neocortical dynamic function and EEG. *The Behavioral and Brain Sciences.* 2000; 23: 371-437.

[52]Müller M, Gruber T, Keil A. Modulation of induced gamma band activity in the human EEG by attention and visual information processing. *International Journal of Psychophysiology.* 2000; 38: 283-299.

[53]Gruber T. Müller MM, Keil A, Elbert T. Selective visual-spatial attention alters induced gamma band responses in the human EEG. *Clinical Neurophysiology.* 1999; 110: 2074-2085.

[54]Rodriguez E, George N, Lachaux J-P, et al. Perception's shadow: long-distance synchronization of human brain activity. *Nature.* 1999; 397: 430-433.

[55]Happé F. Autism: cognitive deficit or cognitive style? *Trends in Cognitive Sciences.* 1999; 3: 216-222.

[56]Singer W. Neuronal synchrony: a versatile code for the definition of relations. *Neuron.* 1999; 24: 49-65.

[57]Tuchman R, Rapin I. Epilepsy in autism. *The Lancet Neurology.* 2002; 1: 352-358.

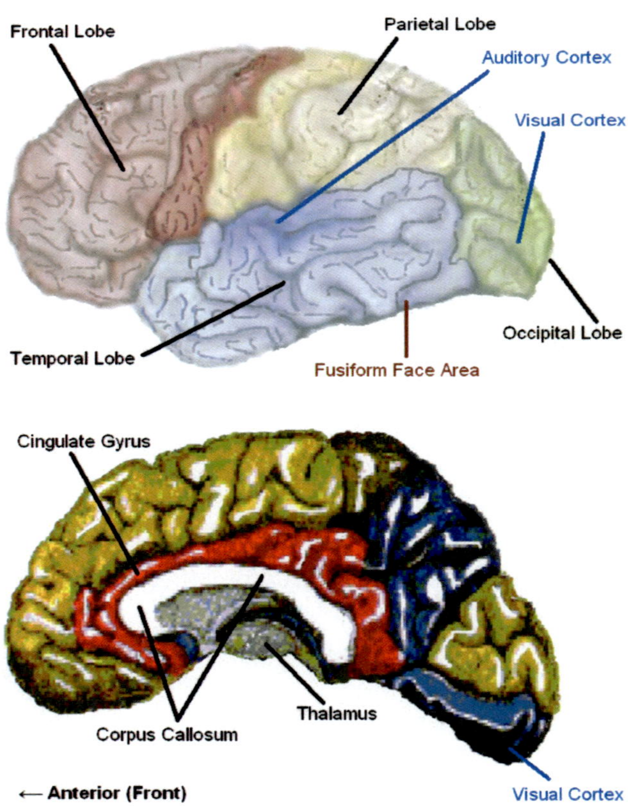

Figure 1 (A) The cortex of the human brain, showing main lobes. (B) The inside of the human brain showing the cingulate gyrus, corpus callosum, and the thalamus, structures important in passing information between areas of the brain.

In: Recent Developments in Autism Research
Editor: Manuel F. Casanova, pp. 127-133

ISBN 1-59454-358-5
© 2005 Nova Science Publishers, Inc.

Chapter V

Gabaergic Dysfunction in Autism

S. Hossein Fatemi*

University of Minnesota,Department of Psychiatry
Division of Neuroscience Research

Autism is a neurodevelopmental disorder with rising prevalence rate of 16–20 per 10,000,[1] characterized by problems in communication, social skills and repetitive behavior and childhood onset.[2] Pathology exists throughout various areas of the brain including frontal, parietal and cerebellar cortices.[27],[4] An interesting recent finding pertains to presence of minicolumnar pathology in the autistic brain.[5] Casanova and coworkers have shown that neocortical minicolumns are narrower in the autistic brain and exhibit less peripheral neuropil space and increased spacing among their constituent cells.[5] These authors have surmised that this form of pathology, by necessity, will impact the GABAergic inhibitory local circuit projections adversely potentially explaining the increased prevalence of seizures in autism.[5] We will also present biochemical data showing that GABAergic dysfunction is also present in autism as reflected by downregulation of various GABAergic interneuron-resident proteins such as Reelin and glutamic acid decarboxylases.

Glutamic acid decarboxylase, is the rate limiting enzyme which is responsible for conversion of glutamate to GABA. In the adult brain, GAD exists in two major isoforms, namely GAD 65 and GAD 67 kDa proteins, which are products of two independently regulated genes located on chromosomes 2 and 10, respectively.[6] GAD 65 enzymatic activity is preferentially distributed to axon terminals, is membrane-bound, and involved in vesiculor synthesis of GABA.[7] GAD 67 is more concentrated in interneurons, is cytoplasmic and involved in nonvesicular GABA release.[8] Measurement of GAD 65 in the autistic cerebellum, showed a reduction of this protein by 50 % ($p < 0.02$) when compared to age matched controls (Table 1).[9] In the same brain area, mean GAD 67 levels dropped by 51 %, albeit nonsignificantly as compared to controls (Table 1).[9] In the parietal cortex, GAD 67 levels dropped by 48 % vs. controls; this reduction did not reach statistical significance (Table 1). GAD 67 levels did drop by 67 % ($p < 0.03$) in the autistic parietal cortex vs. controls (Table 1). Comparison of β-actin levels did not show any significant

* Telephone: 612-626-3633; Fax: 612-624-8935

differences between the two groups. The major deficiencies in levels of GAD 65 and 67 kDa proteins in two important brain areas in autism, may subserve deficiency in availability of GABA affecting important biological functions like learning, locomotor activity, reproduction and circadian rhythms.[10] Additionally, decreases in levels of GAD 65 and 67 kDa proteins in the autistic brain will impact negatively on normal processing of visual, somatic, locomotor and memory information processing and could also explain the observations of increased blood, platelet, and CSF glutamate levels in the autistic patients.[11]–[13] Additionally, deficiency in GABA due to decreased conversion of glutamate, could account for the fact that up to a third of autistic subjects suffer from seizure disorders. Downregulation of GAD 65 and GAD 67 kDa proteins is not limited to autism, and has been demonstrated in schizophrenia[14],[15] and bipolar disorder.[14],[16]

Table 1 Descriptive data for GAD65, GAD67, and β-actin levels

Area	Protein Level	Control		Autistic		Δ	*p*-Value
		Mean	**SE**[1]	**Mean**	**SE1**		
Parietal cortex (Brodmann area 40)	GAD65 (30μg/lane)	4.24	1.0	2.20	2.0	48%↓	n.s.
	GAD67 (30μg/lane)	1.08	3.8	0.42	0.38	61%↓	< 0.03
	β-actin (30μg/lane)	6.4	0.3	6.3	0.5	1.5%↓	n.s.
Cerebellum	GAD65 (30μg/lane)	2.70	0.83	1.4	1.1	50%↓	< 0.02
	GAD67 (30μg/lane)	0.84	0.33	0.43	0.40	51%↓	n.s.
	β-actin (30μg/lane)	7.3	2.9	6.77	0.66	7%↓	n.s.

Reelin is an extracellular serine protease[17] with dual functions during mammalian life; during embryonic period, it is responsible for correct lamination of the brain.[18] In adult life, Reelin subserves cell signalling and synaptic plasticity.[19] The reeler mutant mouse, which carries an autosomal recessive mutation in the reelin (RELN) gene exhibits ataxia and a reeling gait.[20] The reeler brain shows an inverted cortical lamination with abnormal positioning of neurons and aberrant orientation of cell bodies and nerve fibers.[18] There is cerebellar hypoplasia with ectopic Purkinje cells in the homozygous reeler mutant.[21] The RELN gene is localized to chromosome 7 in man.[22] The Reelin protein binds its receptors very-low-density lipo-protein receptor (VLDL-R) and apolipoprotein E2 receptor (APOER2) causing tyrosine phosphorylation of adapter protein disabled-1 (Dab-1)[23] and facilitating the signalling pathway between Reelin and its target cells cortical pyramidal cells.

Several reports have shown decreases in Reelin mRNA and protein in several neuropsychiatric disorders i.e., schizophrenia,[15],[24],[25] bipolar disorder,[25],[26] and major depression,[25],[26] and a variant of lissencephaly.[27] The most recent data, however, show robust reductions in Reelin protein in brain and blood of autistic subjects.[14],[26],[28],[31] Measurement of Reelin 410 kDa glycoprotein expressed as a

[1] SE = standard error of the mean.

function of β-actin in autistic frontal (area 9), parietal (area 40), and cerebellar cortices showed reductions of 67 %, 72 %, and 39 % vs. normal controls, respectively (Table 2).[14] Reelin 330 kDa/β-actin values were also reduced by 80 %, 45 %, and 25 % in frontal ($p < 0.035$), parietal, and cerebellar areas of autistic brains vs. controls respectively (Table 2).[14] Finally, Reelin 180 kDa/β-actin levels dropped by 50 %, 36 % and 27 % in autistic frontal ($p < 0.005$), parietal, and cerebellar ($p < 0.008$) areas vs. controls, respectively (Table 2).[14] Brain levels of β-actin varied minimally and nonsignificantly between groups. Additionally, ratios of Reelin 410 kDa and its isoforms expressed as a function of neuron-specific class III β-Tubulin, a specific marker of neuronal cells, were also reduced proportionally in autistic brain areas 9, 40 and cerebellum vs. controls further supporting the specificity of Reelin reductions in autism.[14]

Table 2 Descriptive data for Reelin/β-actin levels

Area	Protein Level	Control		Autistic		Δ	*p*-Value
		Mean	SE[2]	Mean	SE2		
Cerebellum	Reelin 410/β-actin	0.28	0.10	1.17	0.11	39%↓	< 0.016
	Reelin 330/β-actin	0.04	0.04	0.03	0.04	25%↓	n.s.
	Reelin 180/β-actin	0.70	0.11	0.51	0.24	27%↓	< 0.008
Area 40	Reelin 410/β-actin	0.123	0.09	0.034	0.025	72%↓	n.s.
	Reelin 330/β-actin	0.011	0.027	0.006	0.003	45%↓	n.s.
	Reelin 180/β-actin	0.50	0.14	0.32	0.16	36%↓	n.s.
Area 9	Reelin 410/β-actin	0.30	0.15	0.10	0.10	67%↓	< 0.035
	Reelin 330/β-actin	0.05	0.05	0.01	0.0009	80%↓	< 0.035
	Reelin 180/β-actin	0.60	0.15	0.303	0.190	50%↓	p < 0.005

Fatemi et al.[30] had previously shown that levels of Reelin 410 kDa species were reduced significantly in blood of autistic monozygotic twins and their first degree relatives vs. controls. A further supportive report[31] showed that Reelin 310 kDa isoform was lower in autistic probands having the long GGC repeats (> 12 repeats) vs. matched controls.

The results of genetic association studies concerning involvement of Reelin polymorphisms with autistic disorder is controversial. While two studies support presence of a linkage,[32],[33] four others deny such association.[34]–[37] Despite these controversial genetic studies, several animal studies lend credence to role of Reelin in pathology of autism.[38]–[41]

[2] SE = Standard error of the mean.

Prenatal viral infection in E9 in mice,[39] heterozygoity in a reeler mutant mouse,[38] or prenatal administration of 5-methoxytrypamine in E17 in mice[41] lead to reductions in brain/blood levels of Reelin in the newborn mice.[38],[39],[41] Additionally, examination of brains in the exposed mice, show evidence of neuronal structural deficits similar to that observed in autism[4],[5] linking Reelin deficiency with abnormal brain structure.

In conclusion, the above neuroanatomic, biochemical and genetic data, support GABAergic dysfunction as reflected by GAD 65/67 kDa and Reelin protein deficiencies and existence of minicolumnar pathology in autism. Future studies are needed to provide further support for involvement of GABA system in autism

Acknowledgements

The work of author is supported by grants by Kunin Fund of St. Paul Foundation, The Jonty Foundation and The March of Dimes. The generous use of brain samples by The Autism Tissue Foundation (TARF) and its affiliated brain banks (Harvard, Maryland and Miami University brain banks) is greatly appreciated. I appreciate the secretarial assistance provided by Ms. L. Iversen.

References

[1] Fombonne E. Epidemiological surveys of autism and other pervasive developmental disorders: an update. *Journal of Autism and Developmental Disorders.* 2003;33:265-382.

[2] American Psychiatric Association. *Diagnostic and Statistical Manual of Mental Disorders: DSM-IV.* Washington, DC: APA press; 1994.

[3] Bauman ML, Kemper TL. Histoanatomic observations of the brain in early infantile autism. *Neurology.* 1985;35:866-874.

[4] Bauman ML, Kemper TL. *The Neurobiology of Autism.* 2nd ed. Baltimore, MD: Johns Hopkins University Press; 2004: In press.

[5] Casanova MF, Buxhoeveden DP, Gomez J. Disruption in the inhibitory architecture of the cell minicolumn: implications for autism. *The Neuroscientist.* 2003;9:496-507.

[6] Erlander MG, Tillakaratne NJK, Feldblum S, Patel N, Tobin A. Two genes encode distinct glutamate decarboxylases. *Neuron.* 1991;7:91-100.

[7] Laprade N, Soghomonian JJ. Gene expression of the GAD67 and GAD65 isoforms of glutamate decarboxylase is differently altered in subpopulations of striatal neurosns in adult rats lesioned with 6-OHDA as neonates. *Synaspe.* 1999;33:36-48.

[8] Reetz A., Solimena M., Matteoli M, Folli F, Takei K, De Camilli P. GABA and pancreatic beta-cells: colocalization of glutamic acid decarboxylase (GAD) and GABA with synaptic-like microvesicles suggestes their role in GABA storage and secretion. *The EMBO Journal.* 1991;10:1275-1284.

[9] Fatemi SH, Halt AR, Stary JM, Kanodia R, Schulz SC, Realmuto GR. Glutamic acid decarboxylase 65 and 67 kDa proteins are reduced in autistic parietal and cerebellar cortices. *Biological Psychiatry.* 2002;52;805-810.

[10] Soghomonian JJ, Martin DL. Magnetic resonance imaging study of the brain in autism. *Psychiatry and Clinical Neurosciences.* 1998;52:S219-222.

[11]Pan JW, Lane JB, Hetherington H, Percy AK. Rett syndrome: 1H spectroscopic imaging at 4.1 T. *Journal of Child Neurology.* 1999;14:524-528.

[12]Moreno-Fuenmayer H, Borjas L, Arrieta A, Valera V, Socorro-Candanoza L. Plasma excitatory amino acids in autism. *Investigacion Clinica.* 1996;37:113-128.

[13]Moreno H, Borjas L, Arrieta A, et al. Clinical heterogeneity of the autistic syndrome: A study of 60 families. *Investigacion Clinica.* 1992;33:13-31.

[14]Fatemi SH, Stary JM, Araghi-Niknam M. Egan E. GABAergic dysfunction in schizophrenia and mood disorders as reflected by decreased levels of Reelin and GA-D 65 & 67 kDa proteins in cerebellum. *Schizophrenia Research.* 2004; in press.

[15]Guidotti A, Auta J, Davis JM, et al. Decrease in Reelin and glutamic acid decarboxylase$_{67}$ (GAD$_{67}$) expression in schizophrenia and bipolar disorder: a postmortem brain study. *Archives of General Psychiatry.* 2000;57:1061-1069.

[16]Benes FM, Berretta S. GABAergic interneurons: implications for understanding schizophrenia and bipolar disorder. *Neuropsychopharmacology.* 2001;25:1-27.

[17]Quattrocchi CC, Wannenes F, Persico AM, et al. Reelin is a serine protease of the extracellular matrix. *The Journal of Biological Chemistry.* 2002;277:303-309.

[18]Goffinet AM. An early developmental defect in the cerebral cortex of the Reeler mouse. *Anatomy and Embryology.* 1979;157:205-216.

[19]Costa E, Grayson DR, Guidotti A. Epigentic downregulation of GABAergic function in schizophrenia: potential for pharmacological intervention. *Molecular Interventions.* 2003;3:220-229.

[20]Falconer DS. Two new mutants, "trembler" and "reeler," with neurological actions in the house mouse. *Journal of Genetics.* 1951;50:182-201.

[21]Goffinet AM. Events governing organization of postmigratory neurons: studies on brain development in normal and Reeler mice. *Brain Research.* 1984;319:261-296.

[22]DeSilva U, D'Arcangelo G, Braden VV, et al. The human Reelin gene: isolation, sequencing, and mapping on chromosome 7. *Genome Research.* 1997;7:157-164.

[23]Stockinger W, Brandes C, Fasching D, et al. The Reelin receptor ApoER2 recruits JNK-interacting proteins-1 & -2*. *Journal of Biological Chemistry.* 2000;275:25625-25632.

[24]Impagnatiello F, Guidotti AR, Pesold C, et al. A decrease of Reelin expression as a putative vulnerability factor in schizophrenia. *Proceedings of the National Academy of Sciences of the United States of America.* 1998;95:15718-15723.

[25]Fatemi SH, Earle JA, McMenomy T. Reduction in Reelin immunoreactivity in hippocampus of subjects with schizophrenia, bipolar disorder and major depression. *Molecular Psychiatry.* 2000;5:654-663.

[26]Fatemi SH, Kroll JL, Stary JM. Altered levels of Reelin and its isoforms in schizophrenia and mood disorders. *NeuroReport.* 2001;12:3209-3215.

[27]Hong SE, Shugart YY, Huang DT, et al. Autosomal recessive lissencephaly with cerebellar hypoplasia is associated with human RELN mutations. *Nature Genetics.* 2000;26:93-96.

[28]Fatemi SH, Stary JM, Halt AR, Realmuto GR. Dysregulation of Reelin and Bcl-2 proteins in autistic cerebellum. *Journal of Autism and Developmental Disorders.* 2001;6:529-535.

[29]Fatemi SH, Snow AV, Stary JM, et al. Reelin glycoprotein is reduced in autism. *Biological Psychiatry.* 2004; in press.

[30]Fatemi SH, Stary JM, Egan EA. Reduced blood levels of reelin as a vulnerability factor in pathophysiology of autistic disorder. *Cellular and Molecular Neurobiology.* 2002;22:139-52.

[31]Lugli G, Krueger JM, Davis JM, Persico AM, Keller F, Smalheiser NR. Methodological factors influencing measurement and processing of plasma reelin in humans. *BMC Biochemistry.* 2003;4:9.

[32]Persico A, D'Agruma L, Maiorano N, et al. Collaborative linkage study of autism: Reelin gene alleles and haplotypes as a factor predisposing to autistic disorder. *Molecular Psychiatry.* 2001;6:150-159.

[33]Zhang H, Liu X, Zhang C, et al. Reelin gene alleles and susceptibility for autism spectrum disorders. *Molecular Psychiatry.* 2002;7:1012-1017.

[34]Krebs MO, Betancur C, Leroy S, et al. Absence of association between a polymorphic GGC repeat in the 5′ untranslated region of the Reelin gene and autism. *Molecular Psychiatry.* 2002;7:801-804.

[35]Bonora E, Beyer KS, Lamb JA, et al. Analysis of Reelin as a candidate gene for autism. *Molecular Psychiatry.* 2003;8:885 - 892.

[36]Li J, Nguyen L, Gleason C, et al. Lack of evidence for an association between WNT2 and RELIN polymorphisms and autism. *American Journal of Medical Genetics.* 2004;126B:51-57.

[37]Devlin B, Bennett P, Dawson G, et al. Alleles of a Reelin CGG repeat do not convey liability to autism in a sample from the CPEA Network. *American Journal of Medical Genetics.* 2004;126B:46-50.

[38]Tueting P, Costa E, Dwivedi Y, et al. The phenotypic characteristics of heterozygous reeler mouse. *Neuroreport.* 1999;10:1329-1334.

[39]Fatemi SH, Emamian ES, Kist D, et al. Defective corticogenesis and reduction in Reelin immunoreactivity in cortex and hippocampus of prenatally infected mice. *Molecular Psychiatry.* 1999;4:145-154.

[40]Fatemi SH, Earle J, Kanodia R, et al. Prenatal viral infection leads to pyramidal cell atrophy and macrocephaly in adulthood: implications for genesis of autism and schizophrenia. *Cellular and Molecular Neurobiology.* 2002;1:25-33.

[41]Janusonis S, Gluncic V, Rakic P. Early serotonergic projections to Cajal-Retzius cells: relevance for cortical development. *Journal of Neuroscience.* 2004;24:1652-1659.

In: Recent Developments in Autism Research
Editor: Manuel F. Casanova, pp. 133-143

ISBN 1-59454-358-5
© 2005 Nova Science Publishers, Inc.

Chapter VI

Minicolumnar Pathology in Autism

Manuel F. Casanova [*]
Gottfried and Gisela Kolb Endowed Chair in Psychiatry University of Louisville, Department of Psychiatry, Louisville, KY

Introduction

Autism is a disorder defined by specific qualitative abnormalities in higher order human behavior and higher order cognitive abilities. Many recent advances have characterized the unique features of the behavior in autism and the underlying cognitive deficits. Research has made far less progress in defining the neuroanatomic basis of autism. Neuropathological studies have been confined to fewer than 30 whole brains, limited in scope, and primarily qualitative. The research has found remarkably little considering the devastation of this clinical disorder. Moreover, given the involvement of higher order cognitive abilities and the presence of seizures, researchers have reported a surprising scarcity of abnormalities in the cerebral cortex.[59]

Evidence of abnormalities in cerebral cortex began to emerge with reports of increased total brain volume.[2]-[4] Three recent papers have demonstrated an increase in total cerebral gray /white matter volumes and total cerebellar white matter volume.[5]-[8] These increases resulted from a transient acceleration in postnatal brain growth coinciding with the presentation of the symptoms of autism.[61],[62] This quickening apparently disrupted the developing circuitry underlying the emergence of social, language, communication, and reasoning abilities.

The increase in cerebral white matter volume, though consistent with the increase reported in brain weight, was difficult to interpret until our recent preliminary report of an increase in cortical minicolumns in 3 brain regions from 9 autopsied autistic patients.[11] Cortical minicolumns are smaller and more numerous in autism than in normal controls, indicating an abnormality of neocortical organization. Since several hundred million of these

[*] Tel: (502) 852-4077 FAX: (502) 852-4978, Email: M0CASA02@louisville.edu

minicolumn units are found throughout the cortex, small alterations in the basic template of minicolumns may exert profound effects upon information processing.

Minicolumns are the unit of vertical organization in the cerebral cortex. In the course of evolution, an increase in the numbers of minicolumns has coincided with an even greater increase in white matter. In other words, the proliferation of basic processing units corresponds with an exponential increase in those corticopetal fibers (white matter) needed to maintain connectivity with other cortical regions.[12] This first report of abnormalities in minicolumns provided a neurologically sound localization for deficits in higher order cognitive abilities. It also explained the reported increase in white matter volume and brain weight.

Background

In recent years, neuropathological studies of autism have revealed abnormalities in various brain regions. Bauman and Kemper studied whole hemispheres of 9 cases embedded in celloidin to describe the pathology in both Nissl stained and Golgi impregnated sections.[13]-[23] Bailey et al.[59] added six more cases. Thirteen others have appeared as case reports.[24]-[28] However, many of these earlier cases involved children with associated disorders such as phenylketonuria or fragments of brain tissue.

Kemper and Bauman's studies of nine brains revealed increased cell-packing density and reduced cell size in the amygdala, entorhinal cortex, subiculum, mammillary bodies and septum, and with specific dendritic abnormalities of CA1 and CA4 pyramidal cells. In the cerebellum, both Purkinje and granule cells from neocerebellar cortex show reduced numbers. Similar findings were present in the deep cerebellar nuclei (emboliform, globose and fastigial), where remaining cells were small and pale staining. Of equal importance, brain weight was available for a total of 19 reported cases and was increased by 100–200 g in the autistic children, but did not differ significantly in adult autistic patients. Thus, despite a truncation in dendritic tree development, underdeveloped cells, and a reduction in Purkinje cells, brain weight was increased in the children; furthermore, the cellular changes persisted into adulthood but with "normalized" brain weight. Bailey et al.[59] found no pathological changes in limbic structures but reported abnormalities in cortical lamination, heterotopias, and decreased Purkinje cell counts in all of the 6 specimens they studied. Four of these six cases were megalencephalic, but selection was not unbiased. This was the first study to report abnormalities of the cerebral cortex. It also advocated a central role for the cortex in autism, possibly explaining the seizures and deficits in higher order cognitive abilities in autism. They further proposed that autism involved widespread areas of the brain rather than isolated anatomical structures.[59]

While postmortem studies reported evidence of increased brain weight, clinical studies reported enlarged head circumference.[29]-[33] In analogous fashion, MRI studies have reported increased brain volume.[2]-[4],[6],[34],[35] At least three studies (a total of 172 autistic individuals) demonstrated a postnatal acceleration in brain growth. This quickening resulted in increased brain volume by 2 to 4 years of age in autism, coinciding with the presentation of symptoms.[61] Thereafter, brain growth in the autism population essentially stabilized and "normalized" by adolescence largely as a result of growth in the normal control group.[5],[6],[8] The increase in total brain volume in the autistic children resulted, remarkably, from proportionate increases in cerebral gray matter, cerebral white matter, and cerebellum. The increase in white matter was consistent with the increase in brain weight in children, as myelin adds the most weight to brain in the first years of life. However, why this occurred or existed was left unexplained. No white matter or long tract signs appeared in autism, e.g., scissors-like gait, extensor plantar response. Some have argued that autism is a subcortical white matter disorder similar in concept to subcortical dementia or multi-infarct dementia.

In addition, published and emerging functional imaging studies[36],[37] and saccadic eye movement studies[38],[39] implicated neocortical circuitry and systems. In 2002, we reported an increase in minicolumns in autism that documented substantial neuropathology in the cerebral cortex in autism. It also accounted for both the increase in cortical gray and white matter volumes observed in these patients.[11] Because minicolumns are also a unit of circuitry, the findings would also provide a potential basis for alterations in local and distant cortical connections.

Minicolumns

The minicolumn generally consists of 80–100 neurons that vertically transverse laminas II–VI. Researchers consider it to be a basic anatomical and physiological unit of the cortex.[40]-[49] Jones[42] describes the minicolumn as a unit in which "nerve cells in the middle layers of the cortex, in which thalamic afferents terminate, should be joined by narrow vertical connections to cells in layers lying superficial and deep to them...." Each minicolumn is connected with the thalamus through an afferent system and reciprocal efferents, i.e., pyramidal myelinated bundles. Recurrent collaterals of pyramidal cell axons impose other intrinsic excitatory synaptic actions. These recurrent connections provide linking pathways between columns of similar receptive field modality.

It has been suggested that as brain size increases, the number of neurons that any cell communicates with directly must decrease.[50],[51] This is because the cost of increased wiring and axonal length required to keep neurons at a fixed number of interconnections would be too great. Placing cells into functional units is one way to respond to having individual cells interconnected. An increase in the number of minicolumns (rather than neurons) results in increased connectivity between adjacent and more distant columns. Estimates of cortical interconnectivity for the human brain suggest that each minicolumn is connected to a thousand other modules.[12] In other words, if a fixed percentage of interconnections is maintained with an increasing number of minicolumns, then a larger fraction of the increased brain size is spent wiring the minicolumns.

Some researchers have argued that encephalization is the end result of acquiring supernumerary minicolumns. In other words, the reason why the human brain is a thousand fold bigger than that of mouse lies in the total number of minicolumns.[52] Otherwise there is only two or three fold increase in cortical thickness across mammalian species. An increase in the total number of minicolumns therefore provides a putative explanation to both the gray and white matter observed in the brain of autistic patients.

Minicolumns and Computerized Image Analysis

We apply our minicolumn analysis method[53] to digitized images, yielding measurements of minicolumn width (CW), neuropil space on the periphery of the minicolumn (NS) and within the column (MCS), compactness (RDR), and the gray level index (GLI). The method is briefly recapitulated here.

Neurons are segmented from background by thresholding. Due to variations in staining intensity between different sections, the threshold gray level is determined automatically on a per-image basis. Thresholding by itself tends to fuse closely packed somata into a single object, which the method described below will misinterpret as a single cell. We enhance segmentation, therefore, using the zero-crossing based edge detector of Mehrotra and Zhan[54] to locate boundaries between homogeneous regions in the original image. Pixels on these edges are set to "background" regardless of whether their gray value is above the threshold. Following this step, to exclude glial nuclei and small fragments of perikarya from analysis, objects smaller than a given threshold (15 μm2) are ignored. Another threshold (30 μm2) divides the cells into a larger class that mark minicolumn centers and a smaller class that yields data on column structure and the distribution of neuropil space.

The first stage of the column detection routine divides a region of interest into overlapping horizontal strips. Cell concentration ν is calculated within each strip by kernel smoothing, the kernel width determined heuristically based on the observation that minicolumns are about one cell wide. The second stage of the column detection routine merges columns in overlapping strips (Figure 1); relative cell-density maxima in adjacent strips are linked on a nearest neighbor basis so that the resulting combined areas are maximally vertical. The relative minima on either side of each chain become the left and right boundaries of a polygonal area containing one contiguous aggregate of cells. Aggregates with more than ten cells, allowing for a variety of structure, provide the following data:

1. Minicolumnar width, CW, is the mean left-right dimension of the polygon, where "up" points to the pial surface.
2. Mean interneuronal distance, MCS, is taken over pairs of nearby cells, rigorously defined as cells sharing an edge of the Euclidean minimum spanning tree of the cluster.
3. Peripheral neuropil space, NS, is the width of the cell-poor space on both sides of the minicolumn. Found by subtracting the width of the column core from CW.
4. Compactness, RDR, is the oblongation or ratio of second moments of the cell cluster relative to the oblongation of the polygon.
5. The gray level index, GLI, inside the polygon.

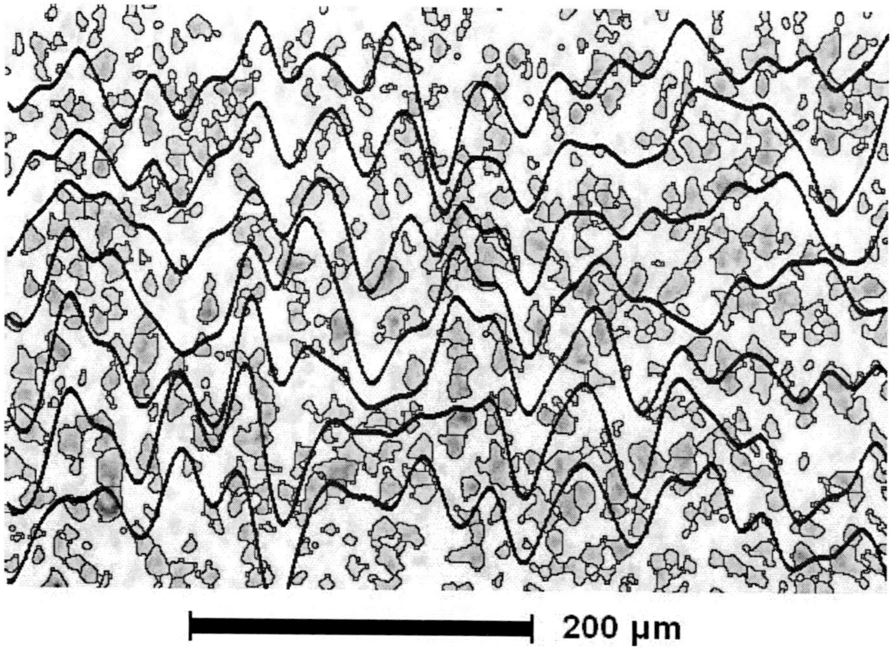

Figure 1.Superimposed on an image of cortical layer III are the boundaries of cells (dark outlines) as determined by the automatic segmentation algorithm, and the resulting cell density profiles at several depths (smooth curves), which determine the estimate of minicolumnar width (CW).

Minicolumns and Pervasive Developmental Disorders of Childhood

Using the above described methodology, we examined three brain regions (one frontal, two temporal) of both hemispheres from nine autism brains and nine controls.[11] Statistical testing used multivariate ANOVA with diagnosis (control or autistic) and Brodmann area 9, 21, and 22, as fixed factors. The Λ test of Wilks revealed significant differences between controls and autistic patients ($p = 0.002$) but the area*diagnosis interaction term was insignificant ($p = 0.388$). This suggests that changes in autism do not vary greatly between the cortical regions examined. Follow-up univariate ANOVAs on each dependent variable revealed significant differences in CW, NS, and RDR. Minicolumns in controls averaged 52.8 μm wide, compared to 46.8 μm in the autistic population, a 13% reduction (Figure 2). Autistic brains also had NS reduced by 23%, 18.7 μm as opposed to 22.8 μm in normals. The columns in autism had a less compact appearance, with a mean RDR of 1.19, while the mean RDR in controls was 1.37, a difference of 12%. Slight differences in MCS and GLI were not significant ($p = 0.538$ and $p = 0.925$, respectively).

The study revealed smaller minicolumns with reduced neuropil space bilaterally in all regions in the brains of autistic patients as compared with controls. Thus, an increased number of minicolumns per given volume of cortex appeared in the brains of autistic patients. Furthermore, four of the nine autistic cases were macroencephalic, with brain weights more than two standard deviations above the means for their corresponding ages.[55]

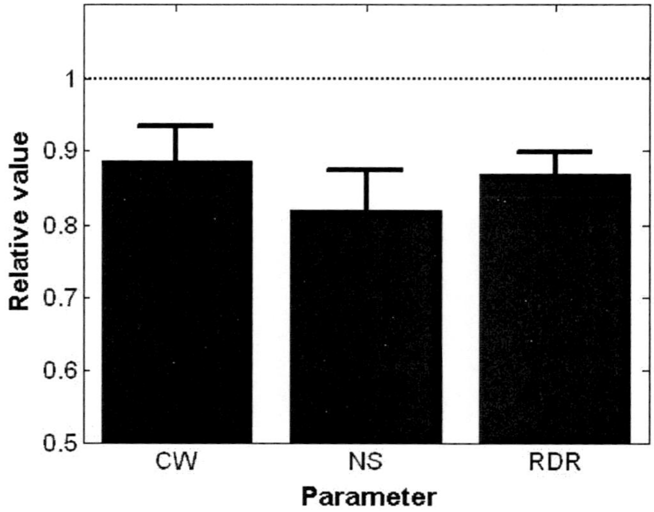

Figure 2.The means of those parameters that differ significantly ($p < 0.01$) in autism are shown here, relative to the mean value in controls (dotted line). Error bars represent one standard error. CW = minicolumn width; NS = peripheral neuropil space; RDR = compactness.

Alteration of columnar organization in brains of autistic patients could be expected to include changes either in cell type, distribution, or size. Previous measurements of neuronal density in one or a few regions in autism reported no significant findings.[24],[25] Thus far, we have obtained similar results: even though minicolumns are more closely packed, they revealed reduced cell density per minicolumn resulting in no overall change in neuronal density.[11],[56]

Our observations have now been extended to patients with Asperger's disorder, considered by many to be a higher functioning autism.[57] We examined two cases with Asperger's syndrome and eighteen controls. We anticipated that the findings in our patients would be qualitatively the same but less severe than those observed in autism. Minicolumns in one patient differed significantly from normals in Brodmann area 22 (part of Wernicke's language region) (p = 0.032, after applying the Bonferroni correction). Specifically minicolumns were smaller and their component cells more dispersed than normal. Other areas examined (9, 22) proved negative. Furthermore the second Asperger's case did not demonstrate significance but changes accrued to aging (79 years) may have obscured minicolumnar abnormalities (i.e., minicolumns become wider and less vertical with aging).[57] The minicolumnar abnormalities observed in Asperger's syndrome, are similar in morphometry but less severe in magnitude and distribution than those previously reported in autism. Further studies are needed using larger series of patients before reaching a final conclusion.

To further investigate the specificity of the reported minicolumnopathies, we investigated other cases in which various etiologies cause a syndrome that closely resembles autism. The first such etiology we identified was untreated phenylketonuria, followed by fetal rubella, fetal cytomegalovirus, and five cases of Rett syndrome. Rett syndrome is classified as a Pervasive Developmental Disorder but is a very different neurological disorder than autism. Although it has midline midbrain and nuclear brainstem abnormalities, its severe cognitive impairments implicate severe cerebral cortical dysfunction. All of these disorders are also typically associated with severe mental retardation. A pilot study of minicolumns in these cases revealed that while they shared a degree of similarity, their minicolumn abnormalities had distinguishable differences from autism. These findings suggest the existence of a family of neocortical disorders involving minicolumnar abnormalities. The minicolumn is a very complex structure and contains many components, only a few of which are measured in Nissl or myelin-stained tissue. Many if not most changes in a minicolumn are not directly apparent in these kinds of studies including details of neurochemistry, unmyelinated fiber bundles, local circuits, synaptic organization, and more. Some of these alterations secondarily affect cell location and cell column size. Therefore, changes that can be described at the level of column width, or the amount of neuropil space in the periphery, can be expected to represent "gross" alterations. This also means that minicolumn size and some other measures of the "gross" anatomy of a minicolumn can be identical at more subtle levels among brains with very different alterations.

Significance of Findings

If the minicolumn is understood as a functional unit within the larger domain of the macrocolumn, several assessments of the data are in order. First, since minicolumns are smaller in all the regions examined in autistic patients, there would be more of them per unit area of cortex. If the brains of autistic individuals were larger than normal, the difference would magnify the impact of smaller columns, resulting in a relative as well as an absolute increase in processing units. Furthermore, unchanged macrocolumn size would rearrange the distribution of afferent input and internal dendritic branching.

Researchers have posited the terminations of thalamocortical and corticocortical projections as the morphological basis of functional columns in somatosensory cortex.[58]-[60] They have been found to be fairly constant in size even across taxa that display differences of several orders of magnitude in brain size.[41],[61] A complex interaction occurs between the size of minicolumns and the brain, depending on the functionality of the area, internal anatomy of the minicolumns, and other considerations.[62] Nonetheless, evolutionary pressures keep column (mini and macro) size essentially constant while increasing total cortical surface area. Without evidence to the contrary, the afferent thalamic terminal input is presumably essentially the same in both autistic and normal brains. Since minicolumns are smaller in the brains of autistic patients, the afferent input will contact more minicolumns than in the normal configuration (Figure 3). In addition, if the brains of normal and autistic patients contain identical dendritic arborization, each dendrite in the autistic patient will contact more minicolumns than in the normal brains. This results in a greater spread of signal and a columnar circuitry pattern that differs from that of the normal brain.

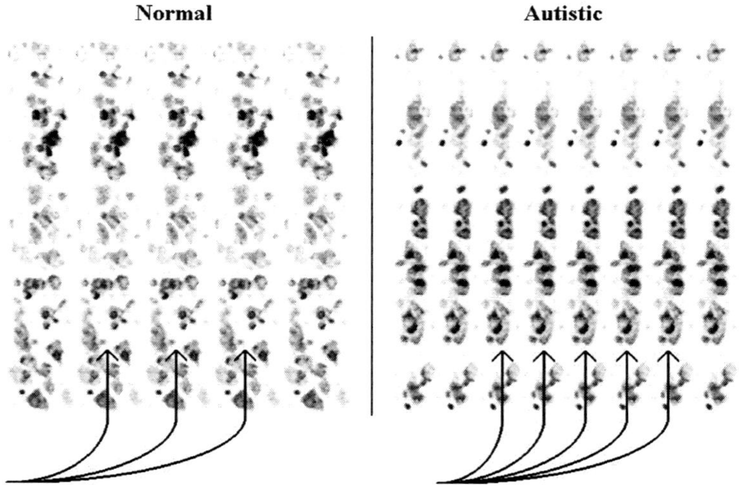

Figure 3.In this schematic illustration of thalamic input in brains of normal and autistic patients, afferent fibers, shown as arrows, innervate a region of cortex 150 μm in diameter in both cases. The same input activates more minicolumns in the autistic person (right) than the non-autistic individual (left), due to the difference in minicolumnar width.

During mammalian evolution, the development of larger brains resulted in more cell columns of similar size. During this slow process, selection pressures ensured that the addition of new cell columns would benefit the organisms or at least not prove maladaptive. In autism an acute and significant increase in processing units occurs in the course of only one generation, resulting in a proliferation of more cell columns and cortical tissue, an acute event that is not the outcome of normal selection pressures. The failure to assimilate supernumerary processing units could result in altered physiological integration of minicolumns, e.g., among themselves (association fibers), or via thalamic innervation.[63] Otherwise, computer modeling suggests that an increase in the number of minicolumns (information processing units) provides for a higher signal-to-noise ratio and improved discrimination.[64]

References

[1] Bailey A, Luther P, Dean A, et al. A clinicopathological study of autism. *Brain.* 1998; 121:889-905.

[2] Filipek P, Richelme C, Kennedy DN, et al. Morphometric analysis of the brain in developmental language disorders and autism. *Annals of Neurology.* 1992; 32:475.

[3] Piven J, Arndt S, Bailey J, Havercamp S, Andreasen NC, Palmer P. An MRI study of brain size in autism. *American Journal of Psychiatry.* 1995; 152:1145-1149.

[4] Piven J, Arndt S, Bailey J, Andreasen NC. Regional brain enlargement in autism: a magnetic resonance imaging study. *Journal of the American Academy of Child and Adolescent Psychiatry.* 1996; 35:530-536.

[5] Aylward EH, Minshew NJ, Field K, Sparks BF, Singh N. Effects of age on brain volume and head circumference in autism. *Neurology.* 2002; 59:158-159.

[6] Courchesne E, Karns CM, Davis HR, et al. Unusual brain growth patterns in early life in patients with autistic disorder: an MRI study. *Neurology.* 2001; 57:245-254.

[7] Herbert MR, Ziegler DA, Deutsch CK, et al. Dissociations of cerebral cortex, subcortical and cerebral white matter volumes in autistic boys. *Brain.* 2003; 126:1182-1192.

[8] Sparks BF, Friedman SD, Shaw DW, et al. Brain structural abnormalities in young children with autism spectrum disorder. *Neurology.* 2002; 59:158-159.

[9] Courchesne E, Carper RA, Akshoomoff NA. Evidence of brain overgrowth in the first year of life in autism. *JAMA: the Journal of the American Medical Association.* 2003; 290:337-344.

[10]Lainhart JE. Increased rate of head growth during infancy in autism. *JAMA: the Journal of the American Medical Association.* 2003; 290:393-394.

[11]Casanova MF, Buxhoeveden DP, Switala AE, Roy E. Minicolumnar pathology in autism. *Neurology.* 2002; 58:428-432.

[12]Hofman MA. Brain evolution in hominids: Are we at the end of the road? In: Falk D, Gibson KR, eds. *Evolutionary anatomy of the primate cerebral cortex.* Cambridge, UK: Cambridge University Press; 2001:113-127.

[13]Bauman ML. Microscopic neuroanatomic abnormalities in autism. *Pediatrics.* 1991; 87:791-796.

[14]Bauman ML, Kemper TL. The brain in infantile autism: a histoanatomic case report. *Neurology.* 1984; 34(Suppl. 1):275.

[15]Bauman ML, Kemper TL. Histoanatomic observations of the brain in early infantile autism. *Neurology.* 1985; 35:866-874.

[16]Bauman ML, Kemper TL. Developmental cerebellar abnormalities: a consistent finding in early infantile autism. *Neurology.* 1986; 36(Suppl. 1):190.

[17]Bauman ML, Kemper TL. Limbic involvement in a second case of early infantile autism. *Neurology.* 1987; 37(Suppl. 1):147.

[18]Bauman ML, Kemper TL. Limbic and cerebellar abnormalities: consistent findings in infantile autism. *Journal of Neuropathology and Experimental Neurology.* 1988; 47:369.

[19]Bauman ML, Kemper TL. Abnormal cerebellar circuitry in autism? *Neurology.* 1989; 39(Suppl. 1):186.

[20]Bauman ML, Kemper TL. Neuroanatomic observations of the brain in autism. In: Bauman ML, Kemper TL, eds. *The neurobiology of autism.* Baltimore, MD: The Johns Hopkins University Press; 1996:119-145.

[21]Bauman ML, Kemper TL. Is autism a progressive process? *Neurology.* 1997; 48(Suppl.):A285.

[22]Kemper TL. Neuropathology of infantile autism. *Journal of Neuropathology and Experimental Neurology.* 1998; 57:645-652.

[23]Raymond GV, Bauman ML, Kemper TL. Hippocampus in autism: a Golgi analysis. *Acta Neuropathologica.* 1996; 91:117-119.

[24]Bailey A, Luthert P, Bolton P, le Couteur A, Rutter M, Harding B. Autism and megalencephaly. *Lancet.* 1993; 341:1225-1226.

[25]Coleman PD, Romano J, Lapham L, Simon W. Cell counts in cerebral cortex of an autistic patient. *Journal of Autism and Developmental Disorders.* 1985; 15:245-255.

[26]Ritvo ER, Freeman BJ, Scheibel AB, et al. Lower Purkinje cell counts in the cerebella of four autistic subjects: initial findings of the UCLA-NSAC autopsy research report. *American Journal of Psychiatry.* 1986; 143:862-866.

[27]Rodier PM, Ingram JL, Tisdale B, Nelson S, Romano J. Embryological origin for autism: developmental anomalies of the cranial nerve motor nuclei. *Journal of Comparative Neurology.* 1996; 370:247-261.

[28]Williams RS, Hauser SL, Purpura DP, DeLong GR, Swisher CN. Autism and mental retardation: neuropathological studies performed in four retarded persons with autistic behavior. *Archives of Neurology.* 1980; 37:749-753.

[29]Davidovitch M, Patterson B, Gartside P. Head circumference measurements in children with autism. *Journal of Clinical Neurology.* 1996; 11:389-393.

[30]Rapin I. *Preschool Children with Inadequate Communication: Developmental Language Disorder, Autism, Low IQ.* London, UK: MacKeith Press; 1996.

[31]Steg JP, Rapoport JL. Minor physical anomalies in normal, neurotic, learning disabled, and severely disturbed children. *Journal of Autism and Childhood Schizophrenia.* 1975; 5:299-307.

[32]Walker HA. Incidence of minor physical anomaly in autism. *Journal of Autism and Childhood Schizophrenia.* 1977; 7:165-176.

[33]Woodhouse W, Bailey A, Rutter M, Bolton P, Baird G, le Couteur A. Head circumference in autism and other pervasive developmental disorders. *Journal of Child Psychology and Psychiatry and Allied Disciplines.* 1996; 37:665-671.

[34]Courchesne E, Muller RA, Saitoh O. Brain weight in autism: normal in the majority of cases, megalencephalic in rare cases. *Neurology.* 1999; 52:1057-1059.

[35]Fombonne E, Roge B, Claverie J, Courty S, Fremolle J. Microcephaly and macrocephaly in autism. *Journal of Autism and Developmental Disorders.* 1999; 29:113-119.

[36]Happé FGE, Brownell H, Winner E. The getting of wisdom: theory of mind in old age. *Developmental Psychology.* 1998; 34:358-362.

[37]Schultz SK, Ho B-C, Andreasen NC. Clinical features characterizing young-onset and intermediate-onset schizophrenia. *Journal of Neuropsychiatry and Clinical Neurosciences.* 2000; 12:502-505.

[38]Sweeney JA, Takarae Y, Macmillan C, Luna B, Minshew NJ. Eye movements in neurodevelopmental disorders. *Current Opinion in Neurology.* 2004; 17:37-42.

[39]Minshew NJ, Luna B, Sweeney JA. Oculomotor evidence for neocortical systems but not cerebellar dysfunction in autism. *Neurology.* 1999; 52:917-922.

[40]Mountcastle VB. Modality and topographic properties of single neurons of cat's somatic sensory cortex. *Journal of Neurophysiology.* 1957; 20:408-434.

[41]Mountcastle VB. The columnar organization of the neocortex. *Brain.* 1997;120:701-722.

[42]Jones EG. Microcolumns in the cerebral cortex. *Proceedings of the National Academy of Sciences of the United States of America.* 2000; 97:5019-5021.

[43]Kaas JH, Nelson RJ, Sur M, Merzenich MM. Organization of somatosensory cortex in primates. In: Schmitt FO, Worden FG, Adelman G, Dennis SG, eds. *The Organization of the Cerebral Cortex.* Cambridge, MA: MIT Press; 1981:237-261.

[44]Favorov OV, Whitsel BL. Spatial organization of the peripheral input to area 1 cell columns, I: the detection of "segregates." *Brain Research.* 1988; 472:25-42.

[45]Favorov OV, Whitsel BL. Spatial organization of the peripheral input to area 1 cell columns, II: the forelimb representation achieved by a mosaic of segregates. *Brain Research.* 1988; 472:43-56.

[46]Favorov OV, Kelly DG. Minicolumnar organization within somatosensory cortical segregates, I: development of afferent connections. *Cerebral Cortex.* 1994; 4:408-427.

[47]Favorov OV, Kelly DG. Minicolumnar organization within somatosensory cortical segregates, II: emergent functional properties. *Cerebral Cortex.* 1994; 4:428-442.

[48]Favorov OV, Kelly DG. Stimulus-response diversity in local neuronal populations of the cerebral cortex. *NeuroReport.* 1996; 7:2293-2301.

[49]Calvin WH. Competing for consciousness: a Darwinian mechanism at an appropriate level of explanation. *Journal of Consciousness Studies.* 1998; 5:389-404.

[50]Deacon TW. Rethinking mammalian brain evolution. *American Zoologist.* 1990; 30:629-705.

[51]Ringo JL. Neuronal interconnection as a function of brain size. *Brain, Behavior and Evolution.* 1991; 38:1-6.

[52]Rakic P, Kornack DR. Neocortical expansion and elaboration during primate evolution: a view from neuroembryology. In: Falk D, Gibson KR, eds. *Evolutionary Anatomy of the Primate Cerebral Cortex.* Cambridge, UK: Cambridge University Press; 2001:30-56.

[53]Buxhoeveden DP, Switala AE, Roy E, Casanova MF. Quantitative analysis of cell columns in the cerebral cortex. *Journal of Neuroscience Methods.* 2000; 97:7-17.

[54]Mehrotra R, Zhan S. A computational approach to zero-crossing-based two-dimensional edge detection. *Graphical Models and Image Processing.* 1996; 58:1-17.

[55]Dekaban AS, Sadowsky D. Changes in brain weights during the span of human life: relation of brain weights to body heights and body weights. *Annals of Neurology.* 1978; 4:345-356.

[56]Casanova MF, Buxhoeveden DP, Switala AE, Roy E. Minicolumnar pathology in the brains of autistic and Asperger's patients. *Neurology.* 2002; 58(Suppl. 3)A2-A3.

[57]Casanova MF, Buxhoeveden DP, Switala AE, Roy E. Asperger's syndrome and cortical neuropathology. *Journal of Child Neurology.* 2002; 17:142-145.

[58]Friedman DP, Jones EG, Burton H. Representation pattern in the second somatic sensory area of the monkey cerebral cortex. *Journal of Comparative Neurology.* 1980; 192:21-41.

[59]Jones EG, Friedman DP, Hendry SH. Thalamic basis of place- and modality-specific columns in monkey somatosensory cortex: a correlative anatomical and physiological study. *Journal of Neurophysiology.* 1982; 48:545-568.

[60]DeFelipe J, Conley M, Jones EG. Long-range focal collateralization of axons arising from corticocortical cells in monkey sensory-motor cortex. Journal of Neuroscience. 1986; 6:3749-3766.

[61]Bugbee NM, Goldman-Rakic PS. Columnar organization of corticocortical projections in squirrel and rhesus monkeys: similarity of column width in species differing in cortical volume. *Journal of Comparative Neurology.* 1983;220:355-364.

[62]Buxhoeveden DP, Casanova MF. The minicolumnar hypothesis in neurosciences. *Brain.* 2002; 125:935-951.

[63]Casanova MF, Buxhoeveden DP, Switala AE, Roy E. Neuronal density and architecture (gray level index) in the brains of autistic patients. *Journal of Child Neurology.* 2002; 17:515-521.

[64]Gustafsson L. Inadequate cortical feature maps: a neural circuit theory of autism. *Biological Psychiatry.* 1997; 42:1138-1147.

In: Recent Developments in Autism Research
Editor: Manuel F. Casanova, pp. 145-170
ISBN 1-59454-358-5
© 2005 Nova Science Publishers, Inc.

Chapter VII

The Use of Animal Models to Understand Autism Spectrum Disorder

Elizabeth M. Powell*
Department of Anatomy and Neurobiology University of Maryland
School of Medicine HSF II S251, Baltimore, MD

Introduction

The human autism spectrum disorder (ASD) encompasses a continuum of behavioral and motor dysfunctions, from the very severe forms associated with medical disorders to the relatively mild types of Asperger syndrome. ASD is a behavioral disorder which is first diagnosed in young children around the age of 1.5 years to 3 years. Now in epidemic numbers, the impact of ASD on society is tremendous, with little available effective pharmaceutical therapy. [1] Animal models of human disease attempt to mimic the deficits or outward symptoms of the disorder. In ASD many of the behavioral deficits may be unique to humans, including language deficits and emotional responses. However, comparative anatomy and behavioral neuroscience has demonstrated that the basic structures and functions of neural pathways are evolutionarily conserved throughout species. Therefore, the challenge is not to model human behavior, such as speech, in animal models but to find the ethological equivalents of the human behavior, and then to investigate perturbations to those systems.

The main dysfunction in ASD is aberrant social interaction. Autistic children display defects in normal play and instead engage in deviant imaginative play. One of the most obvious signs of an autistic-like disorder is lack of empathy and inappropriate social responses, perhaps due to the inability of the brain to integrate circuits for adaptive behavior. [2] Additional symptoms include communication and language deficits, the presence of stereotypies, repetitive and obsessive behaviors and rituals, motor deficits, and narrowly focused interests. Individuals afflicted with ASD have been reported to possess genetic, biochemical, and anatomical aberrations in addition to the behavioral and neurological

* Phone: 410-706-8189; Fax: 410-706-2512; Email: epowe001@umaryland.edu

dysfunction. [3]– [7] Postmortem studies of ASD individuals displayed abnormal arrangements of neurons in the cerebral cortex and decreased numbers of dendritic spines. Both the excitatory glutamate system and the inhibitory GABA system have been implicated as biochemical sources of ASD. [8], [9] Thus, ASD has many components to address in the design of an animal model.

The main question in developing an animal model for any disease is whether the aspects of the disease can be appropriately modeled. [10] The behavioral nature of ASD indicates that non-human primates may provide the most appropriate animal model. Yet, the success of transgenic animals, mainly mice, in mimicking other disease states is enticing. However, it may not be possible to evaluate the key aspects of autism, such as communication, in a non-primate model. [10], [11] Currently, animal models have successfully mimicked different aspects of ASD, but none have shown more than a few of the characteristics. This review will describe the current knowledge of animal behavior and highlight how each model can improve our understanding of normal brain functioning and the dysfunction present in ASD.

Genetic Origins of ASD

The continuum of ASD can be classified into four categories: 1. the classic Kanner type with communication and social dysfunction, coupled with repetitive and obsessive behaviors; 2. Asperger syndrome, with impaired social ability, but otherwise normal or superior cognitive functioning; 3. pervasive developmental disorders not otherwise specified, with milder symptoms or presentation of only some of the behaviors found in the Kanner-type of ASD; and 4. known medical disorders, such as tuberous sclerosis, that display behaviors similar to those observed in Kanner-type autism. The four categories of ASD may represent different disease mechanisms or outcomes of the interaction between genetic and environmental components. Association studies have clearly demonstrated a genetic component of ASD. [12] Twin studies report a concordance rate of 60 %–65 % in monozygotic twins, compared to nearly 0 % in dizygotic twins. [13] In addition, the rate of autism in families with one member having ASD is approximately 100 fold greater than the rate in the general population. [14] Association studies have revealed several candidate loci and genes in families afflicted with ASD of Kanner and Asperger classification and the molecular basis of several known medical disorders.

Single Gene Mutations

Tuberous Sclerosis

Mutations in two highly related tumor suppressor genes, tuberous sclerosis complex 1 (*TSC1*) and tuberous sclerosis complex 2 (*TSC2*), lead to the development of tubers, or benign tumors, in multiple organs, including the temporal lobe of the cerebral cortex. [15] While tuberous sclerosis only comprises a minute fraction of patients with ASD, from 1 %–3 %, patients with tuberous sclerosis have a high incidence of autism, up to 68 %. [12,16] The presence of the tumors is hypothesized to disrupt the formation and maintenance of neural circuitry, leading to the epileptic and autistic disorders. In fact, approximately 30 % of children with ASD also are afflicted with a seizure disorder. Thus, a direct link may exist between ASD and the *TSC1* and *TSC2*.

Several animal models have investigated the roles of *TSC1* and *TSC2* in tumor formation and cancer progression. *TSC1* encodes the protein hamartin, while the product of *TSC2* is tuberin. Hamartin and tuberin interact together to regulate growth. Homozygous null mutations in either *Tsc1* or *Tsc2* in mice are embryonic lethal, but heterozygous animals present with tumors of the kidney and the liver and increased numbers of astrocytes, but no tumors, in the brain. [17] Mice with a deletion of *Tsc1* targeted to the astrocyte population developed electroencephalographically confirmed seizures within the first postnatal month. [18] The Eker rat has a naturally occurring mutation in *Tsc2,* and it develops tubers in multiple organs, including the cerebral cortex. [19] Several transgenic mouse lines have been created to express mutant *Tsc2*, and they display increased cell proliferation. Unfortunately, it is not known whether genetic alterations in *Tsc1* and *Tsc2* lead to behavioral abnormalities. In summary, the cellular defect of tuber growth is recapitulated in some of the mutant rodents, but the subsequent behavioral effects are not yet known.

Fragile X Syndrome

Another genetic defect with a strong correlation to the presentation of ASD is Fragile X Syndrome, which is caused by mutation in the *FMR1* gene. [20] While the actual role of *FMR1* is not yet fully defined, the protein is involved in RNA metabolism. [21] Down-regulation or elimination of the *FMR1* gene product results in mental retardation and in some cases the presentation of ASD symptoms. [22] Thus, while *FMR1* mutations may represent only a subpopulation of the individuals with ASD, deciphering the role of *FMR1* in ASD may increase the understanding of the disorder.

Genetically altered mice that were missing the *Fmrl* gene were hyperactive. They displayed impairment on the Morris water maze indicative of cognitive rigidity, and they demonstrated reduced cognitive flexibility in spatial orientation learning. [23], [24] These cognitive deficits are similar to the repetitive actions and rigid interests in individuals with ASD. The behavioral results in the *Fmrl* mutant mice were dependent upon the genetic background of the mice, indicating the importance of multiple factors in ASD. The *Fmrl* deficiency appeared to be corrected in progeny from the *Fmrl* null mutant mouse crossed with an *Fmrl* over-expressing transgenic mouse, [25] indicating a role for gene therapy in correcting the human Fragile X disorder.

Mice lacking *Fmr2* had a deficit in delay-dependent fear conditioning, a slight deficit in spatial learning on the water maze, and an enhancement in long-term potentiation (LTP) that appeared to be a detriment to learning. [26] Neural anatomical characterization of the underlying circuitry has not been reported, however, dendritic spine abnormalities have been observed, providing addition parallels to ASD. In summary, disruptions in either the *Fmrl* or *Fmr2* genes in mice reduces cognitive flexibility and adaptability in learning paradigms, similar to the rigid behavioral patterns observed in individuals with ASD.

Rett Syndrome

The high prevalence of ASD among males, 4 to 5 times greater than in females, [27] has led researchers to focus on X-linked candidate genes. In addition to *FMR1*, the gene encoding methyl-CpG binding protein (*MeCP2*) is X-linked. Males with mutated *MeCP2* do not survive to term, but females appear normal at birth. [28] Within 6 to 18 months, the onset of

Rett syndrome results in the loss of any previously acquired language and communication skills. The severity and forms of the syndrome range in the affected population, with some individuals exhibiting speech abnormalities, severe cognitive defects, abnormal motor gait, stereotypies such as hand-wringing, and other autistic behaviors. [29] Similar to tuberous sclerosis and Fragile X syndrome, ASD patients diagnosed with Rett Syndrome comprise only a small fraction of autistic population. However, the simplicity of a single gene defect facilitates generation of animal models to study the disorder.

Mutations in *Mecp2* in mice lead to behavioral profiles that are remarkably similar to individuals with Rett Syndrome. Mice harboring a truncated form of *Mecp2* are normal at birth, and after 6 weeks display symptoms. [30] These animals have progressive motor abnormalities, increased anxiety, and stereotypies. Cognition was relatively normal when assessed by the water maze and contextual fear conditioning paradigms. Mice carrying a null mutation in *Mecp2* also appear normal at birth. Motor problems and cognitive defects are first observed at 5 weeks. [31], [32] It has been hypothesized that the postnatal onset of Rett is due to defects in synaptogenesis and abnormal dendritic spine formation, another hallmark of ASD and mental retardation. The deletion of *Mecp2* in the mouse appears to reproduce many of the hallmarks of Rett syndrome and possibly some of the aspects of ASD that are correlated with Rett syndrome.

Linkage and Association Studies

Numerous groups have performed genetic linkage and association studies on families and populations with autistic members. [33] From these studies, in addition to the X chromosome, chromosomes 7 and 15 have been cited as containing candidate loci. In some cases, animal models have been used to evaluate the function of the candidate genes.

Chromosome 15

Several cases of ASD have been reported with abnormalities in the 15q11-q13 locus. [12] Gene expression within the 15q11-q13 locus is very complex, with a high probability of maternal and paternal imprinting and gene duplications. Supernumerary chromosome 15 leads to autistic-like traits, including developmental delay, mental retardation, neurological and behavioral dysfunction. [33] Communication and social interactions are abnormal. Speech may be completely absent or presented as repetitious and echoing. Individuals display hyperactivity, aggression, and the inability to focus their attention. Motor deficits include clumsiness, stereotypies, ritualistic and repetitive behaviors, and self-mutilation. Both Prader-Willi and Angelman syndromes have been mapped to this location, and transgenic mice have been generated that express mutant forms of the candidate genes, providing reagents to study the disorders.

The neuro-endocrine disorder Prader-Willi syndrome is due to the deletion of the paternal allele. Individuals with this disorder have hyperphagia, obesity, psychomotor and mental retardation. While the individual gene is not known, several candidates have been implicated, including *SNURF-SNRPN* [34] and *NECDIN*. [35] Characterization of the null *Necdin* mutant mouse demonstrated enhanced learning and memory on the Morris water maze, [36] which is in contrast to the mental retardation observed in humans. However, there is no data directly linking the *SNURF-SNRPN* and *Necdin* genes to ASD. Therefore, while the genes that cause

Prader-Willi syndrome co-localize within the same chromosomal region as candidates for ASD, it appears that the disorders are distinct.

Angelman Syndrome has been reported to be a result of maternal genetic deficiencies. [37] Afflicted individuals display mental retardation, lack of speech, inappropriate laughter, seizures, and motor dysfunction. A gene encoding the E6-AP ubiquitin-protein ligase, *UBE3A*, is the cause of many of the cases of Angelman Syndrome. Genetically altered mice lacking maternal, but not paternal, *Ube3a* exhibit impaired learning in the context dependent fear conditioning test, decreased long-term potentiation, increased susceptibility to invoked audiogenic seizures, and aberrant motor function. [38] The gender dependence of the phenotype was correlated with the human condition. It should be noted that in one study, there were no mutations found in the coding region of *UBE3A* in the 10 ASD samples. [39] The mutation could however be present in regulatory regions or other genes that control *UBE3A*.

Mutant mice with null mutations in the $GABA_A$ receptor β3 (*GABRB3*), located in the 15q11-q13 locus, also demonstrated behavioral phenotypes suggestive of Angelman syndrome. [40] In addition to being hyperactive and having poor motor coordination, the *GABRB3* knockout mice exhibited abnormal electroencephalographic activity and generalized seizures. [41] Learning and memory was impaired on the step-through passive avoidance and contextual fear conditioning tests. [41], [42] Linkage analysis studies have found correlations between *GABRB3* and ASD in two groups, [43], [44] providing additional support for *GABRB3* as a genetic contributor to ASD.

Chromosome 7

The long arm of chromosome 7 has been cited as a locus for ASD. [45], [46] Several candidate genes are located within this region that directly relate to central nervous system development and function. [47–49] It is noted here that two candidate genes: *FOXP2*, a transcription factor that is implicated in speech and language, [50] and *NrCAM,* a cell adhesion molecule responsible for axonal targeting, [51] may be invaluable in ASD research, but the behavioral phenotypes of transgenic mice have not been assessed. The genes with functions that have been studied in animals include *REELIN*, serotonin receptor 2A (*5-HT2A*), engrailed (*EN2*) and *WNT2/DVL1*.

Reelin

The *reeler* mouse is a naturally occurring mutant that has been studied for decades, both for its abnormal motor phenotype and its inverted cortical and cerebellar laminar structures. Reelin is the product of the *Reeler* gene, and linkage analyses in Italian and American ASD individuals have demonstrated a correlation between polymorphisms in the 5' untranslated region and ASD. [45], [52] The *reeler* mouse displays several characteristics common to ASD including neophobia, cerebellar hypoplasia, impaired learning on the radial arm maze and in fear conditioning tests, social aggression, and abnormal sensorimotor gating or decreased PPI. [53–56] The strong correlation between genetics and behavior in the *reeler* mouse is offset by the lack of the reeler-type of anatomical defect in ASD individuals. Still, the *reeler* mouse provides a valuable tool to study ASD in rodents.

WNT2/DVL1

The *wingless/Wnt* pathway is involved in patterning during fetal development. [57] The *WNT2* gene has been implicated in ASD by both linkage and association studies. [45], [58], [59] The null mutation of *Wnt2* in mice results in 50 % perinatal lethality, due to placentation and vascularization defects. [60] Behavioral studies have not been reported in the surviving mutants. However, mice carrying null mutations for the *Disheveled 1* (*Dvl*1) gene, which is required for signal transduction of the WNTs, demonstrate unique phenotypes. [61]

Anatomically, *Dvl1* knockout mice are indiscernible from their wildtype littermates, and yet the *Dvl1* mutants display aberrant social interaction. [61] Within the setting of group housing, dominance in mice is demonstrated by whisker barbering. Wildtype mice often chew or trim the whiskers and fur of their cagemates. Often the most dominant mouse will barber the whiskers of its cagemates, such that only the dominant mouse retains a full set of whiskers. In cages housing only *Dvl1* null mutant mice, no barbering was observed, and all mice retained full sets of long whiskers. *Dvl1* knockout mice do not huddle together when sleeping, and dams do not form nests for their offspring. In a social dominance test between a wildtype and *Dvl1* mutant mouse, the *Dvl1* mouse always adapted the subordinate role. Sensorimotor gating was attenuated, but motor coordination appeared to be normal in the rotarod and wire suspension tests. No difference was recorded between wildtype and mutant animals in sensitivity to shock. Cognitive functioning, assessed by hippocampal mediated tasks, such as the Morris water maze, appeared to be normal, as were electrophysiological LTP and paired-pulse facilitation assessments. The *Dvl* mutant mouse demonstrates many of the traits found in individuals with high-functioning ASD.

Engrailed 2

The role of the mammalian homolog of the Drosophila *engrailed* gene, *En2,* in ASD is still controversial. *En2* was reported to be genetically linked to ASD45, [62], [63] or not linked to ASD. [64] The knockout *En2* mouse displays morphological abnormalities in the cerebellum. *En2* heterozygous or homozygous null mutant mice have normal motor and habituation to novelty, but show impaired motor learning on the rotarod. [65] The *En2* knockout mouse provides an unusual tool to study cerebellar function, with learning deficits in absence of general motor impairment.

Genetic Mutations in Experimental Animals that Produce ASD-like Dysfunction

The common use of laboratory animals to investigate all aspects of biology, including human disease, has produced a vast literature describing abnormal anatomy, biochemistry, and behavior. In numerous cases, the genetic mutation occurred naturally. The *reeler* mouse is one example of a naturally occurring mutation. However, *reelin*, the mutated gene in the *reeler* mouse, has now been genetically linked to ASD. [52] In other cases, a reverse genetics approach has been employed. In both approaches, the phenotype of the laboratory animal is matched to the characteristics of the human condition. Animal models which display some ASD traits have been identified.

Naturally Occurring Mutations

This review has previously described mutations in *reelin* that yield the *reeler* mouse phenotype and in *Tsc2* that results in the Eker rat. Behavioral differences in voles, guinea pigs, and rodents have been exploited to further understand human psychiatric conditions. To date, no naturally occurring mutations have been reported that lead to behavioral phenotypes in non-human primates.

Social Behavior in Voles

Astute observations between two populations of voles recognized distinct social bonding between the prairie and montane voles. Upon mating, prairie voles form a bond for life and maintain monogamous relationships. [66] In contrast, the montane vole is promiscuous and procreates with numerous partners over its lifetime. A series of biochemical and anatomical studies demonstrated that the spatial expression pattern of the oxytocin and vasopressin receptors in the forebrain regulates the mating patterns and social recognition. [66], [67] Later experiments with genetically modified mice provided additional evidence for a critical for oxytocin in mediating social recognition in all contexts not simply the mating arena. [68]

GS Guinea Pig

A mutant substrain of guinea pigs demonstrated behavioral abnormalities with striking similarities to ASD. The GS guinea pig displayed cerebral cortical and cerebellar anatomical deficits, decreased exploratory behavior, decreased social interactions, motor stereotypies, and motor pathology in cerebellar folia. [69], [70] These characteristics indicated the GS guinea pig as a good model to investigate the cerebellar aspects of ASD. Unfortunately, the GS guinea pig line succumbed to breeding difficulties and the mutation has been lost.

Brattleboro Rat

The Brattleboro rat harbors a natural mutation in the arginine vasopressin (AVP) gene. In absence of AVP, the Brattelboro rat has impaired social recognition and decreased attention and cognition. [71] Administration of exogenous AVP to the dorsolateral septum rescues the social deficit. [71] Brattleboro rats demonstrated a learning deficit in visual attention and cognition. [72] Combined with data from pair bonding in voles, the oxytocin and vasopressin systems appear to be critical in regulating social interactions, additional studies in transgenic mice are described in the next sections.

Genetically Modified Animals

Targeted genetic mutations in rodents have generated animals with numerous anatomical, biochemical and behavioral abnormalities. Many of these genes regulate synaptic transmission or development of neural circuitry, and they have been linked to ASD susceptibility loci.

Oxytocin

Oxytocin is a neuropeptide whose physiological role is classically defined as stimulating smooth muscle contractions during labor and in mammary glands during nursing. The effects of exogenously administered oxytocin are dependent upon the species ant the anatomical location of injection. Pharmaceutical blockade of oxytocin in rats leads to inhibition of the onset of postpartum maternal behavior. [73] Female oxytocin knockout mice (*OTKO*) displayed normal maternal behavior, including nest building, pup retrieval, and grooming, but they were unable to eject milk. [74] The pups emit fewer ultrasonic calls when separated from their mother, [75] suggesting a reduced fear or stress response. Thus, lack of oxytocin may affect early postnatal development.

In the adult, lack of oxytocin is implicated in social dysfunction. *OTKO* mice displayed more aggression than their wildtype littermates in isolation-induced and resident-intruder paradigms. [76] *OTKO* mice are unable to recognize other mice, although this deficit can be rescued by injection of oxytocin into the lateral ventricle. [74] The *OTKO* mice did exhibit normal learning and memory in the water maze and normal olfaction in the hidden food retrieval task. Sensorimotor gating was normal, as were responses to non-social olfactory stimuli. After a social encounter, wildtype and *OTKO* mice showed altered Fos activation in the medial amygdala, the bed nucleus of the stria terminalis, the medial preoptic area, somatosensory cortex, and hippocampus. [77] In summary, oxytocin mediates aspects of social behavior but not non-social actions. A genetic link has been found between the oxytocin receptor and ASD, [78] and children with ASD have significantly lower plasma levels of oxytocin. [79], [80] In addition, intravenous infusion of oxytocin reduced the incidence of repetitive behaviors in adult patients with ASD. [81] Thus, oxytocin appears to have a pivotal role in modulating the behavioral phenotype of ASD.

Arginine Vasopressin (AVP)

Vasopressin is a small nonapeptide that is structurally similar to oxytocin and located adjacent to it on chromosome 20. Similar to oxytocin, vasopressin plays a role in social behavior, as well as regulating blood pressure and fluid homeostasis. [82] Exogenous vasopressin stimulates social interactions in numerous species, including birds, frogs, hamsters and voles. [83], [84] As noted previously, vasopressin and vasopressin receptors regulate the establishment of monogamous pair-bonding among voles. [85] Unique polymorphisms in the *AVP* gene have been found in ASD patients [86] implying *AVP* is a candidate gene in ASD.

Injections of AVP into the lateral ventricles of male rats enhances social recognition, [87] whereas administration of antagonists of the vasopressin (V1a) receptor impairs recognition. [88] Over-expression of the V1a receptor enhances social memory. [89] In males, social recognition is also dependent upon testosterone. [90] With reference to the Brattleboro rat, lack of AVP leads to decreased social recognition, attention and cognition. [72] Similarly, mice lacking the vasopressin V1A receptor have profound impairment in social interaction tasks and decreased anxiety-like behavior, but spatial and non-social learning and memory function appear normal. [91] Thus, AVP modulates social behavior, and alterations in the AVP pathways lead to behaviors that are characteristic of the social deficits observed in ASD.

Gastrin-Related Peptide Receptor (GRPR)

Along the theme that ASD is due to decreased inhibitory tone, loss of gastrin – related peptide receptor leads to reduced inhibition. GRPR is expressed by GABAergic interneurons in the lateral amygdala. Transgenic mice lacking *Grpr* exhibited decreased inhibitory neural transmission, reduced GABA release, as well as increased LTP and persistence in long-term fear memory. [92] Performance on the water maze was normal. In humans, a *GRPR* locus has been identified in a Japanese population with infantile ASD [93] and in a northern European patient. [94] Again, while the *Grpr* null mouse does not provide a model of ASD, it demonstrates some features of the disorder.

Doublecortin (DCX)

ASD is considered a disorder with developmental origins, and thus disruptions in genes that regulate the formation of neural circuitry may lead to neurological and psychological disorders. The doublecortin gene (*DCX*) is X-linked and mediates neuronal migration and lamination in the cerebral cortex and hippocampus. [95] Mutations in *DCX* lead to lissencephaly in males and the formation of a heterotopic band of neurons in the white matter in females. [96], [97] Transgenic *Dcx* null mice did not display the cerebral cortical anatomical defects, but they did show the abnormal hippocampal lamination. [98] Tests of hippocampal mediated functions demonstrated impaired cued and context-mediated fear conditioning. While the long arm of the X chromosome has been implicated in ASD, the role of the doublecortin gene in epilepsy and mental retardation in patients with ASD has now been excluded. Nonetheless, the abnormal hippocampal structure in mice provides a neural substrate for evaluating aberrant circuit formation.

Brain Derived Neurotrophic Factor (BDNF)

Brain derived neurotrophic factor (BDNF) regulates the formation of neural circuitry during the perinatal and postnatal period. BDNF is elevated in neonates and children afflicted with ASD and mental retardation, [99] but not in Rett syndrome. [100] Elevation of BDNF in the brains of mice, in a transgenic over-expressing line, increased the hyperexcitability of the hippocampus and the susceptibility for generalized seizures. [101] The over-expressing *Bdnf* mice also exhibited impaired learning on the passive avoidance test, which is a measure of cognitive flexibility. Genetic linkage studies have not yet revealed *BDNF* as a candidate. Genetic null mutations in *Bdnf* are embryonic lethal, but forebrain-targeted *Bdnf* null mice failed to learn in the Morris water maze and were unable to properly associate cues in fear conditioning or discrimination tasks. [102] Thus decrease in BDNF concentration in the forebrain reduced cognitive flexibility and adaptability, mimicking a characteristic of ASD.

Nicotinic Acetylcholine Receptor Subunit β2 (nAChRβ2)

In the cerebral cortex, nicotine activates prefrontal and cingulate regions and enhances attention and cognition. [103–105] Receptor binding studies have demonstrated decreased nicotinic acetylcholine receptor expression in the cerebral cortex and cerebellum of autistic patients, along with those afflicted with Alzheimer's disease and schizophrenia. [106], [107] The studies also indicate a degree of receptor subunit specificity associated with each condition. In ASD patients, receptors containing the β2 subunit were decreased dramatically. [108], [109] Biochemical and histological localization data from ASD post-mortem tissue provides additional support for the role of *nAChRβ2* in ASD. Thus, a strong correlation exists between reductions in nicotinic receptors and ASD.

In rodents, nicotine stimulates glutamate release from prefrontal cortical areas, [110] regions that are known to regulate attention and cognitive flexibility. In absence of the β2 subunit of the nicotine acetylcholine receptor, the *nAChRβ2* null mice displayed improved spatial learning in a modified cross maze test. However, the *β2* null mutant mice simultaneously exhibited increased navigation and decreased exploratory behaviors in the circular open field test, suggesting altered organization of behavior. [111] The *β2* null mice did not have normal adaptive processing or cognitive flexibility to the altered environment; nor did these mice show sensitization to a new environment. Additional behavioral abnormalities included disturbed social interaction sequences and inability to modify routine behavior when presented with mild conflict. Overall, the behavioral profiles of the *β2* null mice showed many similarities to observations of ASD individuals.

Glutamate Receptor 6 – (Grik2)

Another possible gene candidate for causing altered neurotransmission is *Grik2*, the gene for the kainate glutamate receptor 6, also known as *GluR6*. Linkage studies identified several small nucleotide polymorphisms in *Grik2* in ASD individuals. [112] Transgenic mice lacking *Grik2* are less susceptible to kainate induced seizures. These animals displayed abnormal sensory motor coordination and motivations. [113] Thus, the *Grik2* mice exhibit some features of ASD.

GABA System

Defects in the GABA system have been implicated in several neurological disorders, including epilepsy and ASD [9]. Individuals with ASD have a 50 % reduction in both synthetic GABA enzymes, GAD67 and GAD65, in parietal and cerebellar cortices. [114] The development of the GABA system in the forebrain has been a very active area of research during the last decade. Many of the molecular cues that specify GABAergic neurons or regulate their migration and differentiation have been identified. However, genetically modified mice lacking these cues often die *in utero* or perinatally. One exception is a mouse lacking the urokinase plasminogen activator receptor (*uPAR*) gene. The *uPAR* null mouse appears to have defects in many stages of GABAergic interneuron development, generation, migration and differentiation. The deficits are most likely mediated by hepatocyte growth factor/scatter factor (HGF/SF) through its receptor MET. [115], [116] Anatomical characterization of embryonic, postnatal and adult brains demonstrated a loss of nearly 50 % of the GABAergic cells in the frontal and parietal cortical areas; the cerebellum has not yet been examined. The adult *uPAR* null mouse exhibits spontaneous seizures that were confirmed electroencephalographically, increased anxiety, and decreased social behavior. [116] It is not known how uPAR interacts with molecules in the GABA pathway. No linkage studies indicate that *uPAR* is located within an autism susceptibility locus. However, the *MET* receptor is found within the long arm of human chromosome 7 in the autism susceptibility locus.

Glutamic Acid Decarboxylase (Gad 65)

Complete loss of GABA synthesizing enzymes, glutamic acid decarboxylases 67 and 65, in mice is either neonatal lethal for the *Gad67* gene [117] or leads to incessant generalized seizures for the *Gad65* gene. [118] *Gad65* null mice also show increased anxiety on the elevated zero maze and the light-dark avoidance test. [119] Synaptic plasticity was altered, and long-term depression in visual cortical slices from *Gad65* null mice was significantly weaker than in controls. [120] On a functional level, the loss of *Gad65* leads to improper formation of ocular dominance columns, demonstrating abnormal postnatal neural circuit development. [121]

$GABA_A$ Receptor Subunit β3 (GABRB3)

Further evidence for ASD being a result of insufficient inhibitory neural transmission is provided by studies of the $GABA_A$ receptor subunit β3 (*GABRB3*). A full genome scan linked *GABRB3* to ASD. [45] Genetically altered mice, missing *GABRB3* are hyperactive and hyper-responsive to sensory stimuli. [40] The mutant mice demonstrate motor problems; they have difficulty walking on platforms, the rotarod, and on grids. They are uncoordinated and walk with an unsteady (jerky) gait. The majority of the mutant mice are afflicted with generalized seizures, another common trait in ASD.

GDP Dissociation Inhibitor (α-Gdi1)

The *Gdi1* gene encodes a protein that is a GDP dissociation inhibitor that regulates vesicle fusion and hence synaptic transmission. [122], [123] The gene encodes two forms of the GDI protein, and α-Gdi is the most abundant form in the brain. *Gdi1* has been linked to X-linked mental retardation by several groups, [124–128] but not specifically to ASD. GDI is critical for proper axon outgrowth and formation of neural circuitry. In absence of *Gdi*, lamination in the hippocampus is disrupted and social behavior and some cognitive tasks are impaired. [129] While *Gdi* knockout mice perform similarly to wildtype mice in spatial memory tasks, such as the Morris water maze, they show deficits in short-term memory in the radial arm maze and in the trace but not delay fear-conditioning tests. The *Gdi* knockout mice are less aggressive in the resident-intruder test. The behavioral profile of the *Gdi* null mouse when combined with the genetics studies state a strong case for their involvement in mental retardation. Considering the overlap between mental retardation and ASD, as approximately 70 % of ASD individuals are mentally retarded, it is highly likely that mutations in *Gdi* also contribute to ASD.

Serotonin System

Individuals with ASD have increased plasma and urine concentrations of serotonin (5-HT). [130], [131] Serotonin reuptake inhibitors provide some pharmaceutical relief to the social deficits and repetitive compulsive actions observed in ASD. [132¯134] The role of serotonin in ASD has been a very active focus of research, and possible genetic linkages and associations between the serotonin system and ASD have been widely reported. [62], [135]–[140]

The serotonin transporter gene has been genetically eliminated in mice, and the mice displayed increased anxiety on the elevated zero maze and light-dark avoidance tests. [141], [142] Mice lacking serotonin receptors demonstrated behavioral features common to ASD. Loss of the serotonin 1A receptor may lead to altered emotional states, in particular increased anxiety, although the phenotype is highly dependent upon the background of the mouse strain and the laboratory performing the analysis. [143–145] Lack of the serotonin 2C receptor led to spontaneous epilepsy, increased susceptibility to invoked seizures, increased sensitivity and responsiveness to stress, and repetitive actions and stereotypies. [143], [146]– [148] In summary, alterations in the serotonin system mimic some, but not all, of the features to ASD.

Evironmental Models of ASD

Disease Models

Epidemiological studies demonstrate associations between maternal viral exposure and the frequency of neurological and psychiatric disorders in the offspring. It should be noted that the majority of individuals with ASD do not have a medical history that includes viral infection. The association between ASD and the measles-mumps-rubella vaccine has not been confirmed and is still a controversial topic. [149] On the other hand, maternal influenza infection causes still births and miscarriages, as well as increased risk of schizophrenia and ASD. [150]– [152] Several other viruses, including varicella zoster and diphtheria also have been implicated as the cause of neurological disorders. The common component to all of these infections is the systemic anti-viral response, which often includes release of growth factors and cytokines. Animal models of ASD have used *in utero* and neonatal exposure to viral infections to elucidate possible mechanisms.

Maternal infection of mouse dams with human influenza virus during early development, prior to the formation of the forebrain, induces short-term anatomical and long-term behavioral deficits in the offspring. Postnatal mice exhibited altered neuronal cell density and abnormal generation of the cerebral cortex. Adult mice had increased overall brain size and decreased ventricular area, analogous to human ASD. [153] Affected adult offspring have decreased exploratory behavior, reduced PPI suggesting sensorimotor deficits, and abnormal responses to anti-pyschotic drugs in the PPI paradigm. [154] The affected mice exhibited decreased social interactions. No virus was found in the brains of adult mice that were prenatally exposed to influenza, eliminating the possibility of continual infection. The behavioral dysfunction is hypothesized to be due to activation of the immune system and cytokine and chemokine mediated mechanisms. Additional experiments have demonstrated that the abnormal behavior is not specific to influenza; maternal injection with the chemical compound poly(I:C) evokes an anti-viral response in absence of infection, and leads to similar behavioral dysfunction in the offspring. [155] This animal model provides a paradigm to test prenatal environmental causes of ASD.

Postnatal exposure to viral infections also leads to behaviors that mimic ASD. The most common animal protocol is the inoculation of Borna disease virus intracranially into neonatal rat pups, causing a persistent infection for many weeks. Anatomical and behavioral assessment of adolescent rats (1 month old) demonstrated several features that were analogous to ASD. In one study, infected rats were growth-retarded and unable to walk normally, with delayed righting responses. [156] Abnormal gait was observed in all Borna virus infected rats at one year of age. The infected rats were hyperactive in open field and novel environment tests, and they exhibited increased rearing and sniffing and stereotypic behaviors Anatomical changes included severe cerebral atrophy and cell loss by apoptotic mechanisms. Other reports using the same Borna virus paradigm have shown hippocampal cell loss, impaired spatial learning and memory in the water maze, [157] abnormal social play behavior, [158] increased anxiety, and hyper-reactivity to aversive stimuli. [159] Though the long-term intracranial Borna virus infection paradigm is an experimental tool, with a slight chance of occurrence outside of the laboratory, all of behavior abnormalities mirror the features of ASD.

Maternal Separation Stress

Early hypotheses about the basis of many psychiatric and neurological disorders focused on non-biological origins. Often psychiatric diseases were believed to be a result of poor parenting, including child abuse. [160], [161] Using modern biological and clinical tools, several very recent reports indicate that early life experience contributes to the formation of neural circuitry and behavioral responses. [161]

A commonly studied paradigm of early life stress is short-term maternal separation. Rodent and non-human primate studies have clearly shown a causal relationship between plasma levels of adrenocorticotropic hormone (ACTH), cortisol, and corticotrophin-releasing factor (CRF) and stress. Maternal separation increases levels of all three hormones acutely and up to 24 h post-stress. [162], [163] Increased maternal care giving decreases the levels. Adult rats, that had previously experienced maternal separation stress as neonates, exhibited long-term effects. ACTH and cortisol levels were elevated in response to novel objects and restraint stress. The rats displayed decreased exploration and increased freezing the open field test, and increased acoustic startle response. [164]– [166] Biochemical analysis showed deficits in the GABA system, including decreased densities of benzodiazepam receptors and decreased inhibitory tone. [167] Thus, rats exposed to early life stress display biochemical and behavioral characteristics that parallel individuals with ASD.

External Stimuli

The development of functional neural networks includes a time period of refinement, known as the critical period, when transient connections are either permanently established or abrogated. In the visual system, the diversity of everyday stimuli increases neural activity and the release of BDNF. In classical studies, the absence of stimulus diversity reduces neural activity and has long-lasting effects including loss of binocular vision or recognition of certain patterns. [168], [169] In transgenic animals, the lack of growth factors, such as BDNF, lead to similar outcomes; the critical period does not end, and the neural network is not properly established. [170] In contrast, over-expression of BDNF has the opposite effect, the prematurely high levels of the growth factor cause early termination of the critical period, and improper formation of the neural network. [171] The auditory system follows an analogous developmental pathway, and rats reared in the presence of modulated noise have an impaired ability to distinguish among sounds, an improperly differentiated auditory cortex, and early closure of the critical period, possibly due to increased release of BDNF. [172], [173] The noise reared rats demonstrate abnormal electrical coupling between cortical regions, and are more susceptible to seizure induction. By contrast, constant noise prevents the critical period from ending and also leads to auditory deficits. [174] Individuals with ASD can be hypersensitive and hyper-responsive to sensory cues, caused by malformed cortical networks, possibly due to increased growth factor levels. The animal models with abnormal sensory stimuli can provide a greater understanding of the development of the critical period and consequences of disruptions. [175]

Another form of external stimulus is social interaction. In young and adolescent animals most social interactions are in the form of play. Studies in rats have demonstrated that rough-and-tumble play elicits a laughter-like response, which can be easily measured and correlated to other behavioral measures. [176] Young rats that were exposed to increased play and tickling exhibited an overall increased positive affect and increased attention. [177] Play therapy reduced hyperactivity and increased attention and cognitive flexibility in rats with frontal cortical lesions, in a model of attention deficit/hyperactivity disorder. [178] The results may have been mediated by BDNF. [179] These studies address the development of the neural substrates and possible plasticity of the emotional pathways, and they may provide models of therapies to reverse the social deficits in ASD.

Anatomical and Chemical Lesion Models of ASD

Rodents

Another paradigm to address the question of the neural substrates of neurological and psychiatric disorders is to eliminate a candidate structure or pathway with the goal of recreating the dysfunction. Lesions in the rat amygdala at postnatal day 7 lead to hyperactivity, decreased juvenile play behavior, increased response to stress, and abnormal social behavior. [180] In the same study, lesions in the amygdala in the postnatal 21 day old rat produced only the abnormal social behavior in the adult. Rats with midline lesions of the cerebellar vermis display persevering behavior (cognitive rigidity) and hyperactivity. [181] Thus, alterations in specific structures, such as the amygdala and cerebellum, generate abnormalities that resemble ASD.

The hypothesis that ASD is due to reduced or altered neurotransmission has been tested pharmacologically. Adult mice were rendered hypoglutamatergic by treatment with NMDA receptor agonist MK801 and then evaluated in several tasks. MK801 treatment caused defective habituation, impaired attention, limited ethological measures of grooming, rearing, and explorative digging. [182] Treatment with anti-psychotic agents had varying effects: haloperidol had no effect, but serotonin transporter blockers partially restored some behaviors. In contrast, increasing GABA concentration during development causes cerebellar anomalies with anatomical similarities to children with ASD. [183] Preliminary reports indicate that prenatal valproic acid exposure negatively affects social memory in rats. [184]

Non-Human Primate Lesion Models

While most animal models of ASD are rodents, the behavioral dysfunction in ASD may be best examined the primate. However, only a handful of studies have reported primate behavioral abnormalities that are similar to the deficits witnessed in ASD. Lesions in the amygdala of infant macaques demonstrate abnormal responses to fear and novelty, but social behavior is unaffected. [185], [186] These studies suggest that the anxiety, but not social, component of ASD may be modulated by the amygdala. Bilateral temporal lesions, including the amygdala, in newborn rhesus monkeys initially led to aberrant social and emotional behaviors in the adolescents. [187] But the phenotype was transient, and when the lesioned monkeys reached adulthood, their behavior could not be distinguished from control unlesioned animals. Yet, similar lesions in adult monkeys cause obsessive touching and mouthing of objects. [188] Finally, hippocampal lesions in rhesus monkeys do give rise to socioemotional abnormalities in the adult. [189] Thus, current lesion studies in the primate need to be expanded to gain a further understanding of the neural substrates of social behavior. [190]

Maternal separation studies in non-human primates provide another paradigm for exploring the basis of behavior. Adult rhesus monkeys, who were permanently separated from their mothers at infancy, display increased startle responses (PPI). [191] In another study, maternally-separated adult rhesus monkeys had social and emotional behavior abnormalities. The monkeys demonstrated increased stereotypies, decreased social interactions, and decreased oxytocin concentrations. [192] The long-term consequences of separation stress were similar in non-human primates and rodents.

Future Challenges

The complexity of ASD is uniquely challenging. ASD individuals present deficits in speech and language, yet no other animal can use speech to communicate. Although non-speech forms of communication can be easily assessed in non-human primate models. The social behaviors, cognitive rigidity, and motor deficits in ASD can be more easily mirrored by both rodent and primate models. The development of animal models will need to combine the powerful tools of molecular and cellular biology and genomic research with cognitive neuroscience. [10] To this end, studies have been initiated to investigate differences in gene transcription in temporal lobe structures of maternally separated and maternally raised monkeys. [193] The results from this study and others are eagerly awaited.

References

[1] Gerlai J, Gerlai R. Autism: a large unmet medical need and a complex research problem. *Physiology and Behavior.* 2003; 79:461-470.

[2] Harris JC. Social neuroscience, empathy, brain integration, and neurodevelopmental disorders. *Physiology and Behavior.* 2003; 79:525-531.

[3] Hill EL. Executive dysfunction in autism. *Trends in Cognitive Science.* 2004; 8:26-32.

[4] Casanova MF, Buxhoeveden DP, Switala AE, Roy E. Minicolumnar pathology in autism. *Neurology.* 2002; 58:428-432.

[5] Casanova MF, Buxhoeveden DP, Brown C. Clinical and macroscopic correlates of minicolumnar pathology in autism. *Journal of Child Neurology.* 2002; 17:692-695.

[6] Young JG, Kavanagh ME, Anderson GM, Shaywitz BA, Cohen DJ. Clinical neurochemistry of autism and associated disorders. *Journal of Autism and Developmental Disorders.* 1982; 12:147-165.

[7] Rapin I, Katzman R. Neurobiology of autism. *Annals of Neurology.* 1998; 43:7-14.

[8] Blatt GJ, Fitzgerald CM, Guptill JT, Booker AB, Kemper TL, Bauman ML. Density and distribution of hippocampal neurotransmitter receptors in autism: an autoradiographic study. *Journal of Autism and Developmental Disorders.* 2001; 31:537-543.

[9] Hussman JP. Suppressed GABAergic inhibition as a common factor in suspected etiologies of autism. *Journal of Autism and Developmental Disorders.* 2001; 31:247-248.

[10] Caviness VS. Research strategies in autism: a story with two sides. *Current Opinion in Neurology.* 2001; 14:141-143.

[11]Seong E, Seasholtz AF, Burmeister, M. Mouse models for psychiatric disorders. *Trends in Genetics.* 2002; 18:643-650.

[12]Andres C. Molecular genetics and animal models in autistic disorder. *Brain Research Bulletin.* 2002;57:109-119.

[13]Bailey A, Le Couteur A, Gottesman I, et al. Autism as a strongly genetic disorder: evidence from a British twin study. *Psychological Medicine.* 1995;25:63-77.

[14]Rutter M, Silberg J, O'Connor T, Simonoff E. Genetics and child psychiatry, I: advances in quantitative and molecular genetics. *Journal of Child Psychology and Psychiatry and Allied Disciplines.* 1999; 40:3-18.

[15]Chugani DC, Chugani HT, Muzik O, et al. Imaging epileptogenic tubers in children with tuberous sclerosis complex using alpha- [11C]methyl-L-tryptophan positron emission tomography. *Annals of Neurology.* 1998; 44:858-866.

[16]Smalley SL, Tanguay PE, Smith M,Gutierrez G. Autism and tuberous sclerosis. *Journal of Autism and Developmental Disorders.* 1992; 22:339-355.

[17]Kobayashi T, Minowa O, Kuno J, Mitani H, Hino O, Noda T. Renal carcinogenesis, hepatic hemangiomatosis, and embryonic lethality caused by a germ-line Tsc2 mutation in mice. *Cancer Research.* 1999; 59:1206-1211.

[18]Uhlmann EJ, Wong M, Baldwin RL, et al. Astrocyte-specific TSC1 conditional knockout mice exhibit abnormal neuronal organization and seizures. *Annals of Neurology.* 2002; 52:285-296.

[19]Mizuguchi M, Takashima S, Yamanouchi H, Nakazato Y, Mitani H, Hino O. Novel cerebral lesions in the Eker rat model of tuberous sclerosis: cortical tuber and anaplastic ganglioglioma. *Journal of Neuropathology and Experimental Neurology.* 2000; 59:188-196.

[20]Verheij C, Bakker CE, de Graaff E, et al. Characterization and localization of the FMR-1 gene product associated with fragile X syndrome. *Nature.* 1993; 363:722-724.

[21]Carthew RW. RNA interference: the fragile X syndrome connection. *Current Biology.* 2002; 12:R852-854.

[22]Bailey DB Jr, Hatton DD, Skinner M, Mesibov G. Autistic behavior, FMR1 protein, and developmental trajectories in young males with fragile X syndrome. *Journal of Autism and Developmental Disorders.* 2001; 31:165-174.

[23]Galvez R, Gopal AR, Greenough WT. Somatosensory cortical barrel dendritic abnormalities in a mouse model of the fragile X mental retardation syndrome. *Brain Research.* 2003; 971:83-89.

[24]D'Hooge R, Nagels G, Franck F, et al. Mildly impaired water maze performance in male Fmr1 knockout mice. *Neuroscience.* 1997; 76:367-376.

[25]Peier AM, McIlwain KL, Kenneson A, Warren ST, Paylor R, Nelson DL. (Over)correction of FMR1 deficiency with YAC transgenics: behavioral and physical features. *Human Molecular Genetics.* 2000; 9:1145-1159.

[26]Gu Y, McIlwain KL, Weeber EJ, et al. Impaired conditioned fear and enhanced long-term potentiation in Fmr2 knock-out mice. *Journal of Neuroscience.* 2002; 22:2753-2763.

[27]Jamain S, Quach H, Quintana-Murci L, et al. Y chromosome haplogroups in autistic subjects. *Molecular Psychiatry.* 2002; 7:217-219.

[28]Percy AK. Rett syndrome: current status and new vistas. *Neurologic Clinics.* 2002;20:1125-1141.

[29]Mount RH, Charman T, Hastings RP, Reilly S, Cass H. Features of autism in Rett syndrome and severe mental retardation. *Journal of Autism and Developmental Disorders.* 2003;33:435-442.

[30]Shahbazian M, Young J, Yuva-Paylor L, et al. Mice with truncated MeCP2 recapitulate many Rett syndrome features and display hyperacetylation of histone H3. *Neuron.* 2002;35:243-254.

[31]Chen RZ, Akbarian S, Tudor M, Jaenisch R. Deficiency of methyl-CpG binding protein-2 in CNS neurons results in a Rett-like phenotype in mice. *Nature Genetics.* 2001;27:327-331.

[32]Branchi I, Bichler Z, Berger-Sweeney J, Ricceri L. Animal models of mental retardation: from gene to cognitive function. *Neuroscience and Biobehavioral Reviews.* 2003; 27:141-153.

[33]Lamb JA, Moore J, Bailey A, Monaco AP. Autism: recent molecular genetic advances. *Human Molecular Genetics.* 2000; 9:861-868.

[34]Wirth J, Back E, Hüttenhofer A, et al. A translocation breakpoint cluster disrupts the newly defined 3′ end of the *SNURF-SNRPN* transcription unit on chromosome 15. *Human Molecular Genetics.* 2001; 10:201-210.

[35]Watrin F, Roeckel N, Lacroix L, et al. The mouse Necdin gene is expressed from the paternal allele only and lies in the 7C region of the mouse chromosome 7, a region of conserved synteny to the human Prader-Willi syndrome region. *European Journal of Human Genetics.* 1997; 5:324-332.

[36]Muscatelli F, Abrous DN, Massacrier A, et al. Disruption of the mouse Necdin gene results in hypothalamic and behavioral alterations reminiscent of the human Prader-Willi syndrome. *Human Molecular Genetics.* 2000; 9:3101-3110.

[37]Perk J, Makedonski K, Lande L, Cedar H, Razin A,Shemer R. The imprinting mechanism of the Prader-Willi/Angelman regional control center. *EMBO Journal.* 2002; 21:5807-5814.

[38]Miura K, Kishino T, Li E, et al. Neurobehavioral and electroencephalographic abnormalities in Ube3a maternal-deficient mice. *Neurobiology of Disease.* 2002; 9:149-159.

[39]Veenstra-VanderWeele J, Gonen D, Leventhal BL, Cook EH Jr. Mutation screening of the UBE3A/E6-AP gene in autistic disorder. *Molecular Psychiatry.* 1999; 4:64-67.

[40]Homanics GE, DeLorey TM, Firestone LL, et al. Mice devoid of γ-aminobutyrate type A receptor β3 subunit have epilepsy, cleft palate, and hypersensitive behavior. *Proceedings of the National Academy of Sciences of the United States of America.* 1997; 94:4143-4148.

[41]DeLorey TM, Handforth A, Anagnostaras SG, et al. Mice lacking the β3 subunit of the GABAA receptor have the epilepsy phenotype and many of the behavioral characteristics of Angelman syndrome. *Journal of Neuroscience.* 1998; 18:8505-8514.

[42]DeLorey TM, Olsen RW. GABA and epileptogenesis: comparing gabrb3 gene-deficient mice with Angelman syndrome in man. *Epilepsy Research.* 1999; 36:123-132.

[43]Cook EH Jr, Lindgren V, Leventhal BL, et al. Autism or atypical autism in maternally but not paternally derived proximal 15q duplication. *American Journal of Human Genetics.* 1997;60:928-934.

[44]Maddox LO, Menold MM, Bass MP, et al. Autistic disorder and chromosome 15q11-q13: construction and analysis of a BAC/PAC contig. *Genomics.* 1999; 62:325-331.

[45]Gutknecht L. Full-genome scans with autistic disorder: a review. *Behavior Genetics.* 2001; 31:113-123.

[46]Hutcheson HB, Bradford Y, Folstein SE, et al. Defining the autism minimum candidate gene region on chromosome 7. *American Journal of Medical Genetics.* 2003; 117B:90-96.

[47]Barrett S, Beck JC, Bernier R, et al. An autosomal genomic screen for autism: collaborative linkage study of autism. *American Journal of Genetic Medicine.* 1999; 88:609-615.

[48]Risch N, Spiker D, Lotspeich L, et al. A genomic screen of autism: evidence for a multilocus etiology. *American Journal of Human Genetics.* 1999; 65:493-507.

[49]Philippe A, Martinez M, Guilloud-Bataille M, et al. Genome-wide scan for autism susceptibility genes: Paris Autism Research International Sibpair Study. *Human Molecular Genetics.* 1999; 8:805-812.

[50]Lai CS, Gerrelli D, Monaco AP, Fisher SE, Copp AJ. FOXP2 expression during brain development coincides with adult sites of pathology in a severe speech and language disorder. *Brain.* 2003; 126:2455-2462.

[51]Volkmer H, Leuschner R, Zacharias U, Rathjen FG. Neurofascin induces neurites by heterophilic interactions with axonal NrCAM while NrCAM requires F11 on the axonal surface to extend neurites. *Journal of Cell Biology.* 1996; 135:1059-1069.

[52]Persico AM, D'Agruma L, Maiorano N, et al. Reelin gene alleles and haplotypes as a factor predisposing to autistic disorder. *Molecular Psychiatry.* 2001; 6:150-159.

[53]Fatemi SH. Reelin mutations in mouse and man: from reeler mouse to schizophrenia, mood disorders, autism and lissencephaly. *Molecular Psychiatry.* 2001; 6:129-133.

[54]Tueting P, Costa E, Dwivedi Y, et al. The phenotypic characteristics of heterozygous reeler mouse. *Neuroreport.* 1999;10:1329-1334.

[55]Goldowitz D, Koch J. Performance of normal and neurological mutant mice on radial arm maze and active avoidance tasks. *Behavioral and Neural Biology.* 1986; 46:216-226.

[56]Salinger WL, Ladrow P,Wheeler C. Behavioral phenotype of the reeler mutant mouse: effects of RELN gene dosage and social isolation. *Behavioral Neuroscience.* 2003; 117:1257-1275.

[57]Sussman DJ, Klingensmith J, Salinas P, Adams PS, Nusse R, Perrimon N. Isolation and characterization of a mouse homolog of the *Drosophila* segment polarity gene dishevelled. *Developmental Biology.* 1994; 166:73-86.

[58]Wassink TH, Piven J, Vieland, VJ, et al.Evidence supporting WNT2 as an autism susceptibility gene. *American Journal of Medical Genetics.* 2001; 105:406-413.

[59]Honey GD, Fletcher PC, Bullmore ET. Functional brain mapping of psychopathology. *Journal of Neurology, Neurosurgery and Psychiatry.* 2002; 72:432-439.

[60]Monkley SJ, Delaney SJ, Pennisi DJ, Christiansen JH, Wainwright BJ. Targeted disruption of the Wnt2 gene results in placentation defects. *Development.* 1996; 122:3343-3353.

[61]Lijam N, Paylor R, McDonald MP, et al. Social interaction and sensorimotor gating abnormalities in mice lacking Dvl1. *Cell.* 1997; 90:895-905.

[62]Trottier G, Srivastava L, Walker CD. Etiology of infantile autism: a review of recent advances in genetic and neurobiological research. *Journal of Psychiatry and Neuroscience.* 1999; 24:103-115.

[63]Petit E, Herault J, Martineau J, et al. Association study with two markers of a human homeogene in infantile autism. *Journal of Medical Genetics.* 1995; 32: 269-274.

[64]Zhong H, Serajee FJ, Nabi R, Huq AH. No association between the EN2 gene and autistic disorder. *Journal of Medical Genetics.* 2003; 40:e4.

[65]Gerlai R, Millen KJ, Herrup K, Fabien K, Joyner AL, Roder J. Impaired motor learning performance in cerebellar En-2 mutant mice. *Behavioral Neuroscience.* 1996; 110:126-133.

[66]Young LJ, Winslow JT, Nilsen R, Insel TR. Species differences in V1a receptor gene expression in monogamous and nonmonogamous voles: behavioral consequences. *Behavioral Neuroscience.* 1997;111:599-605.

[67]Insel TR. A neurobiological basis of social attachment. *American Journal of Psychiatry.* 1997;154:726-735.

[68]Pitkow LJ, Sharer CA, Ren X, Insel TR, Terwilliger EF, Young LJ. Facilitation of affiliation and pair-bond formation by vasopressin receptor gene transfer into the ventral forebrain of a monogamous vole. *Journal of Neuroscience.* 2001; 21:7392-7396.

[69]Lev-Ram V, Valsamis M, Masliah E, Levine S, Godfrey HP. A novel non-ataxic guinea pig strain with cerebrocortical and cerebellar abnormalities. *Brain Research.* 1993; 606:325-331.

[70]Caston J, Yon E, Mellier D, Godfrey HP, Delhaye-Bouchaud N, Mariani J. An animal model of autism: behavioural studies in the GS guinea-pig. *European Journal of Neuroscience.* 1998;10:2677-2684.

[71]Engelmann M, Landgraf R. Microdialysis administration of vasopressin into the septum improves social recognition in Brattleboro rats. *Physiology and Behavior.* 1994; 55:145-149.

[72]Jentsch JD, Arguello PA, Anzivino LA. Null mutation of the arginine-vasopressin gene in rats slows attentional engagement and facilitates response accuracy in a lateralized reaction time task. *Neuropsychopharmacology.* 2003; 28:1597-1605.

[73]Insel TR, Gingrich BS, Young LJ. Oxytocin: who needs it? *Progress in Brain Research.* 2001; 133:59-66.

[74]Ferguson JN, Young LJ, Hearn EF, Matzuk MM, Insel TR, Winslow JT. Social amnesia in mice lacking the oxytocin gene. *Nature Genetics.* 2000; 25:284-288.

[75]Winslow JT, Insel TR. The social deficits of the oxytocin knockout mouse. *Neuropeptides.* 2002; 36:221-229.

[76]Winslow JT, Hearn EF, Ferguson J, Young LJ, Matzuk MM, Insel TR. Infant vocalization, adult aggression, and fear behavior of an oxytocin null mutant mouse. *Hormones and Behavior.* 2000; 37:145-155.

[77]Ferguson JN, Aldag JM, Insel TR,Young LJ. Oxytocin in the medial amygdala is essential for social recognition in the mouse. *Journal of Neuroscience.* 2001; 21:8278-8285.

[78]Michelini S, Urbanek M, Dean M, Goldman D. Polymorphism and genetic mapping of the human oxytocin receptor gene on chromosome 3. *American Journal of Medical Genetics.* 1995; 60:183-187.

[79]Modahl C, Green L, Fein D, et al. Plasma oxytocin levels in autistic children. *Biological Psychiatry.* 1998; 43:270-277.

[80]Green L, Fein D, Modahl C, Feinstein C, Waterhouse L, Morris M. Oxytocin and autistic disorder: alterations in peptide forms. *Biological Psychiatry.* 2001; 50:609-613.

[81]Hollander E, Novotny S, Hanratty M, et al. Oxytocin infusion reduces repetitive behaviors in adults with autistic and Asperger's disorders. *Neuropsychopharmacology.* 2003; 28:193-198.

[82]Insel TR, O'Brien DJ, Leckman JF. Oxytocin, vasopressin, and autism: is there a connection? *Biological Psychiatry.* 1999; 45:145-157.

[83]Young LJ. Oxytocin and vasopressin receptors and species-typical social behaviors. *Hormones and Behavior.* 1999; 36:212-221.

[84]Young LJ, Nilsen R, Waymire KG, MacGregor GR, Insel TR. Increased affiliative response to vasopressin in mice expressing the V1a receptor from a monogamous vole. *Nature.* 1999; 400:766-768.

[85]Young LJ, Wang Z, Insel TR. Neuroendocrine bases of monogamy. *Trends in Neurosciences.* 1998;21:71-75.

[86]Kim SJ, Young LJ, Gonen D, et al. Transmission disequilibrium testing of arginine vasopressin receptor 1A (AVPR1A) polymorphisms in autism. *Molecular Psychiatry.* 2002; 7:503-507.

[87]Le Moal M, Dantzer R, Michaud B, Koob GF. Centrally injected arginine vasopressin (AVP) facilitates social memory in rats. *Neuroscience Letters.* 1987; 77:353-359.

[88]Dantzer R, Bluthe RM, Koob GF, Le Moal M. Modulation of social memory in male rats by neurohypophyseal peptides. *Psychopharmacology.* 1987; 91:363-368.

[89]Landgraf R, Frank E, Aldag JM, et al. Viral vector-mediated gene transfer of the vole V1a vasopressin receptor in the rat septum: improved social discrimination and active social behaviour. *European Journal of Neuroscience.* 2003; 18:403-411.

[90]Bluthe RM, Schoenen J, Dantzer R. Androgen-dependent vasopressinergic neurons are involved in social recognition in rats. *Brain Research.* 1990; 519:150-157.

[91]Bielsky IF, Hu SB, Szegda KL, Westphal H, Young LJ. Profound impairment in social recognition and reduction in anxiety-like behavior in vasopressin V1a receptor knockout mice. *Neuropsychopharmacology.* 2004; 29:483-493.

[92]Shumyatsky GP, Tsvetkov E, Malleret G, et al. Identification of a signaling network in lateral nucleus of amygdala important for inhibiting memory specifically related to learned fear. *Cell.* 2002; 111:905-918.

[93]Marui T, Hashimoto O, Nanba E, et al. Gastrin-releasing peptide receptor (GRPR) locus in Japanese subjects with autism. *Brain and Development.* 2004; 26:5-7.

[94]Ishikawa-Brush Y, Powell JF, Bolton P, et al. Autism and multiple exostoses associated with an X;8 translocation occurring within the GRPR gene and 3′ to the SDC2 gene. *Human Molecular Genetics.* 1997; 6:1241-1250.

[95]Francis F, Koulakoff A, Boucher D, et al. Doublecortin is a developmentally regulated, microtubule-associated protein expressed in migrating and differentiating neurons. *Neuron.* 1999; 23:247-256.

[96]des Portes V, Francis F, Pinard JM, et al. *doublecortin* is the major gene causing X-linked subcortical laminar heterotopia (SCLH). *Human Molecular Genetics.* 1998; 7:1063-1070.

[97]Gleeson JG, Allen KM, Fox JW, et al. Doublecortin, a brain-specific gene mutated in human X-linked lissencephaly and double cortex syndrome, encodes a putative signaling protein. *Cell.* 1998; 92:63-72.

[98]Corbo JC, Deuel TA, Long JM, et al. Doublecortin is required in mice for lamination of the hippocampus but not the neocortex. *Journal of Neuroscience.* 2002; 22:7548-7557.

[99]Nelson KB, Grether JK, Croen LA, et al. Neuropeptides and neurotrophins in neonatal blood of children with autism or mental retardation. *Annals of Neurology*. 2001; 49:597-606.

[100]Riikonen R. Neurotrophic factors in the pathogenesis of Rett syndrome. *Journal of Child Neurology*. 2003; 18:693-697.

[101]Croll SD, Suri C, Compton DL, et al. Brain-derived neurotrophic factor transgenic mice exhibit passive avoidance deficits, increased seizure severity and in vitro hyperexcitability in the hippocampus and entorhinal cortex. *Neuroscience*. 1999; 93:1491-1506.

[102]Gorski JA, Balogh SA, Wehner JM, Jones KR. Learning deficits in forebrain-restricted brain-derived neurotrophic factor mutant mice. *Neuroscience*. 2003; 121:341-354.

[103]Levin ED, Bettegowda C, Weaver T, Christopher NC. Nicotine-dizocilpine interactions and working and reference memory performance of rats in the radial-arm maze. *Pharmacology, Biochemistry and Behavior*. 1998; 61:335-340.

[104]Stein EA, Pankiewicz J, Harsch HH, et al. Nicotine-induced limbic cortical activation in the human brain: a functional MRI study. *American Journal of Psychiatry*. 1998; 155:1009-1015.

[105]Dani JA. Overview of nicotinic receptors and their roles in the central nervous system. *Biological Psychiatry*. 2001; 49:166-174.

[106]Graham AJ, Martin-Ruiz CM, Teaktong T, Ray MA, Court JA. Human brain nicotinic receptors, their distribution and participation in neuropsychiatric disorders. *Current Drug Targets in CNS and Neurological Disorders*. 2002; 1:387-397.

[107]Court JA, Martin-Ruiz C, Graham A,Perry E. Nicotinic receptors in human brain: topography and pathology. *Journal of Chemical Neuroanatomy*. 2000; 20:281-298.

[108]Lee M, Martin-Ruiz C, Graham A, et al. Nicotinic receptor abnormalities in the cerebellar cortex in autism. *Brain*. 2002; 125:1483-1495.

[109]Perry EK, Lee ML, Martin-Ruiz CM, et al. Cholinergic activity in autism: abnormalities in the cerebral cortex and basal forebrain. *American Journal of Psychiatry*. 2001; 158:1058-1066.

[110]Lambe EK, Picciotto MR, Aghajanian GK. Nicotine induces glutamate release from thalamocortical terminals in prefrontal cortex. *Neuropsychopharmacology*. 2003; 28:216-225.

[111]Granon S, Faure P,Changeux JP. Executive and social behaviors under nicotinic receptor regulation. *Proceedings of the National Academy of Sciences of the United States of America*. 2003; 100:9596-9601.

[112]Jamain S, Betancur C, Quach H, et al. Linkage and association of the glutamate receptor 6 gene with autism. *Molecular Psychiatry*. 2002; 7:302-310.

[113]Mulle C, Sailer A, Perez-Otano I, et al. Altered synaptic physiology and reduced susceptibility to kainate-induced seizures in GluR6-deficient mice. *Nature*. 1998; 392:601-605.

[114]Fatemi SH, Halt AR, Stary JM, Kanodia R, Schulz SC, Realmuto GR. Glutamic acid decarboxylase 65 and 67 kDa proteins are reduced in autistic parietal and cerebellar cortices. *Biological Psychiatry*. 2002; 52:805-810.

[115]Powell EM, Mars WM, Levitt P. Hepatocyte growth factor/scatter factor is a motogen for interneurons migrating from the ventral to dorsal telencephalon. *Neuron*. 2001; 30:79-89.

[116]Powell EM, Campbell DB, Stanwood GD, Davis C, Noebels JL, Levitt P. Genetic disruption of cortical interneuron development causes region- and GABA cell type-specific deficits, epilepsy, and behavioral dysfunction. *Journal of Neuroscience.* 2003; 23:622-631.

[117]Asada H, Kawamura Y, Maruyama K, et al. Cleft palate and decreased brain gamma-aminobutyric acid in mice lacking the 67-kDa isoform of glutamic acid decarboxylase. *Proceedings of the National Academy of Sciences of the United States of America.* 1997; 94:6496-6499.

[118]Kash SF, Johnson RS, Tecott LH, et al. Epilepsy in mice deficient in the 65-kDa isoform of glutamic acid decarboxylase. *Proceedings of the National Academy of Sciences of the United States of America.* 1997; 94:14060-14065.

[119]Kash SF, Tecott LH, Hodge C, Baekkeskov S. Increased anxiety and altered responses to anxiolytics in mice deficient in the 65-kDa isoform of glutamic acid decarboxylase. *Proceedings of the National Academy of Sciences of the United States of America.* 1999; 96:1698-1703.

[120]Choi SY, Morales B, Lee HK, Kirkwood A. Absence of long-term depression in the visual cortex of glutamic acid decarboxylase-65 knock-out mice. *Journal of Neuroscience.* 2002; 22:5271-5276.

[121]Hensch TK, Fagiolini M, Mataga N, Stryker MP, Baekkeskov S, Kash SF. Local GABA circuit control of experience-dependent plasticity in developing visual cortex. *Science.* 1998; 282:1504-1508.

[122]Gilbert PM, Burd CG. GDP dissociation inhibitor domain II required for Rab GTPase recycling. *Journal of Biological Chemistry.* 2001; 276:8014-8020.

[123]Luan P, Balch WE, Emr SD, Burd CG. Molecular dissection of guanine nucleotide dissociation inhibitor function *in vivo*: Rab-independent binding to membranes and role of Rab recycling factors. *Journal of Biological Chemistry.* 1999; 274:14806-14817.

[124]Kohn M, Steinbach P, Hameister H, Kehrer-Sawatzki H.A comparative expression analysis of four MRX genes regulating intracellular signalling via small GTPases. *European Journal of Human Genetics.* 2004; 12:29-37.

[125]Cox JJ, Holden ST, Dee S, Burbridge JI, Raymond FL. Identification of a 650 kb duplication at the X chromosome breakpoint in a patient with 46,X,t(X;8)(q28;q12) and non-syndromic mental retardation. *Journal of Medical Genetics.* 2003; 40:169-174.

[126]Boda B, Mas C, Muller D. Activity-dependent regulation of genes implicated in X-linked non-specific mental retardation. *Neuroscience.* 2002; 114:13-17.

[127]Castellvi-Bel S, Mila M. Genes responsible for nonspecific mental retardation. *Molecular Genetics and Metabolism.* 2001; 72:104-108.

[128]D'Adamo P, Menegon A, Lo Nigro C, et al. Mutations in GDI1 are responsible for X-linked non-specific mental retardation. *Nature Genetics.* 1998; 19:134-139.

[129]D'Adamo P, Welzl H, Papadimitriou S, et al. Deletion of the mental retardation gene Gdi1 impairs associative memory and alters social behavior in mice. *Humans Molecular Genetics.* 2002; 11:2567-2580.

[130]Cook EH, Leventhal BL. The serotonin system in autism. *Current Opinion in Pediatrics.* 1996; 8:348-354.

[131]Herault J, Petit E, Martineau J, et al. Serotonin and autism: biochemical and molecular biology features. *Psychiatry Research.* 1996; 65:33-43.

[132]Gordon CT, State RC, Nelson JE, Hamburger SD, Rapoport JL. A double-blind comparison of clomipramine, desipramine, and placebo in the treatment of autistic disorder. *Archives of General Psychiatry*. 1993;50:441-447.

[133]Hollander E, Phillips AT, Yeh CC. Targeted treatments for symptom domains in child and adolescent autism. *Lancet*. 2003; 362:732-734.

[134]McDougle CJ, Naylor ST, Cohen DJ, Volkmar FR, Heninger GR, Price LH. A double-blind, placebo-controlled study of fluvoxamine in adults with autistic disorder. *Archives of General Psychiatry*. 1996; 53:1001-1008.

[135]Nabi R, Serajee FJ, Chugani DC, Zhong H, Huq AH. Association of tryptophan 2,3 dioxygenase gene polymorphism with autism. *American Journal of Medical Genetics*. 2004; 125B:63-68.

[136]Anderson GM. Genetics of childhood disorders, XLV: autism, part 4: serotonin in autism. *Journal of the American Academy of Child and Adolescent Psychiatry*. 2002; 41:1513-1516.

[137]Conroy J, Meally E, Kearney G, Fitzgerald M, Gill M, Gallagher L. Serotonin transporter gene and autism: a haplotype analysis in an Irish autistic population. *Molecular Psychiatry* 6 January 2004. Available at: <http://www.nature.com/cgi-taf/DynaPage.taf?file=/mp/journal/vaop/ncurrent/abs/4001459a.html&dynoptions=doi1082650661>.

[138]Persico AM, Pascucci T, Puglisi-Allegra S, et al. Serotonin transporter gene promoter variants do not explain the hyperserotoninemia in autistic children. *Molecular Psychiatry*. 2002; 7:795-800.

[139]Lamb JA, Parr JR, Bailey AJ, Monaco AP. Autism: in search of susceptibility genes. *Neuromolecular Medicine*. 2002; 2:11-28.

[140]Kim SJ, Cox N, Courchesne R, et al. Transmission disequilibrium mapping at the serotonin transporter gene (SLC6A4) region in autistic disorder. *Molecular Psychiatry*. 2002; 7:278-288.

[141]Bengel D, Murphy DL, Andrews AM, et al. Altered brain serotonin homeostasis and locomotor insensitivity to 3, 4-methylenedioxymethamphetamine ("Ecstasy") in serotonin transporter-deficient mice. *Molecular Pharmacology*. 1998; 53:649-655.

[142]Holmes A, Lit Q, Murphy DL, Gold E, Crawley JN. Abnormal anxiety-related behavior in serotonin transporter null mutant mice: the influence of genetic background. *Genes Brain Behavior*. 2003; 2:365-380.

[143]Heisler LK, Chu HM, Tecott LH. Epilepsy and obesity in serotonin 5-HT2C receptor mutant mice. *Annals of the New York Academy of Sciences*. 1998; 861:74-78.

[144]Olivier B, Pattij T, Wood SJ, Oosting R, Sarnyai Z, Toth M. The 5-HT(1A) receptor knockout mouse and anxiety. *Behavioural Pharmacology*. 2001; 12:439-450.

[145]Groenink L, van Bogaert MJ, van der Gugten J, Oosting RS, Olivier B. 5-HT1A receptor and 5-HT1B receptor knockout mice in stress and anxiety paradigms. *Behavioural Pharmacology*. 2003; 14:369-383.

[146]Chou-Green JM, Holscher TD, Dallman MF, Akana SF. Repeated stress in young and old 5-HT(2C) receptor knockout mice. *Physiology and Behavior*. 2003; 79:217-226.

[147]Chou-Green JM, Holscher TD, Dallman MF, Akana SF. Compulsive behavior in the 5-HT2C receptor knockout mouse. *Physiology and Behavior*. 2003; 78:641-649.

[148]Brennan TJ, Seeley WW, Kilgard M, Schreiner CE, Tecott LH. Sound-induced seizures in serotonin 5-HT2c receptor mutant mice. *Nature Genetics*. 1997;16:387-390.

[149] DeStefano F, Thompson WW. MMR vaccine and autism: an update of the scientific evidence. *Expert Review in Vaccines.* 2004; 3:19-22.

[150] Brown AS, Cohen P, Harkavy-Friedman J, et al. Prenatal rubella, premorbid abnormalities, and adult schizophrenia. *Biological Psychiatry.* 2001; 49:473-486.

[151] Brown AS, Schaefer CA, Wyatt RJ, et al. Maternal exposure to respiratory infections and adult schizophrenia spectrum disorders: a prospective birth cohort study. *Schizophrenia Bulletin.* 2000; 26:287-295.

[152] Ciaranello AL, Ciaranello RD. The neurobiology of infantile autism. *Annual Review of Neuroscience.* 1995; 18:101-128.

[153] Fatemi SH, Earle J, Kanodia R, et al. Prenatal viral infection leads to pyramidal cell atrophy and macrocephaly in adulthood: implications for genesis of autism and schizophrenia. *Cellular and Molecular Neurobiology.* 2002; 22:25-33.

[154] Shi L, Fatemi SH, Sidwell RW, Patterson PH. Maternal influenza infection causes marked behavioral and pharmacological changes in the offspring. *Journal of Neuroscience.* 2003; 23:297-302.

[155] Patterson, PH. Maternal infection: window on neuroimmune interactions in fetal brain development and mental illness. *Current Opinion in Neurobiology.* 2002;12:115-118.

[156] Hornig M, Weissenbock H, Horscroft N, Lipkin WI. An infection-based model of neurodevelopmental damage. *Proceedings of the National Academy of Sciences of the United States of America.* 1999; 96:12102-12107.

[157] Rubin SA, Sylves P, Vogel M, et al. Borna disease virus-induced hippocampal dentate gyrus damage is associated with spatial learning and memory deficits. *Brain Research Bulletin.* 1999; 48:23-30.

[158] Pletnikov MV, Rubin SA, Vasudevan K, Moran TH, Carbone KM. Developmental brain injury associated with abnormal play behavior in neonatally Borna disease virus-infected Lewis rats: a model of autism. *Behavioural Brain Research.* 1999; 100:43-50.

[159] Pletnikov MV, Rubin SA, Schwartz GJ, Moran TH, Sobotka TJ, Carbone KM. Persistent neonatal Borna disease virus (BDV) infection of the brain causes chronic emotional abnormalities in adult rats. *Physiology and Behavior.* 1999; 66:823-831.

[160] Leckman JF, Herman AE. Maternal behavior and developmental psychopathology. *Biological Psychiatry.* 2002; 51:27-43.

[161] Heim C, Nemeroff, CB. The role of childhood trauma in the neurobiology of mood and anxiety disorders: preclinical and clinical studies. *Biological Psychiatry.* 2001; 49:1023-1039.

[162] Pihoker C, Owens MJ, Kuhn CM, Schanberg SM, Nemeroff CB. Maternal separation in neonatal rats elicits activation of the hypothalamic-pituitary-adrenocortical axis: a putative role for corticotropin-releasing factor. *Psychoneuroendocrinology.* 1993; 18:485-493.

[163] Dent GW, Okimoto DK, Smith MA, Levine S. Stress-induced alterations in corticotropin-releasing hormone and vasopressin gene expression in the paraventricular nucleus during ontogeny. *Neuroendocrinology.* 2000; 71:333-342.

[164] Liu D, Caldji C, Sharma S, Plotsky PM, Meaney MJ. Influence of neonatal rearing conditions on stress-induced adrenocorticotropin responses and norepinepherine release in the hypothalamic paraventricular nucleus. *Journal of Neuroendocrinology.* 2000; 12:5-12.

[165] Caldji C, Diorio J, Meaney MJ. Variations in maternal care in infancy regulate the development of stress reactivity. *Biological Psychiatry*. 2000; 48:1164-1174.

[166] Plotsky PM, Meaney MJ. Early, postnatal experience alters hypothalamic corticotropin-releasing factor (CRF) mRNA, median eminence CRF content and stress-induced release in adult rats. *Brain Research: Molecular Brain Research*. 1993; 18:195-200.

[167] Caldji C, Francis D, Sharma S, Plotsky PM, Meaney MJ. The effects of early rearing environment on the development of GABAA and central benzodiazepine receptor levels and novelty-induced fearfulness in the rat. *Neuropsychopharmacology*. 2000; *22*: 219-229.

[168] Leventhal AG, Hirsch HV. Effects of early experience upon orientation sensitivity and binocularity of neurons in visual cortex of cats. *Proceedings of the National Academy of Sciences of the United States of America*. 1977; 74:1272-1276.

[169] Sengpiel F, Kind PC. The role of activity in development of the visual system. *Current Biology*. 2002; 12:R818-826.

[170] Huang ZJ, Kirkwood A, Pizzorusso T, et al. BDNF regulates the maturation of inhibition and the critical period of plasticity in mouse visual cortex. *Cell*. 1999; 98:739-755.

[171] Hanover JL, Huang ZJ, Tonegawa S, Stryker MP. Brain-derived neurotrophic factor overexpression induces precocious critical period in mouse visual cortex. *Journal of Neuroscience*. 1999; 19:RC40.

[172] Chang EF, Merzenich MM. Environmental noise retards auditory cortical development. *Science*. 2003; 300:498-502.

[173] Maffei L. Plasticity in the visual system: role of neurotrophins and electrical activity. *Archives of Italian Biology*. 2002; 140:341-346.

[174] Zhang LI, Bao S, Merzenich MM. Disruption of primary auditory cortex by synchronous auditory inputs during a critical period. *Proceedings of the National Academy of Sciences of the United States of America*. 2002; 99:2309-2314.

[175] Rubenstein JL, Merzenich MM. Model of autism: increased ratio of excitation/inhibition in key neural systems. *Genes Brain Behavior*. 2003; 2:255-267.

[176] Panksepp J, Burgdorf J. 50-kHz chirping (laughter?) in response to conditioned and unconditioned tickle-induced reward in rats: effects of social housing and genetic variables. *Behavioural Brain Research*. 2000; 115:25-38.

[177] Panksepp J, Burgdorf J. "Laughing" rats and the evolutionary antecedents of human joy? *Physiology and Behavior*. 2003; 79:533-547.

[178] Panksepp J, Burgdorf J, Turner C, Gordon N. Modeling ADHD-type arousal with unilateral frontal cortex damage in rats and beneficial effects of play therapy. *Brain and Cognition*. 2003; 52:97-105.

[179] Gordon NS, Burke S, Akil H, Watson SJ, Panksepp J. Socially-induced brain 'fertilization': play promotes brain derived neurotrophic factor transcription in the amygdala and dorsolateral frontal cortex in juvenile rats. *Neuroscience Letters*. 2003; 341:17-20.

[180] Wolterink G, Daenen LE, Dubbeldam S, et al. Early amygdala damage in the rat as a model for neurodevelopmental psychopathological disorders. *European Neuropsychopharmacology*. 2001; 11:51-59.

[181]Bobee S, Mariette E, Tremblay-Leveau H, Caston J. Effects of early midline cerebellar lesion on cognitive and emotional functions in the rat. *Behavioural Brain Research.* 2000; 112:107-117.

[182]Nilsson M, Waters S, Waters N, Carlsson A, Carlsson ML. A behavioural pattern analysis of hypoglutamatergic mice: effects of four different antipsychotic agents. *Journal of Neural Transmission.* 2001; 108:1181-1196.

[183]Ingram JL, Peckham SM, Tisdale B, Rodier PM. Prenatal exposure of rats to valproic acid reproduces the cerebellar anomalies associated with autism. *Neurotoxicology and Teratology.* 2000; 22:319-324.

[184]Brost DR, Cross JD, Hollerman JR. Social recognition memory following prenatal valproic acid: an animal model of autism. Paper presented at: Society for Neuroscience Annual Meeting; 2003; New Orleans, LA.

[185]Amaral DG, Bauman MD, Schumann CM. The amygdala and autism: implications from non-human primate studies. *Genes, Brain and Behavior.* 2003; 2:295-302.

[186]Amaral DG, Bauman MD, Capitanio JP, et al. The amygdala: is it an essential component of the neural network for social cognition? *Neuropsychologia.* 2003; 41:517-522.

[187]Bachevalier J. Brief report: medial temporal lobe and autism: a putative animal model in primates. *Journal of Autism and Developmental Disorders.* 1996; 26:217-220.

[188]Meunier M, Nalwa V, Bachevalier J. Reactions to familiar and novel objects in infant monkeys with neonatal temporal lesions. *Hippocampus.* 2003; 13:489-493.

[189]Bachevalier J, Malkova L, Mishkin M. Effects of selective neonatal temporal lobe lesions on socioemotional behavior in infant rhesus monkeys (*Macaca mulatta*). *Behavioral Neuroscience.* 2001; 115:545-559.

[190]Machado CJ, Bachevalier J. Non-human primate models of childhood psychopathology: the promise and the limitations. *Journal of Child Psychology and Psychiatry and Allied Disciplines.* 2003; 44:64-87.

[191]Winslow JT, Noble PL, Lyons CK, Sterk SM, Insel TR. Rearing effects on cerebrospinal fluid oxytocin concentration and social buffering in rhesus monkeys. *Neuropsychopharmacology.* 2003; 28:910-918.

[192]Parr LA, Winslow JT, Davis M. Rearing experience differentially affects somatic and cardiac startle responses in rhesus monkeys (*Macaca mulatta*). *Behavioral Neuroscience.* 2002; 116:378-386.

[193]Hemby SE, Sanchez MM, Winslow JT. Functional genomics approaches to a primate model of autistic symptomology. *Journal of Autism and Developmental Disorders.* 2001; 31:551-555.

In: Recent Developments in Autism Research
Editor: Manuel F. Casanova, pp. 171-193
ISBN 1-59454-358-5
© 2005 Nova Science Publishers, Inc.

Chapter VIII

Neural Network Modeling of Autism

Lennart Gustafsson*
Luleå University of Technology,
S-971 87 Luleå, Sweden
ph. +46 920 491321, fax +46 920 492082
Andrew P. Papliński†
Computer Science and Software Engineering
Monash University, Vic 3800, Australia
ph. +61 3 9905 3242, fax +61 3 9905 5146

Abstract

Neural network models comprise models of neurons, both their firing characteristics and their plasticity characteristics and of the connectivity between the neuron in a neural circuit. The models are used in computer simulations and, because of the size and complexity of the central nervous system, are greatly simplified in all these aspects. A brief overview of such models is presented. A number of attempts to explain aspects of autism, in particular poor generalization and good discrimination, have been made, employing neural network models. These attempts are briefly presented and the biological relevance of the models is discussed. Finally, simulations of learning processes subjected to abnormalities in attention shifting using self-organizing neural networks are presented. It is shown that when attention shifting is restricted by familiarity preference exact learning of objects with little variability occurs, arguably a characteristic of autism, and how early intervention in this learning process can result in normal learning of a broad range of objects.

Key Words: Neural networks, autism, modeling

1 Introduction

A great deal is known about neurons, their internal structure and processes, how they are interconnected and how these connections change over time. This knowledge makes it possible to calculate with some degree of accuracy the efferent (output) signal along a neuron's axon, given the afferent (input) signals that reach synapses on the dendritic tree.

*E-mail address: Lennart.Gustafsson@sm.luth.se
†E-mail address: app@csse.monash.edu.au

Given that we can calculate the activity of a single neuron and knowing how neurons are connected to each other we can also, in principle, calculate the overall neural activity in an area of e.g. neocortex.

The human central nervous system (CNS) contains a large number of neurons and many more connections between these neurons. These numbers vary greatly between individuals and at stages of any individual's life. For neocortex figures of more than ten billion neurons (10^{10}) and more than a hundred thousand billion (10^{14}) connections, or synapses, are often given. It is, however, not necessary to take all neural activity in neocortex into account in order to say something interesting about the activity within one area or a smaller neural structure within an area. This is because neocortex is compartmentalized into specialized areas and has several levels of organization.

Even if not all the neural activity in neocortex has to be taken into consideration when we wish to calculate the activity in a small part of neocortex the number of neurons is still staggering—tens of thousands of neurons in a square millimeter. And a square millimeter is indeed a very small part of neocortex. It is obvious that we cannot manage simultaneous input/output relations among many thousand neurons in any other way than by using a computer.

Some researchers use parallel processing supercomputers and can study nervous systems of simpler organisms, e.g. lampreys, see Lansner et al.,[1] on a high organizational level or even in their entirety. Other researchers design models which have been very greatly simplified in all respects—synapse function, synapse plasticity, connectivity and number of neurons—and hope to say something interesting about mammals and especially humans from these models. The validity of the results depends, of course, on how judiciously the models are designed. The ultimate task of running a model of the entire human CNS with all its complexities at all levels is beyond the capacity of any supercomputer at the present, but there is no compelling reason to believe it will remain so for all future.

The first goal in this chapter is to acquaint the reader with some standard models of biological neural circuits. These models are sometimes called artificial neural networks, but a shorter form is gaining usage and we will call them neural networks.

The second goal of this chapter is to discuss some attempts that have been made to use such neural networks to explain autism. We believe it is wise at this time to pursue the study of autism with different neural network models. If, as there is ample reason to believe, see e.g. Gillberg and Coleman,[2] there are multiple etiologies for autism, it is entirely plausible that several different neural network models will remain relevant as our understanding of autism widens and deepens.

We agree with Douglas and Martin[3] who state that "... it would be rash to press their [models which differ in important respects from biology] analogy to cortical circuits too far. Nevertheless, the potential usefulness of network models that are biologically based cannot be overestimated." It should be understood, however, that the use of neural networks will not provide "proof" of anything, but that a number of hypotheses or theories can be generated and these in turn can be subjected to neurophysiological and neuropsychological tests. Neural networks can also be used to test existing hypotheses and to strengthen or weaken them. Neural networks are emerging as a useful tool in research, but are not a final judge.

Have neural networks proven their worth in any biological context? Yes, results obtained from neural networks have shown a remarkable likeness with experimentally found neural activity in animal sensory cortices, see e.g. Ritter et al.[4].

Our presentation of neural networks is on a conceptual level. We have found a mathematical treatment to be beyond the scope of this chapter and instead we give references to suitable texts for the reader who wishes to pursue a study of neural networks.

2 A Generic Neuron's Input/Output Characteristics and its Modeling

There are many different types of neurons in the CNS but most neural networks have only one neuron model—a generic neuron is modelled. In Figure 1 such a generic neuron is shown.

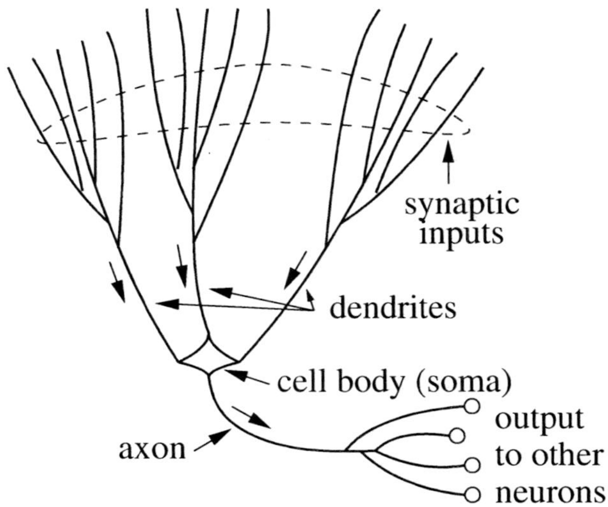

Figure 1: A generic neuron

There is a dentritic tree where afferent signals reach the neuron through a number of synapses. From the cell body or soma, an axon will carry one efferent signal to the dendritic trees of many other neurons. This efferent signal is the result of the cell's processing of all the afferent signals. The signal has the form of trains of spikes of voltages as illustrated in Figure 2.

There is a minimum frequency of such spikes—obviously there cannot be fewer than zero spikes per second—and there is a maximum frequency since there is a refractory period after a spike during which a new spike cannot be generated. A neuron is said to be firing when it produces trains of spikes of voltages. The simplest model of a single neuron

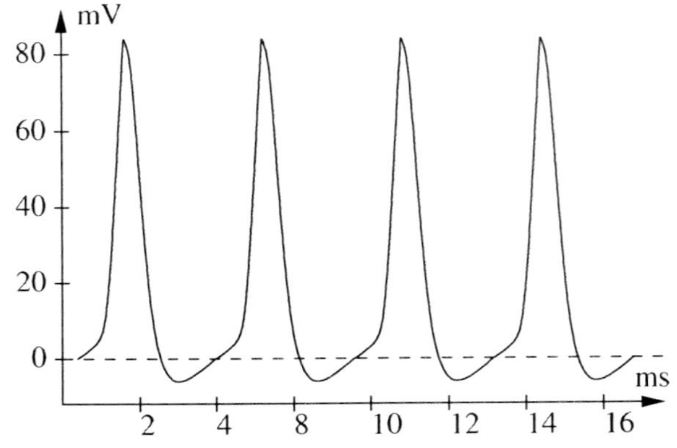

Figure 2: Train of spikes of voltages

is shown in two possible forms in Figure 3. Each synapse is a junction where an afferent signal enters a dendrite. The afferent signals are aggregated along the dendrite to form the postsynaptic activity. The postsynaptic activity is typically a weighted sum of the afferent signals. This postsynaptic activity is then limited in the neuron body to ensure that the efferent signal stays between some minimum and maximum values. Often, but not always, the signals are modelled as voltage levels rather than as frequencies of spikes of voltages. These levels of voltages are simply the averages of the spikes—a high frequency train corresponds to a high voltage level. All neuron models used in the attempts to model autism use voltage levels rather than spikes of voltages. This is done in order to simplify the models, of course. A critical question will then be: does this mean that these models will loose the possibility to display characteristics which are fundamentally important in autism? There is no definitive answer to this question today.

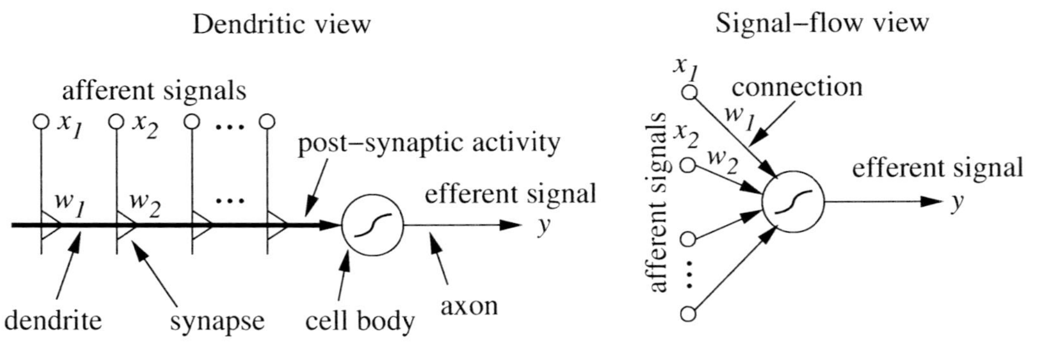

Figure 3: Two representations of a single neuron: left—dentritic form, right—signal-flow form.

3 Neurons Connected into Circuits and Neural Network Models

Neurons form circuits with different characteristics in different parts of the CNS. In cerebral cortex the neurons form a thin sheet, of typically a tenth of an inch thickness. The sheet consists of six layers with different types of neurons in different layers. The interconnections between neurons, both local and far-reaching, are arranged so that the different layers provide different types of connectivity.

The anatomy of cortex is known in much detail but in most neural networks no attempt has been made to model all the complexities of the cortical sheet. Some neural networks yield results where the neural activity show striking resemblance with that measured in animal experiments, whereas others are not designed to yield such similarities. It seems obvious that for modeling biological neural circuits, the interconnections in the neural network should be modelled on biological neural circuits. Models may, and for practical reasons must be, simplified, but what is modelled should be biologically motivated.

The rest of this section contains some mathematical terminology that might be unknown to some readers. The following sections on modeling autism with neural networks will be intelligible without a full understanding of this terminology.

There are two basic building blocks of the neural networks which have been employed in modeling autism: a layer of neurons, and a competitive layer. A layer of neurons is presented in Figure 4.

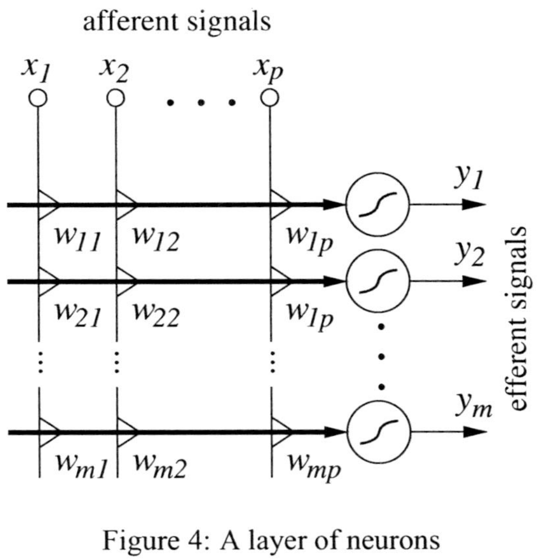

Figure 4: A layer of neurons

The layer is created from single neurons as shown in Figure 3. There are p afferent signals connected to synapses of m neurons. Each synapse stores one parameter, a weight w_{ij}, which is used to form a postsynaptic signal as a weighted sum of the afferent signals.

A competitive layer is shown in Figure 5.

In a competitive layer the efferent signals are fed back to the competing neurons and form the local self-excitatory and lateral inhibitory connections. The self-excitatory con-

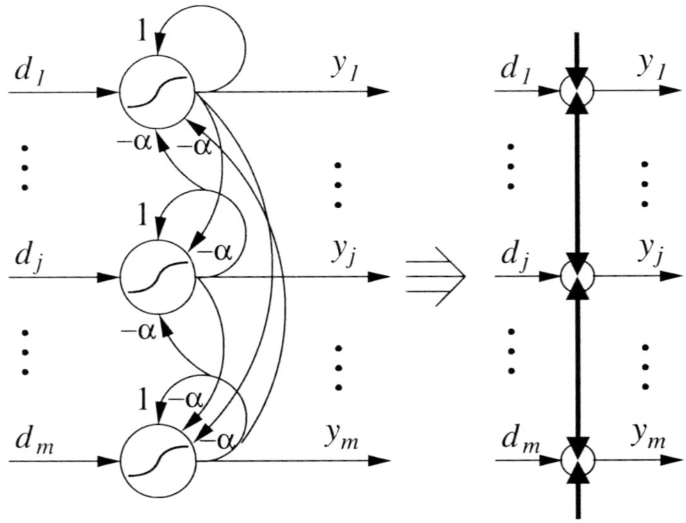

Figure 5: Two views of a competitive layer of neurons.

nections are marked with "1" and the inhibitory connections with "$-\alpha$." As the result of the competition the output of the neuron with the largest input signal (the "winner") is enhanced, whereas all other outputs are suppressed.

Interconnection of layers of neurons forms a multilayer feedforward neural network or multilayer perceptron (MLP). In Figure 6 two views of a two-layer perceptron are shown.

Multilayer feedforward neural networks are often called backpropagation networks due to a popular learning algorithm.

Self-Organizing Maps (SOMs) are competitive neural networks in which neurons are organized in a one- or two-dimensional lattice (grid) representing the **feature space**. In Figure 7 we present an example of a self-organizing map consisting of $m = 12$ neurons in which the **input space** is three-dimensional $(p = 3)$ and the **feature space** is two-dimensional.

The first section of the network is a distance-measure layer of neurons consisting of $m = 12$ dendrites each containing $p = 3$ synapses excited by 3-D input signal vectors $\mathbf{x} = [x_1\ x_2\ x_3]$ and characterised by the weight vector $\mathbf{w}_i = [w_{i1}\ w_{i2}\ w_{i3}]$. The distance-measure layer calculates the distances d_i between each input vector $\mathbf{x}$ and every weight vector $\mathbf{w}_i$. This distance information, $(d_1, \ldots, d_m)$ is passed to the competition layer, the MinNet in Figure 7, which calculates the minimal distance $d_k = \min d_i$ in order to establish the position of the winning neuron k. The competition is implemented through the lateral inhibitory and local self-excitatory connections between neurons in the competitive layer. In addition, every neuron is located at $l = 2$-dimensional lattice and its position is specified by an l-dimensional vector $\mathbf{v}_i = [v_{i1}\ v_{i2}]$.

The synaptic weight vectors, $\mathbf{w}_i$, and the vectors of topological positions of neurons, $\mathbf{v}_i$, are grouped into the weight and position matrices, W, V, respectively.

Signal-flow diagram:

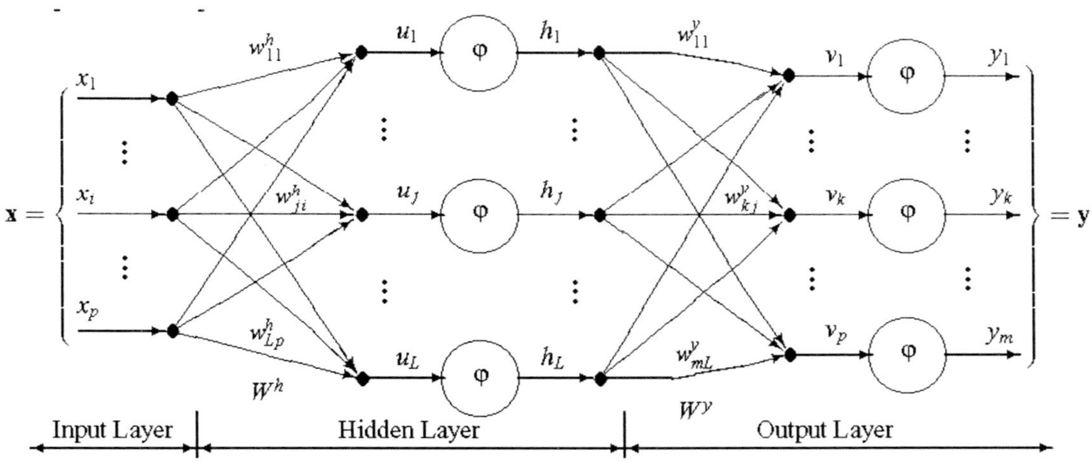

$$u_j = W_j^h \cdot \mathbf{x}\ ; \quad h_j = \varphi(u_j)\ ; \quad v_k = W_k^y \cdot \mathbf{h}\ ; \quad y_k = \varphi(v_k)$$

Dendritic diagram:

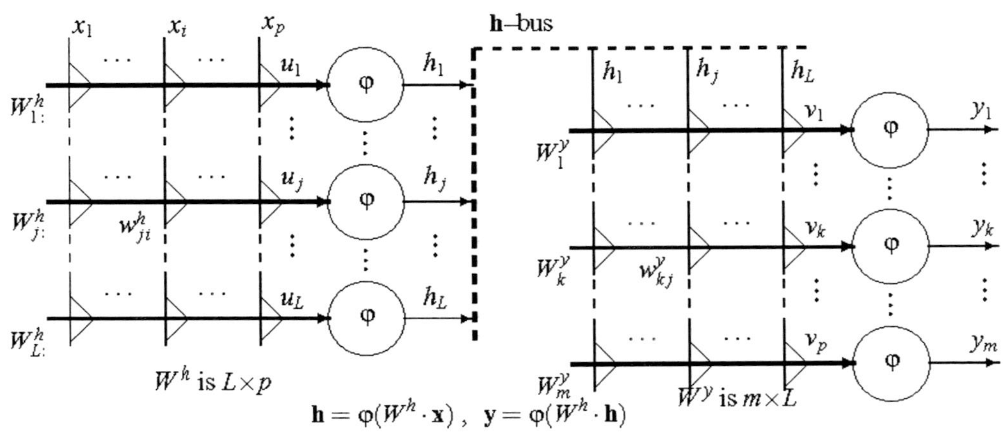

Figure 6: Various representations of a Two-Layer Perceptron

4 Learning is Modification of Synapses

Perceptions, thoughts, emotions, motor action are all manifestations of neural activity, the firing of many neurons. Learning is the process by which the neurons change their proper-

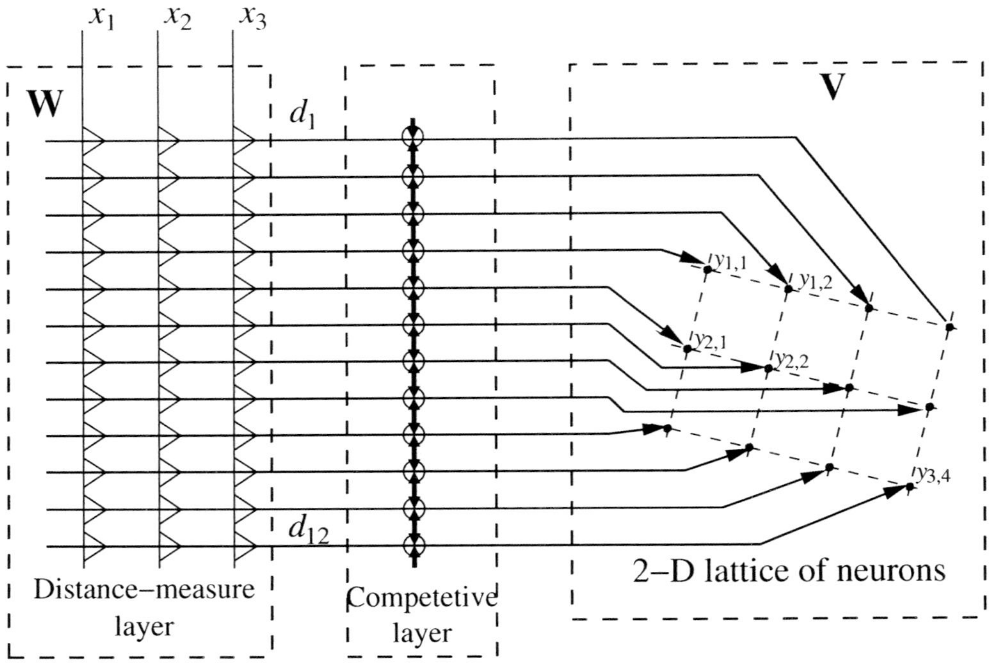

Figure 7: A 2-D SOFM with $p = 3$; $m = [3\ \ 4]$; $l = 2$.

ties so that new or modified patterns of neural activity become possible. It is the efficacies or strengths of the synapses which define the possible neural activities and it is changes in these synapses which constitutes learning.

What could be the mechanism that changes synapses in such a constructive manner as to make learning possible? Hebb suggested in 1949[5] in a famous statement that

> "When an axon of cell A is near enough to excite a cell B and repeatedly or persistently takes part in firing it, some growth process or metabolic changes take place in one or both cells such that A's efficiency as one of the cells firing B, is increased."

It has since been shown that the strengthening of synapses is not sufficient to make learning possible, there must also be a mechanism which weakens synapses. A modified statement which takes this into account is: When the firings of two neurons are correlated then a synapse connecting them is strengthened but if the firings are not correlated then a synapse connecting them is weakened.

Learning according to this statement is called Hebbian learning and it has been demonstrated in the CNS. In order to employ Hebbian learning in a computer simulation it must be formulated in mathematical language. Such formulations have reached a high degree of sophistication but we do not need to go into these details here.

During the 1990's it became clear that a modification of a synapse is not only dependent on the activity of two neurons (the presynaptic and the postsynaptic neuron) but also on the activities of neurons in a neighborhood. A diffusive agent, nitric oxide, was found to be emitted from firing neurons and spread in a neighbourhood, strengthening some synapses and weakening others in that neighbourhood, see e.g. Prast.[6]

Hebbian learning is a time consuming form of learning and much more efficient strategies for learning in a neural network have been designed. Again a question arises: will the results of simulations of learning be valid for biological learning if other, more efficient strategies for synapse strength modifications are employed? Kohonen[7] has presented some computational results that answer this question in the affirmative, but caution should be exercised.

5 Learning in Neural Networks

There are three main paradigms for learning in neural networks, supervised learning, unsupervised learning or self-organization, and reinforcement learning. Arguably the last two are of biological relevance. It is, however, the first two that have been employed in modeling of autism.

In supervised learning a stimulus is entered to a neural network and the resulting output is measured and compared to a target, or desired output, for that particular stimulus. If, as can be expected particularly in an early phase of the learning process, the output is not close to the target, the synapse weights of the neural network are altered to bring the output closer to the target. An algorithm lets a computer calculate suitable changes of all the synapses. This process is repeated thousands of times with different stimuli. Even though this may be an effective learning process it is difficult to see a biological parallel to this calculation of synapse weights by the computer.

In unsupervised learning, or self-organization, the network just strengthens (compare Hebbian learning!) the tendencies present in the network in its initial state and seemingly magically adapts to the stimuli, meaning that the weights of synapses for one neuron or one group of neurons will adapt to and match the characteristics of one category of stimuli. A neuron's output is maximized when its input is the stimuli which it has adapted to. Other categories of stimuli will have other neurons adapted to them. The resulting neural networks are often called feature maps. Feature maps are important in sensory cortices.

In reinforcement learning a resulting output from a neural network is evaluated from some response from the environment as "good or bad." The neural network changes its synapse weights in some non-deterministic way and if the result is good then these changes will be strengthened, and if they are bad, they will weaken. This learning has biological relevance and was understood in psychology before neural networks had been conceived. Thorndike's "law of effect" from 1911[8] offers this formulation of reinforcement learning:

> "Of several responses made to the same situation, those which are accompanied or closely followed by satisfaction to the animal will, other things being equal,

be more firmly connected with the situation, so that, when it recurs, they will be more likely to recur; those which are accompanied or closely followed by discomfort to the animal will, other things being equal, have their connections with that situation weakened, so that, when it recurs, they will be less likely to occur. The greater the satisfaction or discomfort, the greater the strengthening or weakening of the bond."

6 Cohen's Model of Autism

Cohen was first[9, 10] to present explanations of characteristics in autism, based on the theory of neural networks. If a neural network has an excess of neurons and synapses for a given task it will learn every required response to the presented inputs exactly but will perform poorly on inputs which are slightly different than the learned inputs. Overfitting to learned inputs is the opposite of generalization and renders a neural network useless. A correctly dimensioned neural network has a sufficient number of neurons and synapses to learn the required response to the presented inputs but only in an approximate way. The advantage that stems from this is that it will also give good responses to inputs which have not been presented during learning but are similar to the ones which have been learned. Such a correctly dimensioned neural network has the capacity to learn to generalize well, a fundamentally important quality of neural networks. In Figure 8 the neural network's response to inputs presented during training and "new" inputs are shown.

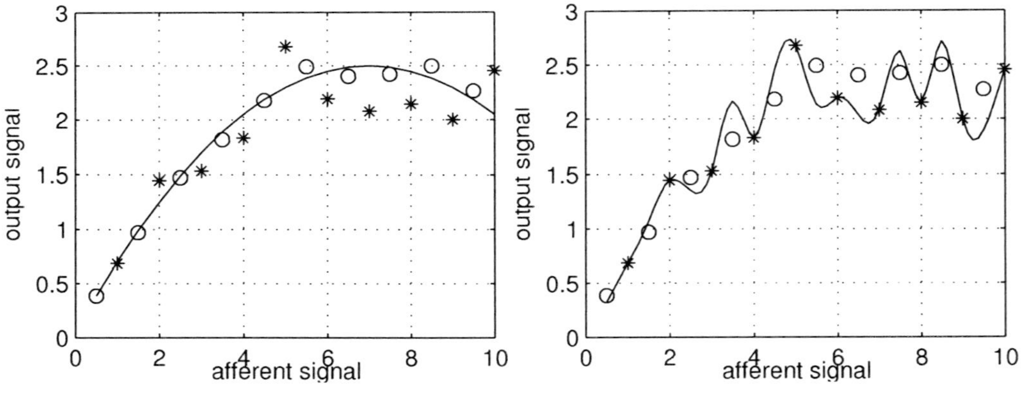

Figure 8: Left figure shows a good fit to the test set and mediocre fit to training set. Right figure shows a poor fit to the test set but perfect fit to the training set.

Noting that parts of the brain, notably the amygdala and hippocampus, have been found to contain more neurons in brains from some individuals with autism than in normal cases, Cohen hypothesizes that this can cause autism with its characteristics of exact learning of facts and poor generalization. Cohen also argues that these characteristics in turn may also cause a demand for sameness, a cardinal feature in autism.

The case illustrated in Figure 8 has a one-dimensional input and a one-dimensional response or output. This is of course because this case can be easily visualized. Realistic situations which entail many-dimensional inputs and outputs cannot be visualized but it is known from neural network theory that a neural network will loose its capacity to generalize if is over-sized also in these more realistic situations.

Cohen uses a multilayer feed-forward backpropagation network such as the one presented in Figure 6 and suggests that even though these networks "are not similar in all respects to biological nervous systems, they mimic some of their properties and may help to explain the properties of real nervous systems." Testing Cohen's hypothesis on other artificial neural network structures more similar to biological nervous systems, in particular to those present in the amygdala and the hippocampus, is needed.

7 Gustafsson's Model of Autism

Starting from a statement by Hermelin[11] that "autistic children do not tend to integrate current experience with schemas and representations stored from previous sensory impressions," Gustafsson[12] presented another model based explanation of autism. Cortical feature maps, specifically characterized by narrow neural columns, is argued to explain basically the same characteristics in autism, good discrimination but poor generalization skills, that Cohen had focussed.

Mountcastle[13] had much earlier stated that (referring to cerebral cortex): "Whatever the level in the processing hierarchy, and the particular task there is a common architecture: the neural columns (mini- and macrocolumns)." It has been established that neurons in a minicolumn have similar but not identical sensitivities to stimuli. Gustafsson argues that narrow columns with fewer than normal neurons would be responsive to a narrower than normal range of stimuli and therefore exhibit good discrimination at the cost of poor generalization.

There was no experimental support for this idea in 1997, but in 2002 Casanova et al.[14] reported that they had found an abnormal columnar organization (narrow and many minicolumns) in autism. What could cause this abnormal columnar organization?

The artificial neural network Gustafsson discusses in his arguments from 1997 is a self-organizing map with lateral excitatory and inhibitory feedbacks (both biologically motivated) in which synapses change according to Hebb's law. In such one-layered neural networks groups of neurons all of which are active upon presentation of one class of stimuli, such as a phoneme in speech, also emerge as a result of self-organization. These neural groups have the same function, albeit much simplified, as the neural columns in cortex. In the following we will assume that these one-layered neural groups may represent the six-layered neural columns in cortex and, in agreement with common usage, call them neural columns.

The width of these neural columns emerging in the model depends on the balance of excitatory and inhibitory effects as illustrated in Figure 9. It has long been known that[15] too little excitatory effect and too much inhibitory effect both result in narrow columns.

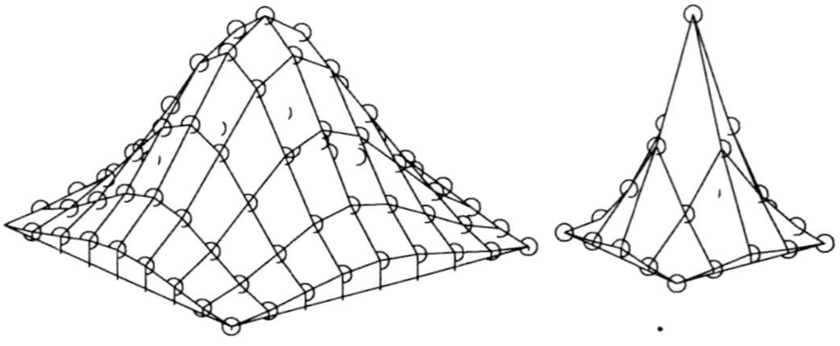

Figure 9: Left figure shows "normal" activity column resulting from good balance of excitatory and inhibitory lateral feedback. Right figure shows narrow activity column resulting from poor balance—weak excitatory/strong inhibitory lateral feedback

It is, however, not clear whether any such imbalance exists in autism. One argument against high inhibitory effects raised by Casanova et al.[16] is the relatively high co-morbidity of autism with epilepsy. Increasing the level of GABA is a well-established therapy against epileptic seizures. GABA is an inhibitory neurotransmitter and one would expect this to aggravate autism, if the hypothesized excessive lateral inhibition would hold. This is, however, not the case. In the case of co-morbid autism and epilepsy the hypothesized excessive lateral inhibition is obviously not convincing. The hypothesis might of course hold in the majority of cases of autism with no co-morbid epilepsy.

It is possible, of course, that the simple neural network model chosen by Gustafsson with its emergent neural columns does not adequately represent the columnar structure with both mini- and macrocolumns in cortex. If this is so, then causes for the narrow minicolumns in autism might not be possible to obtain from neural network theory, applying this model. See also Casanova[16] for a discussion on this issue.

Searches for a genetic linkage to autism have shown that it is not a "single-gene disorder" but rather that multiple, possibly interacting, genes are involved in causing autism, see Yonan.[17] Therefore it is reasonable to search for complementary explanations for narrow minicolumns. Two such alternative/complementary explanations have been presented by Gustafsson.[18, 19]

8 Are Narrow Neural Columns in Autism an Effect of a Serotonin Abnormality?

Although no strong candidate-genes for autism have been found, the linkage studies have indicated a serotonin transporter gene as the most consistent genetic linkage to autism.[17] A serotonin abnormality in the CNS has also been found in autism. In early development children with autism have been found to have a lower capacity to produce serotonin than normal children, but maintain this capacity while it declines in normal children.[20]

Serotonin has more than one role in the CNS, an early role being in synaptogenesis in sensory cortices.[21, 22] The barrel fields in rats are decreased if serotonin levels are lowered.[23]

If serotonin plays a similar role in early development in humans, then the reported initial low capacity for producing serotonin could contribute in causing narrow cortical columns and thus conceivably autism.

We have good reason to believe that a serotonin abnormality contributes in causing autism and the narrow neural columns implicated in autism. The genetic studies suggest that we should try to find complementary mechanisms. Neural network theory proves helpful in this search.

9 A Neural Network Theory Finding: Insufficient Nitric Oxide Causes Narrow Neural Columns

It is well established that nitric oxide plays an important role in synaptic plasticity, both for long term potentiation and long term depression, see e.g. Prast.[6] There are also results that suggest that nitric oxide is important in the metasynaptic columnar organization of cortex.[24]

The influence of nitric oxide on synaptic plasticity has been included into the mathematical models of synaptic modification, employed in neural network modeling. Simulations with such models have shown that a stable neural columnar structure emerges when the neural network self-organizes.[25, 26] Mathematical analysis of such self-organization has yielded as a correlate that the width of the neural columns depends on the production of nitric oxide during self-organization—low levels of nitric oxide results in narrow neural columns.[27, 28]

Results from two simulations of self-organization with nitric oxide as a mediator are shown in Figure 10.

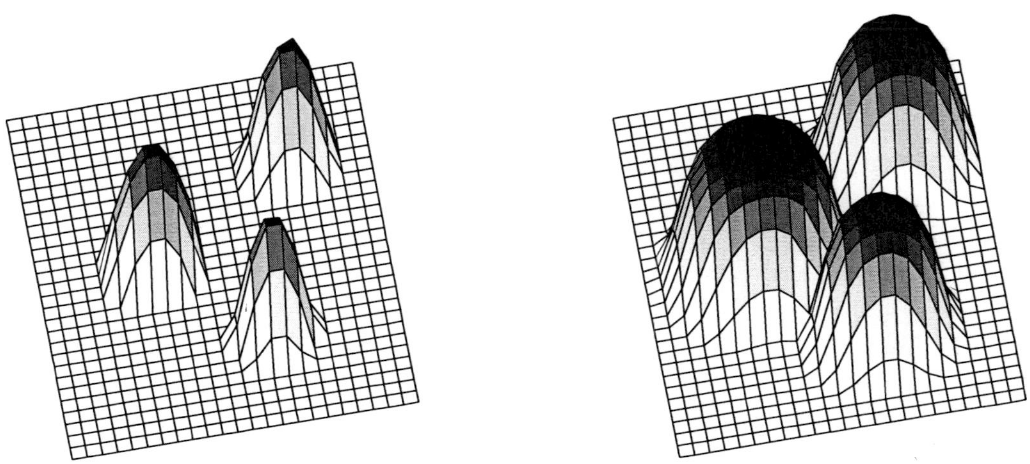

Figure 10: Narrow and wide neural columns driven by the nitric oxide level. In the left figure the nitric oxide level is low and in the right it is high.

All factors except production of nitric oxide, were the same in the two simulations. The result from theory on the dependence of the neural column width on the level of nitric oxide is clearly illustrated.

It has been hypothesized by Gustafsson[18] that insufficient production of nitric oxide could cause the narrow neural columns implicated in autism. Further aspects of this hypothesis are discussed in the following.

It is well known that vision is relatively spared in autism. This could then, according to the hypothesis, be explained if nitric oxide does not play a role in the columnar organization in visual cortex and there are results that suggest this to be the case.[24] In animal experiments it has also been directly demonstrated that visual discrimination and also other visual capacities are not affected by inhibition of nitric oxide.[29]

Nitric oxide has in animal experiments been demonstrated to have effects also in regard to epilepsy, but the effects are surprising: nitric oxide has been found to be both a proconvulsant and an anticonvulsant.[30, 31, 32] Nitric oxide has three different origins in the CNS, neuronal nitric oxide synthase (nNOS), endothelial nitric oxide synthase (eNOS), and inducible nitric oxide synthase (iNOS). Selective inhibition of nNOS makes it more difficult to induce epilepsy but inhibition of eNOS makes it easier to induce epilepsy. This would indicate that insufficient nNOS could contribute in causing autism without co-morbid epilepsy while insufficient eNOS could contribute in causing autism with co-morbid epilepsy. iNOS appears to be similar to nNOS in this respect.

10 Does Columnar Structure in Neural Networks Represent Columnar Structure in Cortex?

There is presently no definitive answer to the question what might cause narrow minicolumns in autism. In neural networks of the self-organizing kind neural columns do emerge, both as a result of lateral excitatory and inhibitory feedback and as a result of the influence of a diffusive messenger, assumed to be nitric oxide. It is, however, not certain that this emergence of neural columns models the columnar structure in cortex. The latter contains two levels, the minicolumns and the macrocolumns.

In the self-organizing neural networks discussed above there is no given initial structure. The columnar structure emerges to fulfill the functional requirements to represent different classes of the stimuli presented to the network.

In cortex there is an initial structure in the form of ontogenetic columns,[33] not stimulus-driven but prenatally formed. If the functional minicolumns are the same as the ontogenetic columns, then the synaptic plasticity of the neurons in the minicolumn allows for tuning the minicolumn to a given stimulus, but the minicolumn itself would not be an emergent structure, as the columns are in the neural network models.

Can the results obtained from a model which is not initially constrained by grouping neurons together in columns be of interest for understanding the development of cortex and the activities in minicolumns? One obvious possibility is that the development of a neural column of the model represents the tuning of the neurons in the minicolumn to a particular stimulus with some limited variability. This is all the more natural an interpretation since both the lateral inhibitory feedback surrounds the minicolumn[16] and the activity of nitric oxide is prominent along the minicolumnar periphery.[24]

A narrow neural column in the model would correspond to the case where few neurons in the minicolumn get tuned to the stimulus. The total neural activity from such a minicolumn as a response to a stimulus would then be lower than normal. The total number of neurons in the minicolumn would set an upper limit to the width of the neural columns formed in the model—larger widths could not then be interpreted in a meaningful way.

A correspondence between the neural network column and the cortical macrocolumn should not be ruled out, however. The basket cells are inhibitory interneurons that reach across a macrocolumn and the diffusion of nitric oxide and its sphere of influence is estimated to reach a distance exceeding 150 mm, i.e. covering several minicolumns.[34] Both these properties of cortex can be included in a self-organizing neural network and result in neural columns much wider than the minicolumn, possibly corresponding to the macrocolumn. The shape of the macrocolumns of sensory cortices may be determined by information from sensory inputs rather than being prenatally formed as the minicolumns, for a review see Catania.[35] In this respect the macrocolumns of cortex correspond to the neural network columns.

It should be noted that Casanova et al.[16] argue that the increased number of minicolumns in autism may have its origin in a disruption in the early prenatal development and that the larger number of minicolumns rather than their width is important in causing autism.

11 McClelland's Model of Autism

In 2000 McClelland, like Cohen and Gustafsson before, takes hyperspecificity, or poor generalization in autism as the starting point for a discussion drawing on insights from design of neural networks that can group similar objects into one category when they are sufficiently close but distinguish between objects which should form different categories.[36]

The balance between generalization and discrimination is of paramount importance in the design of neural networks. McClelland suggests that one technique employed in the design of neural networks to facilitate discrimination, conjunctive coding, might be utilized also in the central nervous system. McClelland further suggests that

> "in the brains of children with autism, they may be predisposed to use an excessively conjunctive form of neural coding [...] This could prevent them from exploiting overlap in cases where overlap leads to the useful ability to generalize. Instead, it would leave the child with the ability to learn associations to particular, specific inputs and without the ability to extend what they have learned to other similar experiences."

McClelland does not suggest any biological mechanism which would provide for this conjunctive coding and identifying such a mechanism will require further work, preferably employing neural networks which more closely model parts of the central nervous system than the traditional feed-forward networks discussed by McClelland do.

12 The Temporal Binding Deficit Hypothesis of Autism

It has been known for more than a hundred years that cerebral cortex has functionally specialized areas. These areas have extensive two-way connections and simultaneous neural activity in several areas may constitute e.g. the neural response to a complex object. It is then of course necessary that the connections between the areas involved function properly. In 2002 Brock et al. suggest that the different areas may work well seen as single entities but do not function properly together and therefore do not integrate different properties of, e.g. a complex object, well.[37] This would offer a neural explanation of the weak central coherence theory of autism, proposed in 1989 by Frith.[38]

The hypothesis is not based on neural networks, rather on biological and behavioural arguments, but the authors compare this hypothesis with the three models based on neural networks presented above and stress that whereas these models are relevant within areas, i.e. they are local models, the binding deficit hypothesis is of a global character. This hypothesis needs to be investigated experimentally but it is of a kind which could also be advantageously studied by employing neural networks.

13 Learning under Attention Shifting Restrictions Shows Autistic Characteristics

Attention abnormalities, among them attention shifting abnormalities, are common in autism. The nature of the restricted attention shifting is not agreed upon, however. One school of thought, led by Courchesne,[39, 40, 41, 42, 43, 44] suggests that there is a general attention shifting impairment caused by the deficit in number of Purkinje cells in the cerebellum, an almost universal finding in autism. A number of researchers, among them Dawson et al.,[45] Pascualvaca et al.,[46] and Minshew et al.,[47] hold a different opinion—there is a higher executive function impairment which restricts attention shifting. Some of these authors argue that people with autism tend to not shift attention to a source of stimuli which they expect to be novel, they are influenced by novelty avoidance or familiarity preference. This of course can be seen as a consequence of the insistence on sameness which Leo Kanner in 1943 found to be a prominent feature of autism.[48]

Gustafsson and Papliński have translated this scientific debate into a test, employing neural networks.[49, 50] They present stimuli from two different sources to a Kohonen[51] self-organizing map such as presented in Figure 7, which during learning adapts to the stimuli from one or both sources. It should be stressed that the neural networks are assumed to be completely adequate for the task they are presented with, it is only the attention shifting which shows any abnormality.

The simulation employs three different modes of attention shifting when a stimulus is presented by the source momentarily not attended to. Normal learning is understood to mean that attention is then unconditionally shifted—normal learning is understood to be novelty seeking. Attention will shift but only with a low probability in the case of a general attention shift impairment.

The case of attention shifting restricted by familiarity preference is more complicated. In the beginning of the learning process both sources are unfamiliar to the self-organizing map and attention is shifted unconditionally. Then as familiarity develops the shifting will show a statistical bias towards the most familiar source. Finally, if both sources become familiar to the map, attention will shift unconditionally.

The results have so far, without exception, yielded maps of the same character for normal learning and learning when attention shifting is restricted by a general attention shifting impairment. Learning when attention shifting is restricted by familiarity preference yields maps characterized by detailed learning of the source which exhibits the least variability among its stimuli. This is detailed learning in narrow fields, a learning with arguably autistic characteristics.

This should not be seen as a proof that the general impairment in attention shifting hypothesis is invalid, there are many more comprehensive simulations that must be done before such a statement could be warranted.

In the simulations presented below the two sources contained stimuli, or objects, that were for one source a number of animals (mammals, birds, fish, reptiles) and for the other source a number of felines. Naturally the feline source has much less variability than the general animal source. In Figure 11 we show the resulting maps consisting of 16 neurons, arranged in a 4×4 matrix, and how they have adapted to the different stimuli. Each stimulus is shown at the neuron which has adapted best to that stimulus. Since there are more stimuli than neurons in this case, some stimuli will share a neuron.

In Figure 11**a** a typical map resulting from normal learning and from learning with a general attention shift impairment is shown. This map shows a very economic use of the neural capacity to represent all stimuli. Stimuli which are not similar to any others, like the gray whale and the anaconda have "their own" neurons with exact adaptation (the number after each stimulus is a measure of the adaptation with a smaller number being better). Stimuli which are similar, like the great cats share one neuron. Some neurons have not been identified with any stimuli. This is a common situation—some neurons are "dead," i.e. they have not adapted to any stimulus, while others have but not as well as those identified with the stimuli.

In Figure 11**b** a typical map resulting from learning with attention shifting restricted by familiarity preference is shown. Here the map has ceased shifting attention to the source containing general animals, devoting almost all the neural capacity to the feline source, learning its stimuli very well, in this case exactly.

Even though these simulations employ neural networks to yield the maps shown above, there is also a rule driven part of the system which is simulated. The attention shifting rules are written to agree in character with experimentally verified behaviour but they are not modelled as neural networks. In autism attention shifting is, of course, also caused by

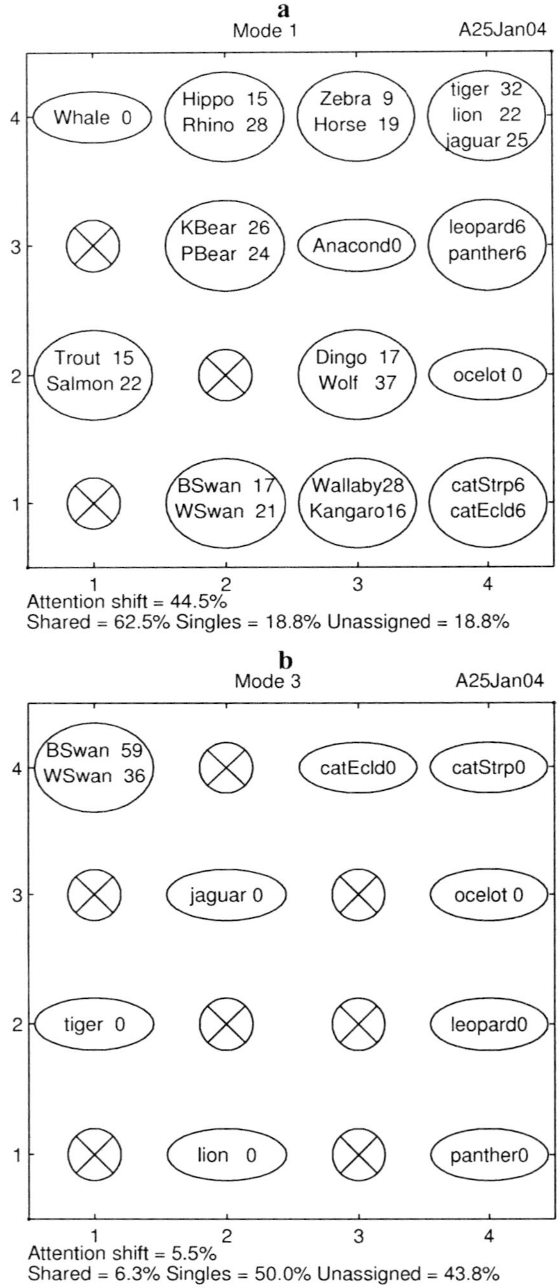

Figure 11: The feature maps developed in the **a**. novelty seeking, and **b**. attention shifting restricted by familiarity preference learning modes. The shaded ovals represent the network response to a test animal

neural activity. A complete neural model of autism based on attention shifting restricted by familiarity preference will demand a non-trivial research effort.

14 Simulating a Scheme for Early Intervention in Autism

The process that leads to exact learning of the source with the least variability when attention shifting is restricted by familiarity preference can be observed—when an attention shift to the alternate source is rejected we understand that source is the least familiar of the sources.

It is then conceivable that we can overexpose the neural network to stimuli from that source to compensate for this relative unfamiliarity. This compensatory action will very possibly have to be repeated but can lead to a map which learns both sources with a resulting map which is identical to that obtained in normal learning. The learning process is, however, entirely different.

In Figure 12 we show two diagrams, representing different aspects of the same learning process.

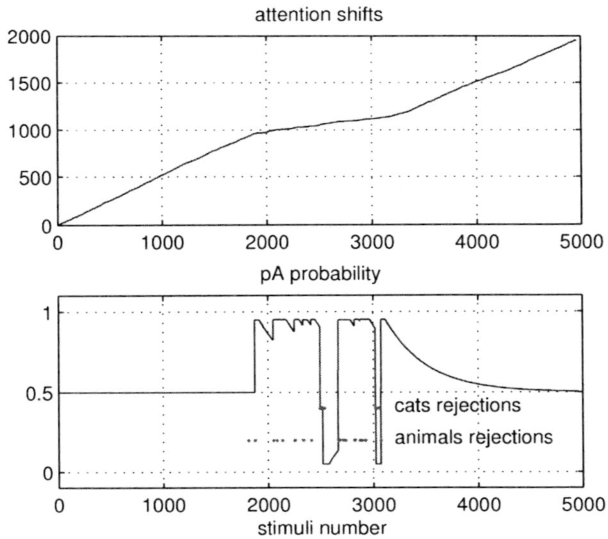

Figure 12: Early intervention. The pA probability is the probability that the next stimulus presented will be chosen from the source containing general animals. The lower row of rejection states indicates when attention shifting to the source containing general animals has been rejected and the upper row of rejection states indicates when attention shifting to the source containing felines has been rejected.

In the top diagram we see how the number of attention shifts initially grows linearly and then grows less rapidly as familiarity preference starts to play a role in the learning process. Finally the number of attention shifts again grows linearly, as rapidly as in the initial stage, this is after the neural network has become familiar with both sources.

The intervention activity which makes it possible for the neural network to develop into a normal map is shown in the lower diagram in Figure 12. The probability for presenting a new stimulus from the source with general animals is in the initial stage constant and such that each individual stimulus has an equal chance for presentation, regardless of source. When familiarity with the feline source start to manifest itself through fewer attention shifts to the source with general animals, then the probability for presenting a stimulus from the source with general animals is immediately and drastically changed. After some such large changes of probability have passed the neural network has become familiar with both sources and no more intervention is necessary.

15 Suggestions for Further Reading

A reader who is willing to face some mathematics can find a great many books and journal papers on neural network theory. Some of this literature is devoted to the study of biological nervous systems and to "mind modeling." We will here make two suggestions which for the most part demand high school mathematics or first year college calculus and algebra.

Neural Networks and Brain Function by Rolls and Treves[52] gives an overview of different neural network architectures and discusses their usefulness in explaining function in different parts of the CNS, such as sensory cortices, hippocampus etc.

Rethinking Innateness: A Connectionist Perspective on Development (Neural Networks and Connectionist Modeling) by Elman et al.[53] argues strongly for the importance of the environment, as taken in by the senses, in the development and organization of cerebral cortex and uses neural networks broadly in the argumentation.

Acknowledgements

This work is part of a cooperation between Luleå University of Technology, Luleå, Sweden and Monash University, Australia. We wish to express our appreciation to the financial support from Stiftelsen Einar och Ragnhild Lundströms minne, Sweden. We would like to thank Professor Manuel Casanova, Juan Trippe and Andrew Switala from University of Kentucky for helpful discussions.

References

[1] Lansner A., Hellgren Kotaleski J., Grillner S. Modeling of the spinal neuronal circuitry underlying locomotion in a lower vertebrate. *Annals of the New York Academy of Sciences* 1998; **860**:239–249.

[2] Gillberg C., Coleman M. *The Biology of the Autistic Syndromes*. 3rd ed. Cambridge, UK: Cambridge University Press; 2000.

[3] Douglas R., Martin K., Neocortex. In: Shepherd GM, ed. *The Synaptic Organization of the Brain*. 4th ed. Oxford, UK: Oxford University Press; 1998:459–509.

[4] Ritter H., Martinetz T., Schulten K., *Neural Computation and Self-Organizing Maps*. Reading, MA: Addison-Wesley; 1992.

[5] Hebb D.O. *The Organization of Behavior: A Neuropsychological Theory*. New York, NY: Wiley; 1949.

[6] Prast H., Philippu A., Nitric oxide as modulator of neuronal function *Progress in Neurobiology* 2001; **64**:51–68.

[7] Kohonen T., *Self-Organising Maps*. 2nd ed. Berlin, Germany: Springer-Verlag; 1995.

[8] Thorndike E.L., *Animal Intelligence*. Darien, CT: Hafner; 1911.

[9] Cohen I.L., An artificial neural network analogue of learning in autism *Biological Psychiatry* 1994; **36**:5–20.

[10] Cohen I.L., Neural network analysis of learning in autism. In: Stein D, Ludick J, eds. *Neural Networks and Psychopathology*. Cambridge, UK: Cambridge University Press; 1998:274–315.

[11] Hermelin B., Images and language. In: Rutter M, Schoppler E, eds. *Autism: A Reappraisal of Concept and Treatment*. New York, NY: Plenum; 1978:141–154.

[12] Gustafsson L., Inadequate cortical feature maps: a neural circuit theory of autism *Biological Psychiatry* 1997; **42**:1138-1147.

[13] Mountcastle V.B., Modality and topographic properties of single neurons of cat's somatic sensory cortex. *Journal of Neurophysiology* 1957; **20**:408–434.

[14] Casanova M.F., Buxhoeveden D.P., Switala A.E., Roy E., Minicolumnar pathology in autism. *Neurology* 2002; **58**:428–432.

[15] Kohonen T., *Self-Organising Maps*. Berlin, Germany: Springer-Verlag 1987.

[16] Casanova M.F., Buxhoeveden D.P., Gomez J., Disruption in the inhibitory architecture of the cell minicolumn: implications for autism. *The Neuroscientist* 2003; **6**:496-507.

[17] Yonan A.L., Palmer A.A., Smith K.C., et al., Bioinformatic analysis of autism and positional candidate genes using biological databases and computational gene network prediction. *Genes, Brain and Behavior* 2003; **2**:303–320.

[18] Gustafsson L., Neural network theory and recent neuroanatomical findings indicate that inadequate nitric oxide synthase will cause autism. In: Pallade V., Howlett R.J., Jain L.C., eds. *Knowledge-based Intelligent Information and Engineering Systems*. Berlin, Germany: Springer-Verlag; 2003:1109-1114.

[19] Gustafsson L., Comment on "Disruption in the inhibitory architecture of the cell minicolumn: implications for autism." *The Neuroscientist* 2004; 17:49-54.

[20] Chugani D.C., Muzik O., Behen M., et al. Developmental changes in brain serotonin synthesis capacity in autistic and nonautistic children. *Annals of Neurology* 1999; **45**:287–295.

[21] Cases O., Seif I., Grimsby J., et al. Aggressive behaviour and altered amounts of brain serotonin and norepinphrine in mice lacking MAOA. *Science* 1995; **268**:1763–1766.

[22] Bennet-Clarke C.A., Leslie M.J., Lane R.D., Rhoades R.W., Effect of serotonin depletion on vibrissae-related patterns in the rat's somatosensory cortex. *Journal of Neuroscience* 1994; **14**:7594–7607.

[23] Cases O., Vitalis T., Seif I., De Maeyer E. Sotelo C., Gaspar P., Lack of barrels in the somatosensory cortex of monoamine oxidase A-deficient mice: role of a serotonin excess during the critical period. *Neuron* 1996; **16**:297–307.

[24] Csillik B., Nemecsok J., Boncz I., Knyihar-Csillik E., Nitric oxide synthase and the acetylcholine receptor in the prefrontal cortex: metasynaptic organization of the brain. *Neurobiology* 1998; **6**:383–404.

[25] Gally J., Montague P., Reeke G. Jr., Edelman G., The NO hypothesis: possible effects of a short-lived, rapidly diffusible signal in the development and function of the nervous system. *Proceedings of the National Academy of Sciences of the United States of America* 1990; **87**:3547–3551.

[26] Montague P., Gally J., Edelman G., Spatial signaling in the development of neural connections. *Cerebral Cortex* 1991; **1**:199–220.

[27] Krekelberg B., Taylor J., Nitric oxide in cortical map formation. *Chemical Neuroanatomy* 1996; **10**:191–196.

[28] Krekelberg B., Taylor J., Nitric oxide: what can it compute? *Network: Computation in Neural Systems* 1997; **8**:1–16.

[29] Tobin J., Gorman L., Baxter M., Traystman R., Nitric oxide synthase inhibition does not impair visual or spatial discrimination learning. *Brain Research* 1995; **694**:177–182.

[30] Homayoun H., Khavandgar S., Namiranian K., Gaskari S.A., Dehpour A.R., The role of nitric oxide in anticonvulsant and proconvulsant effects of morphine in mice. *Epilepsy* 2002; **48**:33–41.

[31] Leite J.P., Chimelli L., Terra-Bustamante V.C., et al. Loss and sprouting of nitric oxide synthase neurons in the human epileptic hippocampus. *Epilepsia* 2002; **43**:235–242.

[32] Milatovic D., Gupta R.C., Dettbarn W.D., Involvement of nitric oxide in kainic acid-induced excitotoxicity in rat brain. *Brain Research* 2002; **957**:330–337.

[33] Rakic P., Specification of cerebral cortical areas. *Science* 1988; **241**:170–176.

[34] Wood J., Garthwaite J., Models of the diffusional spread of nitric oxide: implications for neural nitric oxide signalling and its pharmacological properties. *Neuropharmacology* 1994; **33**:1235–1244.

[35] Catania K.C., Barrels, stripes, and fingerprints in the brain: implications for theories of cortical organization. *Journal of Neurocytology* 2002; **31**:347–358.

[36] McClelland J.L., The basis of hyperspecificity in autism: a preliminary suggestion based on properties of neural nets *Journal of Autism and Developmental Disorders* 2000; **30**:497–502.

[37] Brock J., Brown C.C., Boucher J., Rippon G., The temporal binding deficit hypothesis of autism. *Development and Psychopathology* 2002; **14**:209–224.

[38] Frith U., *Autism: Explaining the Enigma*. Oxford, UK: Basil Blackwell; 1989.

[39] Courchesne E., Townsend J.P., Akshoomoff N.A., et al., A new finding: Impairment in shifting attention in autistic and cerebellar patients. In: Broman SH, Grafinan J., eds. *Atypical Cognitive Deficits in Developmental Disorders: Implications for Brain Function.* Hillsdale, NJ: Erlbaum; 1994:101–137.

[40] Courchesne E., Townsend J.P., Akshoomoff N.A., et al. Impairment in shifting attention in autistic and cerebellar patients. *Behavioral Neuroscience* 1994; **108**:848–865.

[41] Courchesne E., Akshoomoff N.A., Townsend J.P., Saitoh O., A model system for the study of attention and the cerebellum: infantile autism. In: Karmos G, Molnár M., Csépe I., Desmedt J.E., eds. *Perspectives of Event-Related Potentials Research* Amsterdam, The Netherlands: Elsevier; 1995:315–325.

[42] Courchesne E., Deciphering the puzzle: unusual patterns of brain development in autism. Paper presented at: Inaugural World Autism Congress; 2002; Melbourne, Australia.

[43] Townsend J.P., Harris N.S., Courchesne E., Visual attention abnormalities in autism: delayed orienting to location. *Journal of the International Neuropsychological Society* 1996; **2**:541–550.

[44] Townsend J.P., Courchesne E., Covington J., et al., Spatial attention deficits in patients with acquired or developmental cerebellar abnormality *Journal of Neuroscience* 1999; **19**:5632–5643.

[45] Dawson G., Meltzoff A.N., Osterling J., Rinaldi J., Brown E., Children with Autism Fail to Orient to Naturally Occurring Social Stimuli *Journal of Autism and Developmental Disorders.* 1998; **28**:479–485.

[46] Pascualvaca D.M., Fantie B.D., Papageorgiou M., Mirsky A.F., Attentional capacities in children with autism: is there a general deficit in shifting focus? *Journal of Autism and Developmental Disorders* 1998; **28**:467–478.

[47] Minshew N.J., Luna B., Sweeney J.A., Oculomotor evidence for neocortical systems but not cerebellar dysfunction in autism *Neurology* 1999; **52**:917–922.

[48] Kanner L., Autistic disturbances of affective contact. *Nervous Child* 1943; **2**:217–250.

[49] Gustafsson L., Papliński A.P., Preoccupation with a restricted pattern of interest in modelling autistic learning In: Pallade V, Howlett RJ, Jain LC, eds. *Knowledge-based Intelligent Information and Engineering Systems*. Berlin, Germany: Springer-Verlag; 2003:1122–1129.

[50] Gustafsson L., Papliński A.P., Self-organization of an artificial neural network subjected to attention shift impairments and novelty avoidance: implications for the development of autism *Journal of Autism and Developmental Disorders* 2004; **34**:1–10.

[51] Kohonen T., *Self-Organising Maps*. 3rd ed. Berlin, Germany: Springer-Verlag; 2001.

[52] Rolls E.T., Treves A., *Neural Networks and Brain Function*. Oxford, UK: Oxford University Press; 1998.

[53] Elman J.L., Bates E.A., Johnson M.H., Karmiloff-Smith A., Parisi D., Plunkett K., *Rethinking Innateness: A Connectionist Perspective on Development*. Cambridge, MA: MIT Press; 1997.

In: Recent Developments in Autism Research
Editor: Manuel F. Casanova, pp. 195-209

ISBN 1-59454-358-5
© 2005 Nova Science Publishers, Inc.

Chapter IX

Autism Research: Future Directions

Eric London
Director of Medical Affairs for the National Alliance for Autism Research

Over the past decade, in my capacity as the program chair for the National Alliance for Autism Research (NAAR), I have had the exciting and stimulating task of reading approximately 600 research proposals submitted to our small grants program. These grants are intended for innovative pilot studies in the field of autism spectrum disorders (hereinafter, collectively "autism"). I have therefore been afforded an interesting vantage point to observe the scientific direction of autism-related research. Over the years, there have been several waves of new applications which reflect one or another new finding in the neurosciences. The hope is that the finding will have a relationship to autism. Unfortunately, it is a rare event if one of these newly described genes or peptides can be shown to have any nexus with the disorder. Many of the grant proposals are technology driven. That is, a new technique or the latest generation of a technology comes into being offering the possibility of learning about some aspect of the science not available even a year earlier. Of course, some of these techniques do bear fruit and others fail to assist us. Another theme seen frequently in the proposal submissions is to apply to autism a new biologic finding that has been correlated with a similar disease. Examples of this are the MECP2 gene which is associated with Rett's syndrome[1] or the bornavirus which might be associated with schizophrenia.[2] Similar to the interest in new technologies, these types of studies offer the potential for opening up new vistas although, thus far, this strategy has not yielded breakthroughs for autism.

Through the ideas encompassed in these proposals, certain scientific directions seem to be emerging. As is true in all forms of scientific research, the proposals and ideas are driven as much by the pragmatic question of what can be done as by the more fundamental question of what we need to learn. The sad reality is that we are not able at this time to answer some of these fundamental questions because we lack the technical ability to do the research. There is, however, a finite set of tasks which could improve the infrastructure for the research community and thereby facilitate more of the research to be accomplished. Therefore, rather than address the specific genes, proteins or clinical observations which may be the next steps in autism research, let us consider the fundamental administrative and infrastructure issues and how attending to these will guide the future of autism science. Also to be considered are some of the fundamental assumptions upon which autism research is based.

Collaborative vs. Individual Science

Over the past decade there have been some notable shifts in how autism research is organized and supported. To begin with, it is only since 1997 that that there has been significant funding for autism research from the advocacy community. During the same period of time the National Institutes of Health funding of autism research has jumped from about 3 million dollars to over 70 million dollars per year.[3] Although this is still a small amount of funding compared to other diseases of similar prevalence and morbidity, it represents a significant increase for this field. The increase in funding has, for the first time, enabled pilot studies to be undertaken and facilitated the training of fellows. Young scientists now can see a future in dedicating their research careers to autism.

A central issue in the organization of all contemporary research is the tension between encouraging large, well planned research collaborations versus the support of individual scientists engaging in their own projects. This tension is by no means a simple issue.

There are clear advantages in promoting collaborative work. Large numbers of subjects can be studied in a timely fashion. Various investigators can bring their unique expertise into the collaborations to synergistic effect, thereby increasing the sophistication of the effort. Wasteful duplication and competition for its own sake can be avoided. Difficult issues can be agreed upon by consensus rather than having individual investigators defining their own parameters.

There are, nonetheless, drawbacks to large collaborations also. While "consensus science" may be efficient for accomplishing work, it also has the tendency to force large number of investigators to proceed in lockstep. If the group consensus is incorrect, the whole field may proceed in the wrong direction. Creativity can potentially be suppressed by encouraging those with outlying ideas to conform to group norms. A separate issue—but one that is extremely important to the researchers themselves—is that our academic institutions are set up to reward those who distinguish themselves in a sort of "star" system. Each university and each department chairman is looking for the "best" and the "brightest." Young investigators who subsume their individual efforts into large collaborations may be committing professional suicide. It is just much more difficult to distinguish oneself academically if a large part of your *oeuvre* is being planned and carried out in concert with others.

Therefore, in autism research, the question remains: what would be the optimal way to design a balance between collaborative work and individual creativity? It would behoove us as a field to clearly address this issue.

In autism research, a field which had but a few dedicated investigators only ten years ago,, the leaders in the field often come from the same background. In fact, many of the current leaders have been trained in the same labs. This tends to promote an inbred set of beliefs and values. Others with opposing ideas can rather easily be "frozen" out of a leadership role. This is quite dramatic as one considers that there are whole scientific disciplines which appear not to have yet been integrated into the large collaborations. The most glaring examples of this are the developmental biologists who remain largely unengaged in autism research despite the clear relevancy to autism of abnormal brain development. The major collaborations can consume very large percentages of the resources available for research. It is unlikely that the integration of outside ideas and disciplines will occur naturalistically from within the collaborations. Therefore, without conscious encouragement from agencies such as the NIH or the research advocacy groups, the growth of the field will be significantly hindered.

In the past decade, we have witnessed the formation of large collaborations in autism research. This was pioneered by the NIH with their Collaborative Programs of Excellence in Autism (CPEAs) collaboration.[4] This program—initiated in 1997 and now in its second 5 year cycle—includes 11 sites. Although each site is individually and competitively funded, as time passes the collaborative nature of the programs is strengthened. The CPEAs have taken on the task of defining common measures and began to expand studies from individual projects to the larger consortium. In addition, this collaboration is being joined by the NIH's STAART (Studies to Advance Autism Research and Treatment) centers.[5] The goal of collaboration is further being facilitated by a Data Coordinating Center funded by the NIH. By using this infrastructure, these NIH-funded sites as well as other investigators can expand their work into a larger context and ask research questions which previously were not able to be addressed. Another large collaboration already under way is the Center for Disease Control and Prevention-funded CADDRE (Centers for Autism and Developmental Disabilities Research and Epidemiology) program[6]—a collaboration of five sites working collaboratively to study autism epidemiologically. This program will assemble a population based sample of individuals with autism, developmentally atypical and normal controls. The CADDRE program was designed to work as a tightly grouped collaboration, despite the ability of each site to pilot some topics of individual interest.

There are two other large collaborative efforts which deserve mention. One is the NAAR Autism Genome Project.[7] Autism is widely believed to be the most heritable of the complex brain disorders[8],[9]; nevertheless, as is the case in other psychiatric diseases, there has been little success in isolating the genes which are involved.[10],[11] As each of the genetics research groups came to the conclusion that they alone would be unable to identify the genes, an interest developed to work collaboratively with one another. At the NIH's Autism Summit in 2003, NAAR announced a "collaboration of collaborations" comprised of nearly all of the world's autism genetics groups which have accumulated a significant amount of autism "sib pairs." In 2004, this collaboration initiated a genome wide screen with approximately 1200 sib pairs—more than three times the previously largest scan.[12] Subsequent phases of the NAAR Autism Genome Project—a public-private partnership of NAAR, NIH, and foreign governments—are anticipated to undertake the "fine mapping" to identify autism susceptibility genes.

Another public-private collaboration in formation is one to study the high risk baby siblings of already diagnosed autistic children.[7] Due to the rather large reoccurrence rate in families with one diagnosed child, it is estimated that between 3 % and 6 % of siblings will also be diagnosed with autism.[13] Furthermore, the estimate is that as many as 30 % of the siblings will have symptoms consistent with the broader genetic phenotype.[59] These newborns offer the opportunity to study autism in ways never before possible. This would include earlier diagnosis, longitudinal studies of the biological and cognitive development of the child, observation of environmental influences on development, and the impact of earlier interventions. Due to the precious opportunity presented by each of the infant siblings, it was believed that these studies should be undertaken collaboratively to maximize the research's potential.

The increase in availability of post-mortem autism brain tissue is yet another example of the impact of cooperative efforts to improving the research infrastructure. Until very recently there were but a handful of studies on postmortem brain tissue from individuals with autism.[22] While there was near unanimous consensus that further study of brain tissue was invaluable, there was a severe scarcity of post-mortem brain tissue from autistic individuals. It was a formidable task for any one investigator to accumulate the necessary tissue to undertake research. In 1997, however, the Autism Tissue Program (ATP) was initiated to raise awareness within the autism community of the critical importance of brain tissue to autism research and to distribute contributed post-mortem tissue to scientists based on competitive review of research proposals by the ATP's Tissue Advisory Board.[16] There have now been 28 different groups who have received tissue from the ATP.[17] In a similar vein, although a less scarce commodity, gene banks such as the Autism Genetics Resource Exchange[18] have now made DNA readily available to scientists who otherwise may not have the resources or ability to accumulate the samples for themselves. Both of these efforts have made it possible to undertake autism research much more expeditiously and opened the field to a new group of scientists interested in autism research.

The Autism Phenotype

The most strikingly important issue in autism research is the need to better define the disease we call "autism." The failure to do so could be the rate limiting step in our ability to make progress in understanding and treating the disorder. Ironically, this is an area of concern which has already engaged a good amount of the thinking and research. This topic is so important that it warrants a brief digression into how we have arrived at our current predicament.

Autism, like all mental disorders (as defined by the DSM), are phenomenologically based diagnoses. That is to say, we define autism based on observable and reproducible behavioral phenomena. The problem with this (which we share with the other psychiatric illnesses) is that these behaviors are generally the "end points" of extremely complex biological systems. Historically, the field of psychiatry began with empirically based diagnoses.[19] However, the field of psychoanalysis also relied heavily on speculations and hypotheses of the underlying mechanisms which created mental illness. The popularity of these hypotheses and their integration into mainstream psychiatry too often led to false conclusions regarding the etiologies of various psychiatric diseases. During World War II, a movement was started to systematize the diagnostic schema in psychiatry. This resulted in a handbook known as the Diagnostic and Statistical Manual of Mental Disorders (DSM) first published in 1952 with a second revision (DSM II) published in 1968. Although the idea behind the DSM was to create valid and reproducible diagnostic criteria, in fact, these first two attempts were not successful. They were relatively simple and designed by a small group of clinicians who basically drew on their own clinical experiences that were undoubtedly influenced by the prevailing psychoanalytic theories of the times. In 1972, the DSM-III task force was appointed to attempt the very bold step of defining diagnoses as objectively as possible.[19]

Looking back, the dramatic change represented by this paradigm shift can be appreciated. Psychoanalytic hypotheses were derived from single case studies. Causality was often assumed to occur from “unconscious” thoughts which could lead to the symptoms psychiatrists observed.. Diagnoses such as “homosexual panic”[20] were explained by stating that the individual unconsciously feared his or her homosexual impulses causing a breakdown in their defense mechanisms and leading to psychiatric symptoms. Schizophrenia was caused by the “double bind” placed upon the child by his mother.[21] In an especially tragic way, autism was thought to be caused by a “refrigerator mother”—a mother who lacked the empathetic skills needed for nurturing thereby resulting in the child’s extreme inward focus and producing the symptoms of autism.[22]

It may seem remarkable to the 21st century reader that such theories were accepted etiologic hypotheses as late as the 1970’s, but I can testify that this was still being taught in psychiatric residency programs into the late 1970’s. Diagnosis was more of an art than a science. In practice, psychiatrists would make diagnoses based on their own fondness for the theories rather than any objective criteria. Large studies proved that even the most severe psychiatric illnesses were not being diagnosed with any acceptable reliability.

It is against this backdrop that the field of psychiatry made a very difficult decision which resulted in the DSM III. That was to recognize that the etiologies of the psychiatric illnesses were just not known. They then switched to the phenomenologically based diagnosis system which we have today. In need of a more scientific and reliable system of diagnosis, a large sacrifice was made. This was to accept diagnosis possibly devoid of any etiologic basis.. It is this very compromise which may, ironically, be hindering the ability to advance our knowledge of the field.

Using our current phenomenologically based diagnosis, it is very likely that there could be numerous entry points whereby disease states could cause the same endpoint of behavior. This, in reality, would make the disorder currently called “autistic disorder” and the related “pervasive developmental disorders” an umbrella for several etiologically based diseases. The associations made will vary depending on the subjects selected in any particular study. In other words, it is most likely that what we are calling “autism” is more than one disease with several distinct etiologies. Clearly, each time a study encompasses a group of subjects and defines them as having “autism” based on current research criteria, we have to realize the likelihood that we have a heterogeneous group.[23]

Subtypes

How future research efforts should address this predicament is not entirely clear. Several methodologies have been suggested. The simplest is to define subgroups. Unfortunately, this has been a difficult task. It has proved very difficult to say which characteristics are etiologically related to the disease and which are incidental. For example, for decades we have known that there is an association between autism and hyperserotonemia. The hyperserotonemia is also statistically associated with family members who are unaffected. The possibility remains that this is an incidental finding and not etiologically related to autism. Would there be a value in separating out those with hyperserotonemia for autism studies? This is not known although the possibilities seem promising.[24],[25]

There have been some recent studies which have shown that some subgroups of autism seem to have a higher associational correlation with certain areas on genome screens. A subgroup of autism which has more "obsessive compulsive" symptoms (insistence on sameness) and another subtype which has more delayed language has been analyzed by several groups and it has been found that there are areas in the genome scans of these groups which show stronger signals.[26],[27],[28]

These are extremely encouraging results and point to the possibility that through the association with specific genes we will be able to work backwards and isolate true etiologic phenotypes. A very large number of individuals with autism would have to be screened in order to have a large enough sample size for each subtype. As the largest genome screen included only 345 sib pairs,[12] this strategy has not been possible. The NAAR AGP will have approximately 1200 sib pairs and plans to study thousands of trios (child with autism and both parents). This will provide sufficient numbers to allow for the subtyping of the autistic phenotype and to correlate that with genome screen. In a disease which is believed to have the highest heritability of all the complex brain disorders, searching for autism susceptibility genes is a task which cannot be overlooked. Ironically, it is possible that a greater value of the project may be providing a "backdoor mechanism" for the validation of autism subtypes.

As a first step in creating subtypes, the AGP collaboration intends to use the most commonly collected data derived from the Autism Diagnosis Observation Scale[29] (the "ADOS"). This data is derived from behaviorally observed phenomena. Although we remain optimistic that this methodology will yield meaningful associations, this is clearly not a certainty. The question arises again as to whether these well defined and reliably described behaviors are common endpoints of many diseases. If so, it may be possible to define a phenotype that is more specific or valid in an etiologic sense.

Biomarkers or Endophenotypes

Infectious diseases are proven using Koch's postulates.[30] Strep throat is known to be caused by streptococcal bacilli only because the bacteria can be grown from a throat swab. Is an analogy to this possible in a developmental brain disease? Effective treatments and prevention are unlikely unless we know etiologies. At this time, the task seems daunting; however, biomarkers hold some large advantages over the phenotypic macros. The most obvious advantage is that they are easier to define and are more reproducible. Especially in light of the research on the broader phenotype and the rather unmistakable heritability of autism, is seems very likely that some primary genetic contribution can be found in both the individual with autism as well as their families.[29]

If we are to look outside of the accepted behavioral macros to define autism, then the concept of endophenotypes must be considered.[32] These traits are intermediate between a gene's effect and the described disease. Endophenotypes often take the form of biomarkers but could also be behavioral. One method might be to focus more on biologically derived markers. Some reasonably good endophenotypes have been described for schizophrenia[33],[34] and other psychiatric illnesses,[35],[36] and it would seem that autism would present even more fertile ground.

Currently, perhaps the most exciting and simple biomarker in autism is the finding of excessive head growth found in the first year of life of children later diagnosed with autism.[61] Although the exact nature of this head (brain) growth is still being clarified, it does offer a significant lead. Other potential biomarkers under investigation include serotonin levels[24] and growth factor levels found in the bloodspots taken from newborns.[38] Various physiologic and structural biomarkers are being investigated using ERP, MRI, fMRI, MEG, PET and other recently developed techniques.[39],[40],[41] The identification of these biomarkers can also serve as valuable footholds in understanding which biologic systems are likely be the most important to study.

Although many autism investigators are well aware of the need to find biomarkers, a structural (administrative) issue which needs to be addressed is that biomarkers will mostly likely be traits which cross current diagnostic lines. These types of studies may be more difficult to get funded. The subject selection criteria would tend to be more difficult to define. Further, the use of appropriate controls becomes of extreme importance. In autism studies done until now, controls are "assumed" to be "normal". In their population based studies, the CADDRE program recently decided to have two groups of controls, one "neurotypical" and the other developmentally delayed but not meeting criteria for autism.[6] Although the latter is a mixed group it will nonetheless give some indication of how common some of the findings are in diseases not defined as autism. Most studies, however, do not have this luxury. Many of the parameters currently being studied in autism are also present in other brain illnesses. An extreme example is the immunological literature. Nearly all psychiatric illnesses have abnormal immune parameters[42] yet this is rarely noted in autism studies, implying that the findings are specific to autism.[43] Investigations of eye movement and facial recognition are other examples.[29],[34],[36] There clearly needs to be more input from investigators of other brain disorders so that these issues are taken into consideration.

Primary vs. Secondary Phenomena

If behavioral or biological markers are to be developed to define a diagnosis, they must be primary to the disease; that is, etiologically involved in the development of the disease. There is substantial evidence that at least some of the abnormalities associated with autism occur early in fetal development.[22],[44],[27] Although there is also evidence that development continues to go askew after birth and probably into the second year of life[61] or even longer, an extremely important question which has rarely been addressed is which abnormalities found in autism are primary and which occur secondarily. It is possible that the original lesion which causes autism then leads to many secondary phenomena.[46],[47] These secondary developmental trajectories could be responsible for some or even most of the autism phenotype. Therefore, it is much less likely that a secondary phenomenon will correlate with a polymorphism in the genome. Hence, a possible explanation for the lack of success thus far in finding genetic linkage in autism (and with the other psychiatric illnesses such as schizophrenia) is our inability to define the primary abnormality which is etiologically responsible for the disease.

Once again the answer to this problem is not obvious. One general solution is to study the disease in subjects as close to the original lesion as possible. It is obviously more likely that the phenotype that we see in a seven-year old has many layers of secondary influences. It seems obvious that the environment including parenting, schooling, diet, disease, medications, and thousands of other influences affect what we become.[48] There is emerging evidence for example, that the ability of the mother to maintain eye contact with the autistic child is somewhat prognostic of language acquisition and presumably brain development.[49] Therefore, to study autism in its "purest" form we would need to study the subjects at the youngest age possible. The practical reality is that up until this point we knew very little about autistic children earlier than at the time of their diagnosis. In clinical practice the average age at diagnosis is about six to seven years.[50],[51] Even with the most optimal screening the current diagnostic criteria does not support diagnosis until the second year of life.[52] The few studies that we do have which have studied autistic children pre-diagnosis have found that there are abnormalities well before the diagnosis is typically made.[53],[54] Knowing the neurobiological findings, we should not, of course, be surprised by this.

In order to address this issue, a new collaboration has been formed putting together investigators who have been studying the high risk baby siblings of already diagnosed autistic children.[7] We believe that the chance of a sibling also receiving a diagnosis of autism is between 3 % and 6 %. This is approximately 50 times higher than a sibling in an unaffected family. The chance of the sibling showing evidence of the broader autistic phenotype is about 30 %. Therefore, we now have a practical way of studying these children prospectively from birth. In fact, it would be advantageous to be able to study these children *in utero*, and this is a challenge which is likely to be met over the next few years.

One example of the advantages of studying autism in very young children is in studying human face processing. We know that individuals with autism process faces in an atypical fashion.[55] On fMRI it has been shown and replicated that autistic individuals do not use the FFA. There is doubt, however, as to whether this is a primary inborn abnormality of neuronal circuitry or whether the FFA is harnessed into this task by the child becoming an expert on faces through intensive practice. Do autistic newborns show a deficit in interest or recognition for faces? Is their processing of faces different than in neurotypical children? Therefore, abnormalities in the FFA would only be a helpful biomarker if this is an inborn abnormality for children with autism. If the newborns facial processing seemed to match the control children then one could assume that the face processing abnormalities are secondary.

Using this high risk baby sibling population, it is possible to obtain samples of biomarkers at birth or even in utero. The postnatal development can, for the first time, be studied prospectively. This could lead to greater understandings of both the primary and secondary deficits and makes it much more likely that we could devise treatment interventions at an early age to potentially interrupt at least the secondary abnormalities. If we have limited research resources, it would appear highly valuable to study prospectively this high risk group rather than the same studies in older children or adults.

Brain Development

Autism is conceptualized as a "developmental disorder" and most investigators believe that autism is produced by errors in the developing brain.[47] Yet despite the simplicity of the above statement, the vast majority of autism research does not address this issue. Rather, the research is almost always a cross sectional view of a finding usually in the older child or adult. The reason for this is again the difficulty in designing studies that investigate brain development. The prospective longitudinal study methodology is, unfortunately, much more expensive and difficult to organize for administrative reasons. Clearly, the major developmental period of the brain occurs *in utero* and during the first few years of life. Most of that time has been inaccessible to investigators who do human studies, up until now. Therefore, to study that period, the very youngest subjects must be ascertained. The high risk baby siblings initiative will provide the ability to longitudinally study these children from birth and, to a more limited extent, even *in utero*. This could open a window on to that period of time of neurodevelopment which has previously not been able to be studied.

The complexity of human brain development is enormous. Which systems to study remains a huge challenge. We are guided by clinical data such as the face recognition paradigm, auditory processing, attention shifting tasks, and a host of other possible studied parameters.[29] Genetics will give us an enormous foothold if genes can be reliably identified.[23]

Animal studies are another method which can provide models for development and give valuable information as to what needs to be studied in human development.[56] This area, unfortunately, has some serious limitations. Many of theses studies have used animal behavior to model the behaviors contained in the autistic symptoms. Unless this is done with extreme rigor, it is likely that the outcome of these studies, although contributing to the base of knowledge in neuroscience, will have little to do with autism.[57],[58] Once again, if the human phenotype is not carefully defined, correlating it with an animal's behavior has little relevance.. Animal studies, for example, have looked at abnormalities in social skills. In reality the deficits in social skills of autistic individuals is first being If not careful labeling these animals as models for autism can be misleading. Further studies might then be based on the assumption that the animal is, in fact, a good model for autism.

In my own informal survey of investigators who have published on behaviorally based animal models, the majority have had little or no experience studying the autistic behavioral phenotype in humans. In addition, there is little contact between these animal researchers and those experienced at clinical research in autism. A simple remedy for this would be for the animal model scientists to have access to and experience with children and adults with autism and to be able to study their behavior. This could either be done at one's own institution or, if the clinical facility is not available, it could be accomplished at a cooperating institution or in the form of a scheduled workshop.

Another type of model is the neuroanatomic model. These models are highly species dependent but nevertheless can provide important clues for human disease. Unfortunately, a similar problem exists in that many of the investigators studying animal models have on a superficial awareness of the human tissue literature. In reality, the human neuroanatomic literature is still quite inadequate. Oversimplified generalizations comparing brain systems between an animal model and autistic brain tissue abound in the literature. There continues to be very little contact between those who do the human neuroanatomy and scientists who undertake animal models. It is only recently that a few programs have begun this type of integration.[59]

In this case a solution seems clear. The funding agencies could call for proposals which require that studies which purport to design animal models of autism include a component which takes the next step and has a strategy for correlating findings with that obtained in humans through tissue, clinical work, or genetic findings. These correlative issues can most effectively be dealt with through collaborations, either large or small. The benefit of these collaborations would truly flow in both directions. Clinicians will be able to guide the basic scientists and evaluate the suitability of the animal models as adequate models for autism. Similarly, by becoming more familiar with neuronal systems and observing the animal behaviors, the clinicians may be able to refine definitions of the phenotype. A similar collaborative relationship must exist between the basic scientists and the human tissue investigators with respect to neuroanatomic modeling. In autism fellowship training programs, students should be exposed to this range of experience regardless of the field in which they later choose to specialize.

Early Fetal Development

Studying children longitudinally from birth will be a huge advantage over the current practice of the cross sectional study of older children and adults.[60] Even more so, the study of pre-natal development will likely yield additional answers we need to know. These early developmental studies are easy to do in animals in the lab but extremely difficult to study in clinical autism in the child or adult. Although it will be necessary to study all facets of pre-natal and postnatal development, there is evidence that very early development holds many of the keys. Much of the existing evidence points to events which appear to occur in the first few weeks of fetal life.[22],[44],[59] Recently, associations have been made with autism and genes which express very early in prenatal life (HOX and ENGRAILED).[61],[62] If these correlations hold, or if similar developmental genes are described, the study of the molecular biology of these genes will be essential. An overwhelming problem exists as we do not know how to study the very early (pre-natal) developmental biologic abnormalities in the human with autism. The solution to the above conundrum will likely raise not only scientific, but also ethical, issues. The major question is how to get this type of tissue to study.

A source of very early tissue with an autistic potential could come from the frozen embryos being stored in fertility clinics. This tissue would then be grown and studied for very early gene expression. Theses embryos would come from couples who already have an autistic child and so the chances of them being genetically "autistic" would (as in the high risk baby sibling program) be 3 % to 6 %, although the likelihood of having some genetic abnormality which could produce the broader phenotype would likely be considerably greater. A major problem with this strategy would be that we would have no way of knowing which of the embryos would develop autism. Perhaps if a genetic profile of autism were to be developed, there might be a way of predicting which embryos were potentially autistic. The neurobiology could then be studied.

Perhaps a more attractive, less ethically fraught method would be the use of multipotent or perhaps pleuripotent precursor cells. At this time embryologic cell lines do not exist which are "genetically autistic." Considering our current state of knowledge, it would seem challenging to know where to find the suitable cells in order to make one. Although there is much controversy in the field, one potential source might be from CNS of postmortem tissue taken from autistic individuals.[63] These cells would provide the great advantage in that we would know that these cells did indeed derive from an individual who was diagnosed with autism. Although the technology for this is yet to be elucidated, the need for this type of research is compelling.

With the right investment in this type of research, the study of the gene functioning in these very immature cells and the epiphenomena which guide development could potentially be studied. Although the straightforward search for abnormal genes in autism is certainly not to be abandoned, it may in the end be imperative to study the actual functioning of the genes to understand the neurobiology of the disease.

Conclusion

In summary, the field of research in autism has progressed significantly over the past decade. Nevertheless, significant challenges remain to be overcome. Along with the science many of these can be conceptualized as issues concerning research infrastructure or administration. The following points should be addressed:

1. The autism phenotype still cannot be taken for granted. An over-reliance on our current concepts could be misdirecting research directions and needs to be guarded against.
2. The formulation of subtypes is of critical importance. These subtypes need to be proven and to be associated with reproducible markers.
3. More basic phenotypes or endophenotypes need to be described. It is more likely that this can be done through studying the youngest children through prospective longitudinal studies. The goal is to identify primary versus secondary phenomena of the disease.
4. More research attention needs to be devoted to the developmental nature of the disease. Brain development, especially early brain development, must be studied. Limitations need to be addressed in a systematic way.
5. Collaborative relationships need to be fostered. Large numbers of subjects, in some cases, is critically important for meaningful results. Databases need to be created and there will need to be wide access within the research community to such data. The combination of expertise of collaborators from different disciplines should be a requirement for many projects and not considered a luxury. However, this must be balanced by a respect for the individual creativity of investigators. A certain percentage of high risk unorthodox ideas must continue to be supported.
6. Biomaterials such as DNA, brain tissue and perhaps progenitor cells should be readily available to advance autism research.

References

[1] Shibayama A, Cook EH Jr, Feng J, et al. MECP2 structural and 3′-UTR variants in schizophrenia, autism and other psychiatric diseases: a possible association with autism. *American Journal of Medical Genetics*. 2004; 128B:50-53.

[2] Lipkin WI, Hornig M. Microbiology and immunology of autism spectrum disorders. In: Bock G, Goode J, eds. *Autism: Neural Basis and Treatment Possibilities*. Chichester, England: John Wiley & Sons; 2003:129-143.

[3] Office of Extramural Research. *Computer retrieval of information on scientific projects.* [electronic resource]. Available at: <http://crisp.cit.nih.gov/>.
[4] National Institute of Child Health & Human Development. *The collaborative programs of excellence in autism (CPEAs).* [electronic resource]. Available at: <http://www.nichd.nih.gov/autism/cpea.cfm>.
[5] National Institute of Mental Health. *Studies to advance autism research and treatment (STAART) network.* [electronic resource]. Available at: <http://www.nimh.nih.gov/autismiacc/staart.cfm>.
[6] National Center on Birth Defects and Developmental Disabilities. *CADDRE: Centers of excellence for autism and developmental disabilities research and epidemiology.* [electronic resource]. Available at:<http://www.cdc.gov/ncbddd/dd/aic/states/default.htm#caddre>.
[7] National Alliance for Autism Research. *NAAR launches largest autism genetics study.* [electronic resource]. Available at:<http://www.naar.org/news/render_pr.asp?intNewsItemID=176>.
[8] Chudley AE, Gutierrez E ,Jocelyn LJ, Chodirker BN. Outcomes of genetic evaluation in children with pervasive developmental disorder. *Journal of Development and Behavioral Pediatrics.* 1998; 19:321-325.
[9] Bailey A, le Couteur A, Gottesman II, et al. Autism as a strongly genetic disorder: evidence from a British twin study. *Psychological Medicine.* 1995; 25:63-77.
[10]Riley BP. Linkage studies of schizophrenia. *Neurotoxicity Research.* 2004; 6:17-34.
[11]Mathews CA, Reus VI. Genetic linkage in bipolar disorder. *CNS Spectrums.* 2003;8:891-904.
[12]Yonan AL, Alarcon M, Cheng R, et al. A genomewide screen of 345 families for autism-susceptibility loci. *American Journal of Human Genetics.* 2003; 73:886-897.
[13]Bolton P, MacDonald H, Pickles A, et al. A case-control family history study of autism. *Journal of Child Psychology and Psychiatry and Allied Disciplines.* 1994; 35:877-900.
[14]Bailey A, Palferman S, Heavey L, le Couteur A. Autism: the phenotype in relatives. *Journal of Autism and Developmental Disorders.* 1998; 28:369-392.
[15]Kemper TL, Bauman ML. Neuropathology of infantile autism. *Journal of Neuropathology and Experimental Neurology.* 1998; 57:645-652.
[16]Pickett J. Current investigations in autism brain tissue research. *Journal of Autism and Developmental Disorders.* 2001; 31:521-527.
[17]Autism Tissue Program. [online resource]. Available at: <http://www.brainbank.org>.
[18]Geschwind DH, Sowinski J, Lord C, et al. The autism genetic resource exchange: a resource for the study of autism and related neuropsychiatric conditions. *American Journal of Human Genetics.* 2001; 69:463-466.
[19]Andreasen NC, Black DW. History of psychiatry. In: *Introductory Textbook of Psychiatry.* Washington, DC: American Psychiatric Press; 1991:3-15.
[20]Chuang HT, Addington D. Homosexual panic, a review of its concept. Canadian Journal of Psychiatry. 1988; 33:613-617.
[21]Bateson G, Jackson D, Haley J Weakland J. Towards a theory of schizophrenia. *Behavioral Science.* 1956; 1:251-264.
[22]Bettelheim B. *The Empty Fortress: Infantile Autism and the Birth of the Self.* New York, NY: The Free Press; 1967.

[23]Folstein SE, Rosen-Sheidley B. Genetics of autism: complex aetiology for a heterogeneous disorder. *Nature Reviews: Genetics*. 2001; 2:943-955.

[24]Mulder EJ, Anderson GM, Kema IP, et al. Platelet serotonin levels in pervasive developmental disorders and mental retardation: diagnostic group differences, within-group distribution, and behavioral correlates. *Journal of the American Academy of Child and Adolescent Psychiatry*. 2004; 43:491-499.

[25]Coutinho AM, Oliveira G, Morgadinho T, et al. Variants of the serotonin transporter gene (SLC6A4) significantly contribute to hyperserotonemia in autism. *Molecular Psychiatry*. 2004; 9:264-271.

[26]Buxbaum JD, Silverman J, Keddache M, et al. Linkage analysis for autism in a subset families with obsessive-compulsive behaviors: evidence for an autism susceptibility gene on chromosome 1 and further support for susceptibility genes on chromosome 6 and 19. *Molecular Psychiatry*. 2004; 9:144-150.

[27]Bradford Y, Haines J, Hutcheson H, et al. Incorporating language phenotypes strengthens evidence of linkage to autism. *American Journal of Medical Genetics*. 2001; 105:539-547.

[28]Shao Y, Raiford KL, Wolpert CM, et al. Phenotypic homogeneity provides increased support for linkage on chromosome 2 in autistic disorder. *American Journal of Human Genetics*. 2002; 70:1058-1061.

[29]Lord C, Risi S, Lambrecht L, et al. The autism diagnostic observation schedule—generic: a standard measure of social and communication deficits associated with the spectrum of autism. *Journal of Autism and Developmental Disorders*. 2000; 30:205-223.

[30]Münch R. Robert Koch. *Microbes and Infection*. 2003;5:69-74.

[31]Dawson G, Webb S, Schellenberg GD, et al. Defining the broader phenotype of autism: genetic, brain, and behavioral perspectives. Development *and Psychopathology*. 2002; 14:581-611.

[32]Gottesman II, Gould TD. The endophenotype concept in psychiatry: etymology and strategic intentions. *The American Journal of Psychiatry*. 2003; 160:636-645.

[33]Benjamin J, Ebstein RP, Belmaker RH. Genes for human personality traits: endophenotypes of psychiatric disorders. In: Benjamin J, Ebstein RP, Belmaker RH, eds. *Molecular Genetics and the Human Personality*. Arlington, VA: American Psychiatric Publishing; 2002:333-344.

[34]Bölte S, Poustka F. The recognition of facial affect in autistic and schizophrenic subjects and their first-degree relatives. *Psychological Medicine*. 2003; 33:907-915.

[35]Rangaswamy M, Porjesz B, Chorlian DB, et al. Resting EEG in offspring of male alcoholics: beta frequencies. *International Journal of Psychophysiology*. 2004; 51:239-251.

[36]Kathmann N, Hochrein A, Uwer R, Bondy B. Deficits in gain of smooth pursuit eye movements in schizophrenia and affective disorder patients and their unaffected relatives. *The American Journal of Psychiatry*. 2003; 160:696-702.

[37]Courchesne E, Carper RA, Akshoomoff NA. Evidence of brain overgrowth in the first year of life in autism. *JAMA*. 2003; 290:337-344.

[38]Nelson KB, Grether JK, Croen LA, et al. Neuropeptides and neurotrophins in neonatal blood of children with autism or mental retardation. *Annals of Neurology*. 2001; 49:597-606.

[39]Goldberg J Szatmari P, Zwaigenbaum L. Diminished serotonin receptor function: a potential endophenotype of autism. Presented at: International Meeting for Autism Research; 8 May 2004; Sacramento, CA.

[40]Dawson G, Webb S, Faja S, Pau M. Face processing is altered in autism families: behavioral and ERP evidence. Presented at: International Meeting for Autism Research; 2004; Sacramento, CA.

[41]Klin A, Jones W, Schultz R, Volkmar F, Cohen D. Defining and quantifying the social phenotype in autism. *The American Journal of Psychiatry*. 2002; 159:895-908.

[42]Arolt V, Rothermundt M, Peters M, Leonard B. Immunological research in clinical psychiatry: report on the consensus debate during the 7th Expert Meeting on Psychiatry and Immunology. *Molecular Psychiatry*. 2002; 7:822-826.

[43]Singh VK, Lin SX, Yang VC. Serological association of measles virus and human herpesvirus-6 with brain autoantibodies in autism. *Clinical Immunlogy and Immunopathology*. 1998; 89:105-108.

[44]Bailey A, Luthert PJ, Dean A, et al. A clinicopathological study of autism. *Brain*. 1998; 121:889-905.

[45]Rodier PM, Ingram JL, Tisdale B, Nelson S, Romano J. Embryological origin for autism: developmental anomalies of the cranial nerve motor nuclei. *Journal of Comparative Neurology*. 1996; 370:247-261.

[46]Silva SC, Correia C, Fesel C, et al. Autoantibody repertoires to brain tissue in autism nuclear families. *Journal of Neuroimmunology*. 2004; 152:176-182.

[47]Rubenstein JL, Merzenich MM. Model of autism: increased ratio of excitation/inhibition in key neural systems. *Genes, Brain, and Behavior*. 2003; 2:255-267.

[48]Rogers SJ. Empirically supported comprehensive treatment for young children with autism. *Journal of Clinical Child Psychology*. 1998; 27:168-179.

[49]Siller M, Sigman M. The behaviors of parents of children with autism predict the subsequent development of their children's communication. *Journal of Autism and Developmental Disorders*. 2002; 32:77-89.

[50]Mandell DS, Listerud J, Levy SE, Pinto-Martin JA. Race differences in the age at diagnosis among medicaid-eligible children with autism. *Journal of the American Academy of Child and Adolescent Psychiatry*. 2002; 41:1447-1453.

[51]Fombonne E, Heavey L, Smeeth L, et al. Validation of the diagnosis of autism in general practitioner records. *BMC Public Health*. 2004; 4:5.

[52]Baghdadli A, Picot MC, Pascal C, Pry R, Aussilloux C. Relationship between age of recognition of first disturbances and severity in young children with autism. *European Child & Adolescent Psychiatry*. 2003; 12:122-127.

[53]Osterling JA, Dawson G, Munson JA. Early recognition of 1-year-old infants with autism spectrum disorder versus mental retardation. *Development and Psychopathology*. 2002; 14:239-251.

[54]Bryson S, Zwaigenbaum L, Brian J, Roberts W, Szatmari P, McDermott C. Temperament in infants later diagnosed with autism. Presented at: International Meeting for Autism Research; 8 May 2004; Sacramento CA.

[55]Schultz RT, Grelotti DJ, Klin A, et al. The role of the fusiform face area in social cognition: implications for the pathobiology of autism. *Philosophical Transactions of the Royal Society of London, Series B: Biological Sciences*. 2003; 358:415-427.

[56]Belmonte MK, Cook EH, Anderson GM, et al. Autism as a disorder of neural information processing: directions for research and targets for therapy. *Molecular Psychiatry*. 2004; 9:646-663.

[57]Flint J. Behavioral phenotypes: conceptual and methodological issues. *American Journal of Medical Genetics*. 1998; 81:235-240.

[58]Garner JP, Meehan CL, Mench JA. Stereotypies in caged parrots, schizophrenia and autism: evidence for a common mechanism. *Behavioural Brain Research*. 2003; 145:125-134.

[59]Rodier PM. Converging evidence for brain stem injury in autism. *Development and Psychopathology*. 2002; 14:537-557.

[60]Akshoomoff N, Pierce K, Courchesne E. The neurobiological basis of autism from a developmental perspective. *Development and Pschopathology*. 2002; 14:613-634.

[61]Gharani N, Benayed R, Mancuso V, Brzustowicz LM, Millonig JH. Assocciation of the homeobox transcription factor, ENGRAILED 2, with autism spectrum disorder. *Molecular Psychiatry*. 2004; 9:540.

[62]Ingram JL, Stodgell CJ, Hyman SL, Figlewicz DA, Weitkamp LR, Rodier PM. Discovery of allelic variants of HOXA1 and HOXB1: genetic susceptibility to autism spectrum disorders. *Teratology*. 2000; 62:393-405.

[63]Xu Y, Kimura K, Matsumoto N, Ide C. Isolation of neural stem cells from the forebrain of deceased early postnatal and adult rats with protracted post-mortem intervals. *Journal of Neuroscience Research*. 2003;74:533-540.

Index

A

aberrant, 109, 128, 145, 149, 150, 153, 158
acetylcholine, 153, 191
adrenocorticotropic hormone, 157
aetiology, 207
allele, 148, 161
amino acids, 131
amnesia, 163
amygdala, 34, 69, 70, 71, 80, 86, 105, 107, 134, 152, 158, 163, 164, 169, 170, 179, 180
anticonvulsant, 183, 192
appearance, 73, 137
arginine, 151, 163, 164
Asperger Syndrome (AS), 8, 9, 10, 11, 13, 15, 98, 143, 168
ataxia, 128
atrophy, 132, 156, 168
attention deficit hyperactivity disorder, 71
autoantibodies, 208
autopsy, 141
autosomal recessive, 128
axon, 127, 155, 171, 173, 177

B

bacteria, 200
basal ganglia, 71, 97
behavior, vii, ix, xi, 32, 47, 53, 76, 78, 79, 83, 91, 100, 106, 127, 133, 142, 145, 146, 149, 150, 151, 152, 153, 154, 155, 156, 158, 159, 160, 161, 163, 164, 166, 167, 168, 170, 199, 203
benign tumors, 146
benzodiazepine, 169
binding, xi, 118, 122, 125, 147, 153, 161, 166, 185, 192
biology, 150, 159, 166, 172, 204
biomarkers, 200, 201, 202
bipolar disorder, 128, 131, 206
birds, 152, 186
blood, 74, 89, 90, 92, 111, 128, 129, 130, 132, 152, 165, 207
blood pressure, 152
body weight, 143
brain growth, 44, 45, 58, 63, 65, 94, 95, 133, 134, 141
brain volume, 44, 57, 58, 59, 60, 61, 62, 64, 65, 66, 67, 68, 69, 70, 71, 72, 74, 76, 89, 92, 94, 96, 133, 134, 140
brainstem, 69, 74, 82, 104, 108, 138
breeding, 151

C

cancer progression, 147
causation, ix, xii, 29, 30
cell line, 204
cell membranes, 91, 92
cell minicolumn, 130, 190
central nervous system, 28, 31, 76, 100, 102, 149, 165, 171, 172, 184, 185
central nervous system (CNS), 27, 28, 31, 48, 76, 100, 102, 149, 161, 165, 171, 172, 173, 175, 178, 181, 182, 183, 184, 185, 189, 204, 206
cerebellum, 34, 45, 68, 69, 71, 72, 85, 86, 87, 90, 91, 96, 97, 98, 104, 107, 127, 129, 131, 134, 135, 150, 153, 154, 158, 185, 192
cerebral blood flow, 84, 85, 86, 87, 89, 104, 105
cerebrospinal fluid (CSF), 128, 170
chicken, 83
chromosomes, 43, 127, 128, 131, 148, 149, 152, 154, 161, 162, 163, 207
cleft palate, 161
clinical examination, 3
clinical trials, viii
cluster of differentiation (CD), 105, 162
cognition, 37, 49, 85, 86, 89, 151, 152, 153, 170, 208

communication, ix, xiii, 8, 22, 32, 47, 52, 54, 72, 84, 87, 92, 112, 120, 127, 133, 145, 146, 148, 159, 207, 208
concentration, 40, 91, 96, 99, 136, 153, 158, 170
congenital, 32, 42
contralateral, 90
controlled study, 167
cornea, 109
corpus callosum, 32, 45, 49, 54, 72, 73, 80, 81, 82, 83, 91, 97, 98, 99, 108, 111, 126
cortex, xi, xii, 39, 40, 67, 68, 69, 72, 74, 82, 85, 86, 87, 88, 90, 91, 94, 95, 96, 103, 104, 106, 108, 109, 110, 111, 114, 125, 126, 127, 128, 131, 132, 133, 134, 135, 137, 139, 140, 141, 142, 143, 146, 147, 152, 153, 156, 157, 164, 165, 166, 169, 175, 180, 181, 182, 183, 184, 185, 189, 190, 191
corticotropin, 168, 169
cortisol, 157
creatinine, 91
cystic fibrosis, viii
cytokines, 156
cytomegalovirus, 138

D

daily living, xi
dementia, 31, 39, 48, 53, 135
demyelination, 102
dendritic cell (DC), 96, 97, 100, 101, 103, 106, 107, 130, 139, 160, 167, 174, 206
depression, 128, 131, 154, 166, 182
developing brain, 202
developmental disorders, vii, xiii, 8, 15, 18, 21, 22, 24, 80, 94, 97, 106, 122, 124, 126, 130, 142, 146, 199, 207
diagnosis, ix, 1, 9, 10, 14, 15, 29, 30, 99, 115, 137, 197, 199, 201, 202, 208
diet, 202
differentiation, 10, 154
diffusion, 58, 73, 76, 77, 78, 79, 80, 81, 93, 99, 100, 101, 102, 103, 104, 108, 184
diphtheria, 156
disability, 17, 30, 31, 41, 46, 48, 85
discomfort, 179
dizygotic twins, 99, 146
DNA, 198, 205
dominance, 38, 40, 41, 121, 122, 150, 154
dorsal, 165
dyslexia, 41, 74

E

echolalia, 52
electroencephalogram, 126
emotions, xii, 42, 86, 105, 114, 118, 177
encephalitis, 31
endocrine, 32, 148
entorhinal cortex, 134, 165
environmental factors, vii, 69
enzymatic activity, 127
enzymes, 127, 154
epidemic, 14, 24, 145
epidemiology, 21, 24, 25, 206
epilepsy, 31, 71, 120, 122, 126, 153, 154, 155, 161, 166, 181, 182, 183
ethnic background, 2
ethnicity, 19, 21
etiology, x, 44, 138, 162
evolution, xi, xii, 103, 134, 140, 141, 143
exogenous, 151
extracellular matrix (ECM), 131

F

false negative, 3
false positive, 19, 81
familial, 41
family history, 18, 37, 94, 206
fat, 109
females, 31, 41, 147, 153
fertility, 19, 204
fertilization, 169
fetus, 41
fiber bundles, 48, 139
fibers, 48, 67, 72, 74, 76, 77, 81, 82, 108, 134, 140
first degree relative, 129
follow-up, 16, 23
frontal lobe, xi, 39, 69, 72, 84, 91, 98, 114, 123

G

gait, 128, 135, 148, 155, 156
gender, xi, 4, 83, 115, 116, 117, 119, 149
gene, 43, 128, 131, 132, 147, 148, 149, 150, 151, 152, 153, 154, 155, 159, 160, 161, 162, 163, 164, 165, 166, 167, 168, 181, 191, 195, 198, 200, 203, 204, 205, 207
gene expression, 163, 168, 204
gene promoter, 167
gene therapy, 147
gene transfer, 163, 164
general practitioner, 25, 208
generalized seizures, 149, 153, 154, 155

genetic defect, 147
genetic factors, 40, 43, 66
genetics, 149, 150, 155, 160, 197, 206
genome, 155, 197, 200, 201
gestation, 64, 71, 72
glands, 151
glatiramer acetate (GA), 97, 131
glial cells, 45, 63, 72
glucose, 89
glycoprotein, 128, 131
gray matter, 67, 68, 69, 70, 72, 74, 96, 135
growth factors, 154, 156, 157, 165, 201

H

head circumference, 44, 57, 58, 59, 60, 62, 63, 64, 65, 66, 94, 134, 140
head injury, 31
hemiplegia, xi
hemisphere, xii, 33, 34, 38, 39, 40, 41, 45, 49, 53, 91, 96
hepatic, 160
hepatocyte, 154
heritability, 73, 200
herpes virus, 208
heterogeneity, 3, 19, 93, 100, 131
heterozygous, 132, 147, 150, 162
histone, 161
homeostasis, 84, 90, 152, 167
homogenous, 79
homozygous, 128, 150
hormone, 168
hormones, 157
host, 19, 203
hydrocephalus, 58
hyperplasia, 76, 96
hypersensitive, 157, 161
hyperventilation, 92
hypoplasia, 128, 131, 149
hypothesis, xi, 10, 14, 18, 19, 21, 34, 45, 49, 53, 107, 118, 121, 125, 143, 158, 180, 181, 182, 185, 186, 191
hypoxia, 92

I

idiopathic, 45, 58, 64, 66, 71, 83
imagination, ix, 8
immune system, 156
immunoreactivity, 131, 132
in vitro, 165
in vivo, 100, 102, 104, 166
indication, 112, 201
inducible protein (IP), 207
infancy, 31, 54, 63, 73, 95, 123, 141, 159, 169
infants, 44, 106, 113, 115, 116, 123, 125, 158, 170, 198, 208
infections, 19, 156, 168
influenza, 156, 168
infrastructure, 195, 197, 198, 205
inhibitor, 90, 155, 166
inoculation, 156
inositol, 92
inspiration, 36
interactions, 22, 47, 81, 90, 148, 151, 152, 156, 157, 159, 162, 165, 168
interleukin (IL), 22
interneurons, 127, 131, 152, 165, 184
intracellular, 166
intravenous (IV), 5, xi, 3, 7, 8, 11, 12, 22, 24, 109, 130, 152

K

kidney, 147
Krabbe disease, 102

L

labor, 84, 151
laminar, 149, 164
Langerhans cells (LC), 104, 193
language, xi, 1, 15, 33, 34, 36, 37, 38, 41, 42, 47, 48, 59, 60, 66, 68, 69, 71, 74, 76, 86, 87, 88, 89, 90, 94, 96, 106, 112, 113, 118, 121, 122, 133, 138, 140, 145, 148, 149, 159, 162, 178, 190, 200, 202, 207
language acquisition, 47, 202
left ventricle, 38
lesions, 158, 160, 170, 201
lifespan, 93
linkage, 27, 43, 54, 129, 132, 148, 149, 150, 153, 154, 162, 181, 201, 206, 207
liver, 147
locus, xi, 43, 148, 149, 152, 154, 164

M

macrocephaly, 44, 54, 58, 59, 60, 62, 63, 66, 70, 71, 74, 75, 94, 95, 97, 132, 142, 168
macrocolumns, 180, 181, 183, 184
magnetic resonance imaging (MRI), 38, 39, 44, 48, 60, 64, 65, 71, 72, 73, 74, 76, 78, 79, 80, 81, 93, 94, 95, 96, 97, 98, 99, 100, 101, 102, 103, 105, 107, 124, 134, 140, 141, 165, 201

magnetic resonance spectroscopy (MRS), 90, 91, 107
males, 21, 29, 31, 41, 60, 63, 67, 69, 71, 74, 80, 117, 147, 152, 153, 160
mammalian brain, 143
mammals, 172, 186
mat, 9, 38, 60, 63, 64, 68, 72, 74, 80, 85, 115, 116, 117, 119, 121, 127, 129, 150, 178, 202
matrix, 78, 186
maturation, 65, 69, 73, 95, 102, 104, 123, 169
measles, 21, 23, 25, 156, 208
medial, 46, 54, 69, 84, 86, 91, 152, 163, 170
median, 2, 3, 4, 169
memory, ix, xi, 27, 28, 29, 33, 34, 35, 36, 37, 39, 40, 41, 42, 43, 45, 46, 48, 50, 51, 52, 54, 85, 88, 105, 106, 112, 122, 128, 148, 149, 152, 155, 156, 158, 164, 165, 166, 168, 170
messenger RNA (mRNA), 128, 169
metabolism, 90, 91, 92, 107, 147
Metachromatic leuklodystrophy (MLD), 119, 121
microcephaly, 58, 62, 66, 96
minicolumns, 45, 127, 133, 134, 135, 136, 137, 138, 139, 140, 181, 183, 184, 191
modelling, 193
moderate, 4, 6, 7, 61, 74, 119
monozygotic twins, 129, 146
morbidity, 181, 196
morphology, 68, 71, 73, 81, 99
Mountcastle, Vernon, 142, 180, 190
mRNA, 128, 169
multi-infarct dementia, 135
multiple factors, 147
multiple sclerosis (MS), 21, 54, 94, 95, 97, 98, 99, 102
multipotent, 204
mumps, 21, 23, 156
music, 31, 32, 33, 37, 38, 40, 42, 50
mutations, 128, 131, 147, 148, 149, 150, 151, 153, 155, 160, 163, 162
myelin, 76, 90, 91, 135, 139

N

neocortex, 67, 96, 97, 142, 164, 172
nerve, xi, 48, 128, 135, 142, 208
nerve fibers, 128
nervous system, 31, 180, 188, 191
neural function, 46
neural networks, 65, 85, 86, 157, 172, 173, 175, 176, 178, 179, 183, 184, 185, 186, 188, 189
neuroimaging, 57, 66, 73, 83, 84, 89, 90, 92, 93, 95, 104, 105
neurons, 34, 45, 51, 89, 90, 91, 110, 112, 118, 121, 128, 131, 135, 142, 146, 153, 154, 161, 164, 169, 171, 172, 173, 174, 175, 176, 177, 178, 179, 180, 183, 184, 186, 190, 192
neuropeptide, 151
neurotransmitters, 84, 90, 92, 159, 181
neurotrophic factors, 165
nicotine, 153
norepinephrine (NE), 52
nucleotide, 154, 166
nucleus, 45, 71, 87, 90, 152, 164, 168

O

obesity, 148, 167
occipital lobe, 67, 80, 88, 91
oculomotor, 72
old age, 142
olfactory, 29, 69, 152
optic nerve, 32

P

pathogenesis, vii, viii, 165
pathology, xi, xiii, 34, 39, 41, 103, 127, 129, 130, 134, 141, 143, 151, 159, 162, 165, 190
pathophysiology, 100, 132
pediatric, 32, 106
peptides, 152, 163, 164, 195
perfusion, 39, 74, 84, 104
perinatal, 150, 153
phenotype, 66, 72, 96, 149, 150, 151, 152, 155, 158, 161, 162, 197, 200, 201, 202, 203, 204, 205, 206, 207, 208
phenylketonuria, 134, 138
phosphorylation, 128
physiology, 165
pigs, 151
pituitary, 32, 168
pituitary gland, 32
placebo, 50, 167
plasma, 132, 152, 155, 157
plasma levels, 152, 157
plasminogen, 154
plasticity, 31, 44, 48, 128, 154, 158, 166, 169, 171, 172, 182, 183
platelet, 128
polymorphism, 167, 201
population, 2, 5, 6, 7, 9, 10, 11, 12, 14, 16, 17, 18, 19, 20, 21, 22, 23, 24, 25, 29, 30, 50, 58, 62, 63, 83, 134, 137, 146, 147, 148, 152, 167, 197, 201, 202

posterior, 40, 66, 68, 73, 82, 85, 86, 97, 108, 110, 113, 115, 116, 119, 122
postnatal, 44, 45, 58, 59, 60, 63, 71, 98, 133, 134, 147, 148, 152, 153, 154, 158, 169, 202, 204, 209
precursor cells, 204
prematurity, 31
prenatal, 34, 40, 41, 130, 156, 158, 170, 184, 204
prevention, 200
primate, 95, 141, 143, 146, 157, 158, 159, 170
probe, 80
prognostic, 202
progression, 39, 48
proliferation, xi, 44, 63, 134, 140, 147
protease, 128, 131
proteins, 127, 128, 130, 131, 147, 149, 155, 160, 161, 164, 165, 195
psychosis, 9, 22
public awareness, 14
public health, vii, viii, 25

R

receptor, 128, 152, 153, 154, 155, 164, 165
receptors, 90, 128, 131, 149, 151, 152, 153, 155, 157, 159, 158, 161, 163, 164, 165, 167, 169, 191, 208
reflexes, 42
regression, 115
reproduction, 128
respiratory, 168
retina, 31
risk factors, 20, 21, 44, 95
RNA, 147, 160
rodents, 147, 149, 151, 153, 158, 159
rubella, 21, 23, 25, 138, 156, 168

S

Savant Syndrome, 5, 27, 29, 30, 43, 44, 46, 52, 53
schizophrenia, xiii, 80, 97, 102, 103, 128, 131, 132, 142, 153, 156, 162, 168, 195, 200, 201, 205, 206, 207, 209
schizophrenic, 207
sclerosis, 8, 21, 59, 60, 71, 97, 146, 148, 160
seizures, 59, 60, 65, 66, 92, 125, 126, 128, 127, 133, 134, 147, 149, 154, 15, 1575, 160, 165, 167, 181
sensitivity, 3, 9, 36, 110, 112, 150, 155, 169
septum, 32, 134, 151, 163, 164
serotonin, 38, 45, 71, 76, 90, 97, 106, 107, 149, 155, 158, 166, 167, 181, 182, 191, 201, 207, 208
short-term memory, 155
sibling, 43, 202, 204
smooth muscle, 151
social impairment, ix, 116
socialization, ix
speech, 38, 41, 74, 87, 88, 95, 115, 116, 145, 148, 149, 159, 162, 180
spine, 147, 148
standard deviation, 60, 61, 63, 66, 87, 137
stereotyping, 36
stimulus, 37, 84, 87, 89, 112, 123, 125, 157, 178, 183, 184, 186, 188, 189
strain, 155, 163
stroke, 31, 48
style, xii, 37, 43, 126
subcutaneous (SC), 54, 102, 130, 165, 208
suicide, 196
synapses, 51, 69, 118, 171, 172, 173, 174, 175, 176, 177, 178, 179, 180

T

tactile, 29
task performance, 85, 105
telencephalon, 165
temporal lobe, 38, 39, 49, 50, 54, 74, 75, 80, 84, 91, 106, 146, 159, 170
testosterone, 31, 40, 41, 152
thinking, ix, xi, 37, 40, 85, 86, 110, 198
threshold, 33, 136
tics, 71, 171
transcription, 149, 159, 161, 169, 209
transduction, 150
transformation, 81
translocation, 161, 164
trauma, 91, 168
tryptophan, 71, 90, 106, 160, 167
tumors, 146, 147
tyrosine, 128

U

urokinase, 154

V

vaccine, 23, 25, 44, 156, 168
vasopressin, 151, 152, 163, 164, 168
ventricles, 69, 152
viral infection, 130, 132, 156, 168
viruses, 156, 168, 208
virus infection, 156
vision, 32, 33, 35, 116, 121, 157, 182